Promoting Health and Academic Success
The WSCC Approach

SECOND EDITION

Promoting Health and Academic Success
The WSCC Approach

SECOND EDITION

David A. Birch, PhD
The University of Alabama, Professor Emeritus

Donna M. Videto, PhD, RMCHES
SUNY Cortland, Professor Emerita

Hannah P. Catalano, PhD, MCHES
University of North Carolina–Wilmington

EDITORS

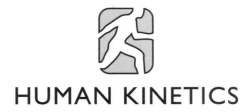

Library of Congress Cataloging-in-Publication Data

Names: Birch, David A., editor. | Videto, Donna M., editor. | Catalano, Hannah P., 1986- editor.
Title: Promoting health and academic success : the WSCC approach / David A. Birch, Donna M. Videto, Hannah P. Catalano, editors.
Description: Second edition. | Champaign, IL : Human Kinetics, 2025. | Includes bibliographical references and index.
Identifiers: LCCN 2023049940 (print) | LCCN 2023049941 (ebook) | ISBN 9781718217140 (paperback) | ISBN 9781718217157 (epub) | ISBN 9781718217164 (pdf)
Subjects: LCSH: School health services--United States. | Health education--United States. | Health promotion--United States. | Academic achievement--Health aspects. | BISAC: EDUCATION / Teaching / Subjects / Health & Sexuality | EDUCATION / Teaching / Methods & Strategies
Classification: LCC LB3409.U5 P76 2025 (print) | LCC LB3409.U5 (ebook) | DDC 371.7/1--dc23/eng/20231114
LC record available at https://lccn.loc.gov/2023049940
LC ebook record available at https://lccn.loc.gov/2023049941

ISBN: 978-1-7182-1714-0 (print)

Copyright © 2025 by David A. Birch, Donna M. Videto, and Hannah P. Catalano
Copyright © 2015 by David A. Birch and Donna M. Videto

Human Kinetics supports copyright. Copyright fuels scientific and artistic endeavor, encourages authors to create new works, and promotes free speech. Thank you for buying an authorized edition of this work and for complying with copyright laws by not reproducing, scanning, or distributing any part of it in any form without written permission from the publisher. You are supporting authors and allowing Human Kinetics to continue to publish works that increase the knowledge, enhance the performance, and improve the lives of people all over the world.

The online learning content that accompanies this product is delivered on HK*Propel*, **HKPropel.HumanKinetics.com**. You agree that you will not use HK*Propel* if you do not accept the site's Privacy Policy and Terms and Conditions, which detail approved uses of the online content.

To report suspected copyright infringement of content published by Human Kinetics, contact us at **permissions@hkusa.com**. To request permission to legally reuse content published by Human Kinetics, please refer to the information at **https://US.HumanKinetics.com/pages/permissions-translations-faqs**.

This book is a revised edition of *Promoting Health and Academic Success: The Whole School, Whole Community, Whole Child Approach*, published in 2015 by David A. Birch and Donna M. Videto.

The web addresses cited in this text were current as of November 2023, unless otherwise noted.

Acquisitions Editor: Bethany J. Bentley; **Managing Editor:** Jacob Roden; **Copyeditor:** Beth Ciha; **Proofreader:** Leigh Keylock; **Indexer:** Dan Connolly; **Permissions Manager:** Laurel Mitchell; **Graphic Designer:** Dawn Sills; **Cover Designer:** Keri Evans; **Cover Design Specialist:** Susan Rothermel Allen; **Photograph (cover):** Reprinted from ASCD, *Whole School, Whole Community, Whole Child: A Collaborative Approach to Learning and Health* (2014).; **Photographs (interior):** © Human Kinetics, unless otherwise noted; **Photo Asset Manager:** Laura Fitch; **Photo Production Manager:** Jason Allen; **Senior Art Manager:** Kelly Hendren; **Illustrations:** © Human Kinetics, unless otherwise noted; **Printer:** Sheridan Books

Printed in the United States of America   10 9 8 7 6 5 4 3 2 1

The paper in this book is certified under a sustainable forestry program.

Human Kinetics
1607 N. Market Street
Champaign, IL 61820
USA

United States and International
Website: **US.HumanKinetics.com**
Email: info@hkusa.com
Phone: 1-800-747-4457

Canada
Website: **Canada.HumanKinetics.com**
Email: info@hkcanada.com

E8890

CONTENTS

Foreword xi
Preface xiii

CHAPTER 1 **Whole School, Whole Community, Whole Child:
A Framework for Health and Academic Success** 1
David A. Birch • Hannah P. Catalano • Donna M. Videto
Evolution of School Health 2
Moving From CSH to WSCC 3
WSCC Resources: Enhancing the Presence of the Model and Supporting WSCC in Practice 5
Summary 7
Learning Aids 8
References 9

CHAPTER 2 **History of WSCC** 11
Diane DeMuth Allensworth • Hannah P. Catalano
First Stage of Health Promotion: Addressing Infectious Diseases 13
Second Stage of Health Promotion: Addressing Individual Behaviors 14
Third Stage of Health Promotion: Addressing the Social Determinants of Health 20
Evolution of the WSCC Model 24
Summary 26
Learning Aids 26
References 27

CHAPTER 3 **Overview of the WSCC Model** 31
Hannah P. Catalano • David A. Birch • Donna M. Videto
WSCC Model Overview 32
The 10 WSCC Components 35
School Health Index 50
Community as an Overarching WSCC Concept 50
Summary 52
Learning Aids 52
References 53

CHAPTER 4	Health and Academic Success	59

Michele Wallen

Health-Risk Behaviors 60
Health and Education in Early Childhood 62
Adverse Childhood Experiences 62
Chronic Absenteeism 63
Making a Difference Through the WSCC Approach 65
Summary 72
Learning Aids 73
References 74

CHAPTER 5	Meeting the Needs of Diverse Students, Families, and Communities	79

Angelia M. Sanders

Students With Disproportionately Poor Education Outcomes 80
Diversity, Equity, and Inclusion 85
Position Statements on Diversity, Equity, and Inclusion 87
Considerations Related to Social Justice–Oriented Schools 89
Promoting Diversity, Equity, and Inclusion Through Cultural Humility 92
Incorporating Diversity, Equity, and Inclusion Into Family Engagement 93
Promoting Diversity, Equity, and Inclusion Through Community Involvement 93
Summary 94
Learning Aids 95
References 96

CHAPTER 6	Developing and Maintaining Collaborations	101

Bonni C. Hodges • Donna M. Videto

School–Family–Community Collaborations 102
Developing Successful Collaborations 103
Supporting Quality Collaborations 105
Barriers and Challenges to Collaboration 107
Recruiting Partners for Collaborations 110
Implementing and Sustaining Collaborations 111
Summary 113
Learning Aids 113
References 115

CHAPTER 7 **Planning and Evaluating WSCC** 117
Donna M. Videto • Bonni C. Hodges
Systematic Planning 118
Creating a Comprehensive Profile for Program Planning 120
Actions for Collecting Needs Assessment Profile Data 123
A Word About Data and Their Use 130
Evaluating WSCC 132
Planning for Program Evaluation 134
Summary 136
Learning Aids 137
References 139

CHAPTER 8 **Implementing WSCC** 141
Donna M. Videto • Hannah P. Catalano • David A. Birch
Step 1: Establish Leadership With a Designated School Health Coordinator 142
Step 2: Secure Administrative Support and Develop a District-Level School Health Council and School Health Teams 145
Step 3: Identify Available Resources in the School, District, and Community 148
Step 4: After Reviewing the Initial Data, Determine the Outcomes of Greatest Priority 149
Step 5: Create an Action Plan Based on Realistic Goals and Objectives Agreed Upon by Partners 150
Step 6: Establish a Realistic Timeline for Implementing Strategies From the Action Plan 153
Step 7: Implement the Plan and Strategies 153
Step 8: Review and Implement the Evaluation Plan 155
Step 9: Provide Professional Development for Faculty and Staff 155
Step 10: Communicate Steps and Successes 157
Summary 157
Learning Aids 158
References 159

CHAPTER 9 Considerations for WSCC in Practice — 161

A Perspective on the Role of State Education Agencies in Promoting WSCC — 162
Rosemary Reilly-Chammat

The Role of the Federal Government in Education 162
The Role of the States in Education 163
Leadership by State Education Agencies in School Health 164
Frameworks to Support the Work: WSCC and the Multitiered System of Supports Framework 166
Future Opportunities 168
References 169

Every School Healthy: An Urban School Case Study — 170
Sue Baldwin • Assunta R. Ventresca

Needs Assessment and District Response 171
Key Stakeholder Engagement 172
Professional Development 173
Implications for School Health 174
References 175

A Synopsis of International Efforts to Improve School Health Programs — 176
Lloyd J. Kolbe

The Need for International Efforts to Improve School Health Programs 176
U.S. and International School Health Program Frameworks 177
International Organizations Working to Improve School Health Programs 178
Journals of School Health 180
The Future of National and International Efforts to Improve School Health Programs 180
Summary 183
References 183

Teacher Education: Preparing Educators for WSCC Engagement — 186
Elisa Beth McNeill

References 189

The Importance of Professional Development — 191
Lori Paisley

WSCC Professional Development 191
Summary 194
References 196

Learning Aids 196

CHAPTER 10 Perspectives on WSCC in Practice 197

The American School Health Association's Perspective on the WSCC Framework 198
Kayce D. Solari Williams • Randi J. Alter

The Role of the American School Health Association in Advancing the WSCC Framework   198
Working Across Disciplines for Student Success   200
The Role of Associations in Advancing WSCC Into the Future   200
References   201

Society for Public Health Education: Champion for Quality School Health Education 202
M. Elaine Auld

The Early Years   203
Ramping Up Efforts   203
WSCC Takes Center Stage   206
Moving Forward   207
References   208

The Whole Campus Model: A WSCC Framework for Health Promotion on College Campuses 210
Bonni C. Hodges • Donna M. Videto • Alexis Blavos

The Whole College Student   211
The Whole Campus Model   212
Summary   217
References   218

The Need for a WSCC-Based School Health Research Agenda 220
Michael J. Mann

The Importance of School Health and School Health Research   220
The Promise of the WSCC Model   221
Outstanding Questions Shaping the Future of WSCC-Based School Health Research   222
The Promise of a WSCC-Based Research Agenda for School Health   223
Elements of an Effective Process   224
Imagining the Future of WSCC   226
Summary   227
References   227

WSCC: A Future Perspective   228
Sean Slade
A Model for Our Times   228
Pandemic as a Cure   228
The Rise of WSCC   229
Where We Are Going   230
A Culture of Well-Being   231
Toward a Healthy Future   232
References   233
Learning Aids   233

Index   235
About the Editors   241
About the Contributors   243

FOREWORD

The well-being of humans is determined by the quality of four systems developed by each nation: (1) public health and health care, (2) education, (3) economic productivity and wealth distribution, and (4) governance. Each system is interdependent upon the others. The world's schools underlie these systems because they materially shape the health, education, productivity, and resulting quality of life of the young people who manifest the futures of their respective nations and of humankind collectively. More than 1.5 billion young people attend primary and secondary schools around the world every school day, 50 million of them within the United States. Research has shown that well-developed school health programs, sometimes called health-promoting schools, could become one of the most effective means nations have of improving both the health and education of their people.

Indeed, human societies over the centuries progressively have developed scientific disciplines, professions, and effective practices to improve the lives of their people. During the past century, school health evolved as a new discipline contemporaneously with the evolution of public health, health care, and education. Scientific journals provided means for school health experts to systematically identify, communicate, and archive carefully reviewed information that could be used by practitioners, researchers, policymakers, and the public to improve both health and education outcomes. Universities employed scholars to amalgamate and use this information; conduct research to assess and increase the effectiveness of programs; and provide undergraduate, graduate, preservice, and in-service training to enable various types of school health professionals to master their practices. However, few modern textbooks have been developed to help organize school health as a scientific discipline and, accordingly, to strengthen professional development and effective practice.

Promoting Health and Academic Success: The WSCC Approach, Second Edition, is one of the most modern, comprehensive, and authoritative textbooks available—online and in print, within the United States and internationally—to help organize the scientific discipline, professional development, and consequent effective practice of school health programs. By using the multicomponent Whole School, Whole Community, Whole Child (WSCC) approach, which is widely used throughout the United States, this textbook purposefully explains the collaborative means available to all who share interdependent responsibilities for improving the health and education of students. These individuals include school administrators and teachers; parents and students; staff of community education, health, and social service organizations; nurses and physicians; counselors, psychologists, and social workers; food service staff; health educators; physical educators and coaches; custodians; safety personnel; legislators; and school health coordinators charged with orchestrating the critical but otherwise scattered efforts of these professionals and community members. This textbook is vital for training each of these individuals and professions and for improving, uniting, and amplifying their respective efforts and voices.

Now more than ever, societies must help schools improve the health and education of their young people. In the United States, students are increasingly more racially, culturally, and economically diverse. Many live in poverty. Many live with only one or neither parent. Many are immigrants, many are transient, many are homeless, and many have special education needs. Many experience one or numerous health threats, including hunger or neglect; asthma; obesity and consequent risk for diabetes, heart disease, and cancer; attention-deficit/hyperactivity disorder or autism spectrum disorder; or hazards in the school environment such as exposure to polychlorinated biphenyls, noroviruses, pesticides, and bullying. During the past several years these often insidious threats have been compounded by the effects of the COVID-19 pandemic, climate change, economic inequities, political divisiveness, gun violence, and international conflicts. These conditions together have generated widespread student anxiety, depression, and suicide. Increasing student absences, declining student performance scores, increasing political pressures on schools, more teachers and administrators leaving the education profession, fewer teachers entering the profession, and more discouraged college teacher preparation faculty threaten our education system as never before. So grave are these threats to education systems around the world that at the 2022 World Health Assembly the United Nations Secretary-General convened the Transforming Education Summit, the very first focus of which was to build "Inclusive, Equitable, Safe and Healthy Schools," which also is the focus of this textbook.

There is much each of us as individuals can do, especially together, to help our young people become healthy, safe, supported, engaged, and challenged to do their very best. I, like others, often look back on my life and ask myself what I could have done better and what I could do now. I commend to you this textbook and these questions.

Lloyd J. Kolbe, PhD

PREFACE

Parents, educators, and community members want children to experience optimal health and academic success. Research clearly demonstrates the relationship between students' health and academic achievement (Bradley & Greene, 2013; Centers for Disease Control and Prevention [CDC], 2022; Kolbe, 2019). Students who are supported by family members, teachers, and other adults and who engage in healthy behaviors at school, at home, and in the community are more likely to come to school focused on learning and ultimately achieve academic success.

Although the relationship between students' health and education is increasingly understood by educators, health professionals, family members, and community members, the capacity of these stakeholders to enhance health and learning is often negatively influenced by limited school resources, issues related to inadequate policies and practices, and the overall school environment. Beyond the school, a range of social issues—such as structural racism and other forms of discrimination, poverty, and community safety concerns—affect both students' health and their learning. These obstacles, within the school and the community, present challenges to both education and health.

In the mid-1980s a model eventually known as the Coordinated School Health (CSH) model was introduced by two leaders in school health, Diane Allensworth and Lloyd Kolbe. This model was designed to coordinate various school programs to promote health and academic success for students. The basic idea behind CSH was that schools should address the health of students through coordinated activities, policies, and programs that involved the following eight components:

- Health education
- Health services
- Physical education
- Nutrition services
- Counseling, psychological, and social services
- Healthy school environment
- Family and community involvement
- Health promotion for staff

Although this model was enthusiastically endorsed by many stakeholders and received national attention, comprehensive implementation of CSH was limited. This lack of acceptance was partially attributed to the perception of CSH as a health model rather than a health and education model (Allensworth, 2015).

In 2014, a new version of coordinated school health and academic success, the Whole School, Whole Community, Whole Child (WSCC) approach, was developed by the CDC and ASCD, a prominent education professional organization. The importance of this higher level collaboration between the education and health communities was captured by Wayne H. Giles, former director of the CDC's Division of Population Health, who stated, "It is time to truly align the sectors and place the child at the center. Both public health and education serve the same students, often in the same settings. We must do more to work together and collaborate" (ASCD, 2014, p. 4).

The WSCC model highlights the idea that healthy students are more likely to be academically successful than students dealing with health issues. From a structural standpoint, the WSCC model places the child at the center and highlights the importance of five Whole Child tenets: healthy, safe, engaged, supported, and challenged. In addition, the concept of community is presented as an overarching feature of the approach (see figure 1.1, p. 4). Included in the WSCC model are the following 10 components:

- Health education
- Physical education and physical activity
- Nutrition environment and services
- Health services
- Counseling, psychological, and social services
- Social and emotional climate
- Physical environment
- Employee wellness
- Family engagement
- Community involvement

The first edition of this book, *Promoting Health and Academic Success: The Whole School, Whole Community, Whole Child Approach* (Birch & Videto, 2015), served as a resource in the transition from CSH to WSCC. The second edition incorporates WSCC knowledge and experience that have been gained since the publication of the first edition of the book in 2015. The current edition has two specific purposes: (1) to serve as a textbook for college and university undergraduate and graduate courses that address WSCC, school health programs, children's health, and topics emanating from the 10 WSCC components and (2) to serve as a resource for state departments of education, state departments of health, school districts, individual schools, and other agencies and organizations involved in initiating, maintaining, and improving efforts in health promotion and academic success for students. The authors who have contributed to this edition of the book have experience as leaders in school health and WSCC at the national, state, and local levels. Several individuals directly involved in the development of the WSCC model are contributors to this edition, including Diane Allensworth, M. Elaine Auld, David Birch, and Lloyd Kolbe. Another contributor, Sean Slade, was a member of the CDC and ASCD core group that provided the leadership for the development and finalization of the model.

Since the publication of the first edition, schools and communities have faced challenges that have had an impact on how schools meet the needs of students. These challenges include the presence of a major communicable disease, COVID-19; school safety issues, especially within the context of several mass shootings in schools; controversy regarding curriculum content and teaching and learning methods related to areas such as social justice and sexuality; racism and other forms of systemic discrimination; students' mental and emotional health; and the well-being of faculty and staff members. We see the WSCC model as a framework for positively addressing these ongoing societal issues through its coordinated structure of various school programs and its inclusive engagement of parents, families, and community members.

The first four chapters in this book provide an overview of the WSCC model, the rationale behind and history of coordinated school health resulting in the evolution to WSCC, a detailed presentation of the WSCC components, and background information on the relationship between students' health and academic success. Chapters 5 to 8 focus on WSCC in practice. Chapter 5 presents important considerations and strategies related to the role of WSCC in addressing the needs of diverse students, families, and communities. The importance of developing and maintaining partnerships is examined in chapter 6. Chapters 7 and 8 provide specific direction related to the planning, implementation, and evaluation of WSCC. Chapters 9 and 10 present the perspectives and practical experiences of WSCC leaders related to support, operationalization, and future considerations related to the model. Application activities at the end of each chapter provide an opportunity to apply information to simulations based on WSCC scenarios.

We believe *Promoting Health and Academic Success: The WSCC Approach, Second Edition*, will be an invaluable resource for college and university faculty members, students, and professionals in education and health who are working with schools and school districts to improve academic achievement and student health. Ultimately, we believe this resource can play an important role in planning, implementing, and evaluating education and health initiatives through the meaningful, coordinated engagement of school administrators, teachers, staff members, parents and other family members, public health professionals, and community members. We believe these initiatives will not only improve health but also increase the likelihood of academic success.

David A. Birch
Donna M. Videto
Hannah P. Catalano

References

Allensworth, D. (2015). Historical overview of coordinated school health. In D.A. Birch & D.M. Videto (Eds.), *Promoting health and academic success: The Whole School, Whole Community, Whole Child approach* (pp. 13-28). Human Kinetics.

ASCD. (2014). *Whole School, Whole Community, Whole Child: A collaborative approach to learning and health.* https://files.ascd.org/staticfiles/ascd/pdf/siteASCD/publications/wholechild/wscc-a-collaborative-approach.pdf

Birch, D.A., & Videto, D.M. (Eds.). (2015). *Promoting health and academic success: The Whole School, Whole Community, Whole Child approach.* Human Kinetics.

Bradley, B.J., & Greene, A.C. (2013). Do health and education agencies in the United States share responsibility for academic achievement and health? A review of 25 years of evidence about the relationship of adolescents' academic achievement and health behaviors. *Journal of Adolescent Health, 52*(5), 523-532. https://doi.org/10.1016/j.jadohealth.2013.01.008

Centers for Disease Control and Prevention. (2022). *Health and academics.* www.cdc.gov/healthyschools/health_and_academics/index.htm

Kolbe, L.J. (2019). School health as a strategy to improve both public health and education. *Annual Review of Public Health, 40,* 443-468. https://doi.org/10.1146/annurev-publhealth-040218-043727

Instructor Resources in HK*Propel*

The following instructor ancillaries are available within the instructor pack in HK*Propel*:

- The instructor guide includes learning objectives, review items, application activities, project-based assignments, and lists of additional resources and further readings. The instructor guide also contains a sample syllabus.
- The presentation package includes approximately 200 slides of text, artwork, and tables from the book that instructors can use for class discussion and presentation. The slides in the presentation package can be used directly within PowerPoint or printed to make transparencies or handouts for distribution to students. Instructors can easily add, modify, and rearrange the order of the slides.

Instructor ancillaries are free to adopting instructors, including an ebook version of the text that allows instructors to add highlights, annotations, and bookmarks. Please contact your Sales Manager for details about how to access instructor resources in HK*Propel*.

Student Resources in HK*Propel*

New to this edition is HK*Propel* access for students. It supplements the textbook with the following online elements:

- Lists of additional resources and further readings are provided for each chapter.
- Review items, application activities, and project-based assignments are also provided for each chapter.

See the card at the front of the print book for your unique HK*Propel* access code. For ebook users, reference the HK*Propel* access code instructions on the page immediately following the book cover.

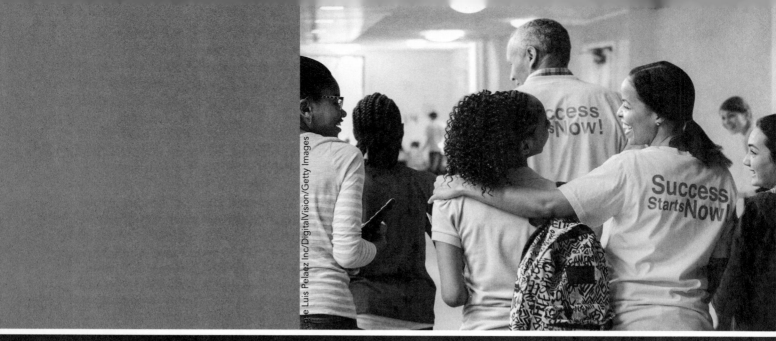

CHAPTER 1

Whole School, Whole Community, Whole Child: A Framework for Health and Academic Success

David A. Birch • Hannah P. Catalano • Donna M. Videto

LEARNING OBJECTIVES

1. Describe the evolution of school health models from the early 20th century to the present time.
2. Summarize the components and structure of the Whole School, Whole Community, Whole Child (WSCC) model.
3. Identify resources that promote and support the WSCC model.

KEY TERMS

American School Health Association (ASHA)
ASCD
CDC Healthy Schools
Coordinated School Health (CSH) model
Division of Adolescent and School Health (DASH)
National Association of Chronic Disease Directors (NACDD)
School Health Index (SHI) Self-Assessment and Planning Guide
Society for Public Health Education (SOPHE)
Stakeholder
Whole Child approach
Whole Child tenets
Whole School, Whole Community, Whole Child (WSCC) model

Since the early part of the 20th century, promoting the health of students has been recognized as a responsibility of schools. The model for school health that was used for most of the 20th century was a three-component model that included health education, the school environment, and health services. In the 1980s Diane Allensworth and Lloyd Kolbe developed an expanded approach, originally known as the Comprehensive School Health model but later called the **Coordinated School Health (CSH) model**, that included eight components. The intent of CSH was that it would serve not only as a vehicle for promoting the health of students but also as a strategy for promoting academic success (Allensworth & Kolbe, 1987). Implementation of CSH in schools, however, was limited (Allensworth, 2015). In 2014, ASCD (formerly known as the Association for Supervision and Curriculum Development) and the Centers for Disease Control and Prevention (CDC) collaborated on the development of a new 10-component framework, the Whole School, Whole Community, Whole Child (WSCC) model (ASCD, 2014). This chapter presents a brief historical overview of school health before the introduction of WSCC. A more detailed history is presented in chapter 2. The primary focus of this chapter is to present an overview of WSCC to introduce the model. The overview includes a description of the model, the 10 components, and the tenets of the Whole Child approach. The model is presented in more detail in chapter 3. In addition to the model overview, examples of WSCC-related activities and resources that have emerged from highly visible national organizations are presented in the chapter.

Evolution of School Health

Promoting the health of students has historically been recognized as a responsibility of schools. In the early part of the 20th century, a primary focus of school health was the prevention of communicable diseases. The model for school health that was used for most of the 20th century was a three-component model that included health education, the school environment, and health services.

In the late 1980s, to provide direction in addressing the health priorities of school-age children, Diane Allensworth and Lloyd Kolbe, prominent leaders in school health, proposed an eight-component model for health promotion, the Comprehensive School Health (CSH) program. The term "comprehensive" was later replaced by "coordinated" when referring to CSH. The eight CSH components were as follows:

- School health services
- School health education
- School health environment
- Integrated school, family, and community health promotion efforts
- School physical education
- School food service
- School counseling
- School site health promotion programs for faculty and staff

The intent was for CSH to serve not only as a vehicle for promoting the health of students but also as a supporting factor for the promotion of academic success (Allensworth & Kolbe, 1987). Students' health and academic success are interdependent. Students who face health challenges such as stress, physical and emotional abuse, aggression and violence, safety concerns, hunger, malnourishment, hyperactivity, lack of sleep, vision problems, asthma, and dental health problems often experience academic issues (Basch, 2011; Kolbe, 2019). Research demonstrates a strong relationship between students' healthy behaviors and academic achievement as indicated by standardized test scores, graduation rates, and attendance (CDC, 2022b).

The importance of CSH was emphasized through the publication of a special issue of the *Journal of School Health* (*JOSH*) in December 1987. Allensworth and Kolbe coauthored the introductory article in the issue, which presented an overview of the new approach to school health and its interdependence with education (Allensworth & Kolbe, 1987). National leaders in the relevant areas were invited to write articles related to each of the eight components.

As CSH moved through the 1990s, the term *comprehensive* was replaced by *coordinated* when referring to CSH. Although CSH received increased national recognition in the late 1980s and funding was provided by the **Division of Adolescent and School Health (DASH)** of the CDC to selected state departments of education and departments of health, implementation in local school districts was less than optimal (Basch, 2011). McKenzie and Richmond (1998) described this dilemma, stating, "The promise of a Coordinated School Health program thus far outshines its practice" (p. 10). More than 10 years later, Basch (2011) provided another perspective by stating, "Though rhetorical support is increasing, school health is currently not a central part of the fundamental mission of schools in America, nor has it been well integrated into the broader national strategy to reduce the gaps in educational opportunity and outcomes" (p. 595). One possible reason for this lack of acceptance was that educators and other **stakeholders** viewed CSH as a health program focused only on health outcomes rather than an initiative that would also contribute to improved academic outcomes (Allensworth, 2015). Further information related to CSH is presented in chapter 2.

Moving From CSH to WSCC

ASCD, a leading education professional organization, has been a leader in the 21st century in illuminating the connection between health and education. In 2007, ASCD implemented its **Whole Child approach**. This approach focuses on the long-term development and success of children rather than only on a narrowly defined version of academic achievement. An important element of the approach is the inclusion of five **Whole Child tenets**: healthy, safe, engaged, supported, and challenged. These tenets were identified as essential for students' health and learning (ASCD, 2014). The Whole Child approach is addressed in more detail in chapter 3.

In 2014, building on both the ASCD Whole Child approach and the original eight-component CSH model, ASCD and the CDC collaborated on the development of a new school health model called the **WSCC model** (ASCD, 2014). The development of the new model involved a core group that provided leadership to the project, a consultation group that developed documents and frameworks related to the new model, and a review group that periodically reviewed and provided feedback on the work of the consultation group. Members of the three groups were selected because of their roles as leaders in both education and health (Lewallen et al., 2015). The WSCC model was introduced at two national conferences, the ASCD conference in Los Angeles in March 2014 and the **Society for Public Health Education (SOPHE)** conference in Baltimore also in March 2014 (Birch & Videto, 2015). WSCC incorporates and builds on both CSH and the ASCD Whole Child approach. The model is designed to promote alignment, integration, and collaboration between education and health and is intended to enhance health outcomes and academic success (ASCD, 2014).

A diagrammatic representation of the overall WSCC model is presented in figure 1.1. As depicted in the figure, the child is the focal point of the model and is placed at the center surrounded by the five Whole Child tenets. Coordinating policy, process, and practice are placed in a ring around the tenets, which signifies the intention of the model to promote both learning and health. An even larger ring consisting of 10 school components surrounds the child, the tenets, and the coordination ring. The 10 components serve as focal points for the full range of learning and health support systems for each child, in each school, in each community. The community is on the periphery of the model, which demonstrates that although the school may be the focal point, it remains a reflection of its community and requires community input, resources, and collaboration to support students. Essentially, school issues are community issues, and community issues are often school issues.

An important aspect of WSCC is the expansion from eight CSH components to 10 WSCC components. One original component, healthy and safe school environment, was expanded into two separate components: physical environment and social and emotional climate. Another original component, family and community involvement, was expanded into two components: community involvement and family engagement (ASCD, 2014). The evolution of the three school health models is presented in chapter 2 (see figure 2.1).

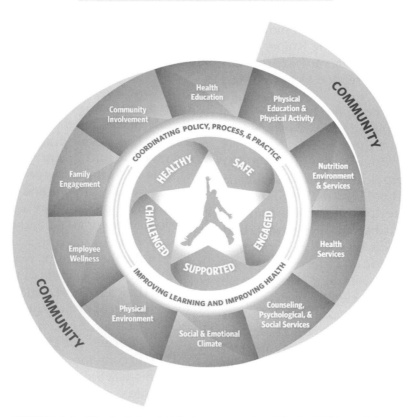

FIGURE 1.1 Whole School, Whole Community, Whole Child model.
Reprinted from ASCD, *Whole School, Whole Community, Whole Child: A Collaborative Approach to Learning and Health* (2014).

Since its introduction in 2014, WSCC has received considerable attention at the state and national levels (King & Lederer, 2019). Because it was developed through collaboration between an education association (ASCD) and a health organization (the CDC), WSCC appears to have more local, state, and national recognition than CSH as both an education model and a health model among schools and organizational stakeholders. In a 2015 special issue of *JOSH* focused on WSCC, Lewallen and colleagues (2015) suggested that the inclusion of both education and health in the model provides a framework for schools to both promote academic achievement and address the numerous individual, school, and community factors that affect students' health. An overview of the special journal issue (H. Hunt, 2015) is presented in the WSCC in Practice sidebar on page 6.

WSCC Resources: Enhancing the Presence of the Model and Supporting WSCC in Practice

Although no research exists that can point with precision to the implementation of WSCC in U.S. schools, the engagement of highly visible national organizations in WSCC-related activities appears to indicate a more prominent presence in education and health for WSCC than CSH. Several WSCC resources have emerged from these activities.

The CDC has developed a range of resources to support the education, public health, and school health sectors in their WSCC-related efforts. **CDC Healthy Schools** provides background information specific to WSCC and information related to children's cognitive, physical, social, and emotional development as it relates to health and learning (CDC, 2022d). Another CDC Healthy Schools resource, the *School Health Index (SHI) Self-Assessment and Planning Guide*, uses the WSCC framework to assess the promotion of health in individual schools through the provision of curriculum analysis tools for both health education and physical education (CDC, 2022a) and background information for best practices for each of the 10 WSCC components (CDC, 2021). CDC Healthy Schools also presents CDC data linking youth health behaviors and academic achievement. A unique interactive CDC tool, Virtual Healthy School, uses familiar school scenes to demonstrate how schools can support their students' health and academic achievement (CDC, 2022c). Additional CDC resources are provided, including evidence-based strategies and promising practices for school health services, nutrition services, and physical education and physical activity and the integration of out-of-school time across the WSCC framework.

The **American School Health Association (ASHA)** has also played an important role in the promotion of WSCC. Through its national conference, webinars, and peer-reviewed publication, *JOSH*, ASHA has provided support and resources to educators and schools in the promotion of health and academic success through the implementation of the WSCC model. The organization's commitment to WSCC is demonstrated through its core values, which emphasize both the linkage between students' health and academic success and the importance of a coordinated approach to school health. In a statement prefacing their core values, ASHA states, "We believe the [WSCC] model is the best representation of a truly collaborative approach to health and learning" (ASHA, 2022, para. 3). One important indicator of ASHA's commitment to WSCC is the November 2015 issue of *JOSH* that focused on the model. More details related to this issue are presented in the WSCC in Practice sidebar on page 6.

SOPHE has also been an important contributor to the national presence of the WSCC model. As part of its efforts to support WSCC, SOPHE, in collaboration with CDC Healthy Schools, engaged 28 school and district staff members and developed a 10-part suite of WSCC training materials called the WSCC Team Training Modules (SOPHE, n.d.). The modules are intended for use by states, districts, or local schools to support school teams in imple-

WSCC IN PRACTICE
2015 Special Issue of the *Journal of School Health*: The Whole School, Whole Community, Whole Child Model

A special issue of *JOSH*, published in November 2015, was developed through a contract with the CDC and the National Association of Chronic Disease Directors (NACDD). The entire issue consists of articles related to the WSCC model. The intent was to introduce WSCC to readers and provide details related to the development, rationale for, and content of the model. The articles in this issue of *JOSH* provide an excellent supplementary resource to the second edition of this book.

The first article in the issue, titled "The Whole School, Whole Community, Whole Child Model: A New Approach for Improving Educational Attainment and Healthy Development for Students" and authored by Theresa C. Lewallen, Holly Hunt, William Potts-Datema, Stephanie Zaza, and Wayne Giles, all CDC staff members in 2015, includes an overview of the development of WSCC and a description of the 10 components that make up the framework of the model. The article concludes by describing WSCC as a comprehensive framework for schools and districts and closes by stating the following:

> *By focusing on children and youth as students, addressing critical education and health outcomes, organizing collaborative actions and initiatives that support students, and strongly engaging community resources, the WSCC approach offers important opportunities for school improvements that will advance educational attainment and healthy development for students (p. 737).*

Other important aspects of the WSCC model are addressed in the remaining articles. The title and authors of each of the remaining articles are as follows:

- "Critical Connections: Health and Academics" (Michael et al., 2015)
- "Lessons Learned From the Whole Child and Coordinated School Health Approaches" (Rasberry et al., 2015)
- "What Have We Learned From Collaborative Partnerships to Concomitantly Improve Both Education and Health?" (Kolbe et al., 2015)
- "How the Whole School, Whole Community, Whole Child Model Works: Creating Greater Alignment, Integration, and Collaboration Between Health and Education" (Chiang et al., 2015)
- "Placing Students at the Center: The Whole School, Whole Community, Whole Child Model" (Morse & Allensworth, 2015)
- "Supporting the Whole Child Through Coordinated Policies, Processes, and Practices" (Murray et al., 2015)
- "A Whole School Approach: Collaborative Development of School Health Policies, Processes, and Practices" (P. Hunt et al., 2015)
- "Building Sustainable Health and Education Partnerships: Stories From Local Communities" (Blank, 2015)
- "Using the Whole School, Whole Community, Whole Child Model: Implications for Practice" (Rooney et al., 2015)

The articles in this issue of *JOSH* were authored by individuals working in diverse roles and settings related to WSCC. The issue presents resources related to the academic and health rationale for WSCC; the components of the model's framework; and important considerations related to planning, implementation, and evaluation. Since the publication of this issue of *JOSH*, a plethora of reports and peer-reviewed articles have been published that address various topics related to WSCC. Many of these are cited in the various chapters in this book. A second special issue of *JOSH* (December, 2020) included two editorials and 14 articles focused on WSCC. The volume of WSCC publications since the introduction of the model in 2015 may be one indicator of an increasing presence of WSCC in schools.

menting the WSCC model and are accessible from the SOPHE website. For its leadership in developing this resource, SOPHE received the ASHA 2021 Whole School, Whole Community, Whole Child (WSCC) Award (SOPHE, 2021). Additional information regarding this resource is provided in a WSCC in Practice sidebar in chapter 3.

Another example of public health engagement with the WSCC model comes from the **National Association of Chronic Disease Directors (NACDD)**. The core membership of NACDD includes U.S. state and territorial directors and their staff members (NACDD, n.d.a). The value placed on WSCC by NACDD is demonstrated through several resources developed by the organization. One NACDD resource, *The Whole School, Whole Community, Whole Child Model: A Guide to Implementation* (NACDD, 2017), is intended to provide guidance to administrators, teachers, school and district staff members, community partners, public health professionals, parents, and other stakeholders interested in moving WSCC forward in communities and schools. NACDD has also developed an online resource called the School Health Resource Guide (NACDD, n.d.b) that can be useful for WSCC activities in a school district or school.

A unique collaborative effort exemplifies the partnership potential of WSCC. The Healthy Schools Toolkit is an extensive WSCC resource funded by the Robert Wood Johnson Foundation, informed by a national advisory committee, and developed in a university and public school partnership between the Brown School at Washington University in St. Louis and two urban school districts, the Saint Louis (Missouri) Public Schools and the Normandy (Missouri) School Collaboration. The toolkit was designed to help school leaders identify methods for building healthier school communities. The kit includes three modules: People, Systems, and Messages. It also includes resources related to WSCC implementation and detailed information generated from WSCC implementation in the Saint Louis and Normandy schools (Washington University in St. Louis, n.d.).

Another valuable resource, the WellSAT WSCC, was developed by the Collaboratory on School and Child Health and the Rudd Center for Food Policy and Obesity, both housed at the University of Connecticut. This school policy evaluation tool was designed to enable school districts to assess the alignment of their policies with the 10 components of the WSCC model. This resource is built on earlier versions of the WellSAT, including one developed in 2019. In regard to assessing policy related to WSCC, the 2019 version assessed only two components of the model: the nutrition environment, and physical education and physical activity (Koriakin et al., 2020). The WellSAT WSCC, a revised version finalized in 2021, expanded the assessment to all 10 component areas of WSCC. This resource provides school districts with a freely accessible tool for assessing the alignment of policies with the WSCC model (University of Connecticut Collaboratory on School and Child Health, n.d.).

Summary

School health has evolved from a focus on health education, the school environment, and health services to the current 10-component WSCC model. This model was developed collaboratively by an education organization (ASCD) and the CDC. This collaboration, along with the WSCC model's focus on the child and the important role of the family, school, and community, has presented opportunities for the education and health sectors to engage as partners in activities to support WSCC and expand the model's sphere of awareness and support. WSCC not only provides a framework for the promotion of academic achievement and health for children and youth but also can provide a space for addressing family, community, and school issues emanating from misinformation, inequity, and social injustices. For WSCC to reach its full potential, stakeholders in schools and communities will need to understand and address the connection between health and learning; place importance on focusing on the needs of the child in addressing this connection; and stress the necessity of collaboration among schools, families, and communities.

LEARNING AIDS

GLOSSARY

American School Health Association (ASHA)—A multidisciplinary organization made up of administrators, counselors, dietitians, nutritionists, health educators, physical educators, psychologists, school health coordinators, school nurses, school physicians, and social workers. ASHA works to lead and engage in efforts to prioritize school-based approaches that promote lifelong health, build a community to support the whole child, and activate champions of school health.

ASCD—Founded in 1943, ASCD (formerly the Association for Supervision and Curriculum Development) is a global leader in developing and delivering innovative programs, products, and services that empower educators to support the success of each learner.

CDC Healthy Schools—A unit in the CDC that works with states, school systems, communities, and national partners to prevent chronic disease and promote the health and well-being of children and adolescents in schools. The WSCC model is the unit's framework for addressing health in schools.

Coordinated School Health (CSH) model—An eight-component model designed to promote health and learning in schools. The eight components were health education, physical education, health services, nutrition services, counseling and psychological services, healthy and safe school environment, health promotion for staff, and family and community involvement. This approach was a forerunner to the WSCC approach.

Division of Adolescent and School Health (DASH)—A unit in the CDC that promotes environments where teens can gain fundamental health knowledge and skills, establish healthy behaviors for a lifetime, connect to health services, and avoid becoming pregnant or infected with HIV or sexually transmitted diseases.

National Association of Chronic Disease Directors (NACDD)—A membership organization composed of chronic disease directors in state and territorial health departments and their staff members and other chronic disease professionals working in state, tribal, and territorial health departments; nonprofits; academia; and private industry. NACDD advocates, educates, and provides technical assistance to inform programming and sustain and grow chronic disease prevention.

School Health Index (SHI) Self-Assessment and Planning Guide—A CDC resource developed in partnership with school administrators and staff, school health experts, parents, and nongovernmental health agencies. The guide provides schools with a self-assessment tool that uses the 10 WSCC components as a framework to examine health and safety policies, programs, and services to provide direction for the development of an action plan for addressing student health.

Society for Public Health Education (SOPHE)—A professional organization for health educators working in all health education sectors and health education students enrolled in professional preparation programs at the undergraduate and graduate levels.

stakeholder—Any individual or organization who is interested or engaged in a school's teaching and learning, students' academic success, and students' overall well-being. Stakeholders include students; parents and family members; teachers; administrators; staff members; community members; members of the business, faith, and law enforcement communities; and elected and nonelected public officials and employees. Stakeholders can also be organizations representing a variety of individuals, professionals, and interest groups.

Whole Child approach—An initiative started in 2007 by ASCD that focuses greater attention on a holistic, well-rounded education that caters to each child's social, emotional, mental, physical, and cognitive development.

Whole Child tenets—The five key principles—healthy, safe, engaged, supported, and challenged—that underlie the WSCC model. The presence of these tenets as experienced by students is critical for promoting their health and academic success. An emphasis on the tenets should be a consideration in the development of the school curriculum and school-related policies, processes, and practices.

Whole School, Whole Community, Whole Child (WSCC) model—A collaborative model for promoting health and academic success. It is an expanded framework of the ASCD Whole Child approach and CSH that integrates components of each approach.

APPLICATION ACTIVITIES

1. You are a peer mentor for students who have just enrolled in your major. During a mid-semester meeting with your mentees, you describe some of the courses that are required for the major. One of your current courses is The Relationship Between Education and Health. The focal point of the course is the WSCC model. As you identify the title of the course, two students ask the following questions: "What is the WSCC model?" and "What is the relationship between education and health?" In the limited time you have for discussion during the meeting, provide one response that addresses both questions. Identify important facts or considerations related to WSCC that you will include in your response.

2. Conduct a literature search of newspapers, magazines, and social media for a story (or several stories) of a student whose academic progress was affected by a health or safety issue. Identify any positive actions that were taken in this situation or make recommendations for how the situation could have been addressed in a more productive way. Consider the role of the WSCC model in your response.

3. Review one of the following two CDC resources presented in the chapter: the *School Health Index (SHI) Self-Assessment and Planning Guide* or Virtual Healthy School. Write a review that provides a brief description of the resource, your thoughts on it as a tool for understanding WSCC, and its potential value for educators and health professionals. Your review should be approximately 500 words.

REFERENCES

Allensworth, D.D. (2015). Historical overview of coordinated school health. In D.A. Birch & D.M. Videto (Eds.), *Promoting health and academic success: The Whole School, Whole Community, Whole Child approach* (pp. 13-28). Human Kinetics.

Allensworth, D.D., & Kolbe, L.J. (1987). The Comprehensive School Health program: Exploring an expanded concept. *Journal of School Health*, 57(10), 409-412.

American School Health Association. (2022). *Priority areas and core beliefs in action—ASHA.* www.ashaweb.org/priority-areas-and-core-beliefs-in-action/

ASCD. (2014). *Whole School, Whole Community, Whole Child: A collaborative approach to learning and health.* https://files.ascd.org/staticfiles/ascd/pdf/siteASCD/publications/wholechild/wscc-a-collaborative-approach.pdf

Basch, C.E. (2011). Healthier students are better learners: A missing link in school reforms to close the achievement gap. *Journal of School Health*, 81, 593-598. https://doi.org/10.1111/j.1746-1561.2011.00632.x

Birch, D.A., & Videto, D.M. (Eds.). (2015). *Promoting health and academic success: The Whole School, Whole Community, Whole Child approach.* Human Kinetics.

Blank, M.J. (2015). Building sustainable health and education partnerships: Stories from local communities. *Journal of School Health*, 85(11), 810-816. https://doi.org/10.1111/josh.12311

Centers for Disease Control and Prevention. (2021). *Components of the Whole School, Whole Community, Whole Child approach.* www.cdc.gov/healthyschools/wscc/components.htm

Centers for Disease Control and Prevention. (2022a). *Assessing school health.* www.cdc.gov/healthyschools/assessment.htm

Centers for Disease Control and Prevention. (2022b). *Health and academics.* www.cdc.gov/healthyschools/health_and_academics/index.htm

Centers for Disease Control and Prevention. (2022c). *Virtual Healthy School.* www.cdc.gov/healthyschools/vhs.htm

Centers for Disease Control and Prevention. (2022d). *Whole School, Whole Community, Whole Child (WSCC).* www.cdc.gov/healthyschools/wscc/

Chiang, R.J., Meagher, W., & Slade, S. (2015). How the Whole School, Whole Community, Whole Child model works: Creating greater alignment, integration, and collaboration between health and education. *Journal of School Health, 85*(11), 775-784. https://doi.org/10.1111/josh.12308

Hunt, H. (Ed.). (2015). The Whole School, Whole Community, Whole Child model [Special issue]. *Journal of School Health, 85*(11). https://onlinelibrary.wiley.com/toc/17461561/2015/85/11

Hunt, P., Barrios, L., Telljohann, S.K., & Mazyck, D. (2015). A whole school approach: Collaborative development of school health policies, processes, and practices. *Journal of School Health, 85*(11), 802-809. https://doi.org/10.1111/josh.12305

King, M.H., & Lederer, A.M. (2019). Coordinated school health initiatives: The rationale for school level implementation—A commentary. *Journal of School Health, 89*(8), 599-602. https://doi.org/10.1111/josh.12784

Kolbe, L.J. (2019). School health as a strategy to improve both public health and education. *Annual Review of Public Health, 40,* 443-468. https://doi.org/10.1146/annurev-publhealth-040218-043727

Kolbe, L.J., Allensworth, D.D., Potts-Datema, W., & White, D.R. (2015). What have we learned from collaborative partnerships to concomitantly improve both education and health? *Journal of School Health, 85*(11), 766-774. https://doi.org/10.1111/josh.12312

Koriakin, T.A., McKee, S.L., Schwartz, M.B., & Chafouleas, S.M. (2020). Development of a comprehensive tool for school health policy evaluation: The WellSAT WSCC. *Journal of School Health, 90*(12), 923-939. https://doi.org/10.1111/josh.12956

Lewallen, T.C., Hunt, H., Potts-Datema, W., Zaza, S., & Giles, W. (2015). The Whole School, Whole Community, Whole Child model: A new approach for improving educational attainment and healthy development for students. *Journal of School Health, 85*(11), 729-739. https://doi.org/10.1111/josh.12310

McKenzie, F.D., & Richmond, J.B. (1998). Linking health and learning: An overview of coordinated school health programs. In E. Marx, S.F. Wooley & D. Northrup (Eds.), *Health is academic: A guide to coordinated school health programs* (pp. 1-11). Teachers College Press.

Michael, S.L., Merlo, C.L., Basch, C.E., Wentzel, K.R., & Wechsler, H. (2015). Critical connections: Health and academics. *Journal of School Health, 85*(11), 740-758. https://doi.org/10.1111/josh.12309

Morse, L.L., & Allensworth, D.D. (2015). Placing students at the center: The Whole School, Whole Community, Whole Child model. *Journal of School Health, 85*(11), 785-794. https://doi.org/10.1111/josh.12313

Murray, S.D., Hurley, J., & Ahmed, S.R. (2015). Supporting the whole child through coordinated policies, processes, and practices. *Journal of School Health, 85*(11), 795-801. https://doi.org/10.1111/josh.12306

National Association of Chronic Disease Directors. (n.d.a). *About NACDD—National Association of Chronic Disease Directors.* https://chronicdisease.org/page/about_nacdd/

National Association of Chronic Disease Directors. (n.d.b). *School health resource guide.* www.nacddresourceguide.org/schoolhealth/

National Association of Chronic Disease Directors. (2017). *The Whole School, Whole Community, Whole Child model: A guide to implementation.* https://chronicdisease.org/the-whole-school-whole-community-whole-child-model-a-guide-to-implementation/

Rasberry, C.N., Slade, S., Lohrmann, D.K., & Valois, R.F. (2015). Lessons learned from the Whole Child and coordinated school health approaches. *Journal of School Health, 85*(11), 759-765. https://doi.org/10.1111/josh.12307

Rooney, L.E., Videto, D.M., & Birch, D.A. (2015). Using the Whole School, Whole Community, Whole Child model: Implications for practice. *Journal of School Health, 85*(11), 817-823. https://doi.org/10.1111/josh.12304

Society for Public Health Education. (n.d.). *WSCC team training modules.* https://elearn.sophe.org/wscc-training-modules

Society for Public Health Education. (2021, July 19). *SOPHE honored with ASHA 2021 Whole School, Whole Community, Whole Child (WSCC) Award.* www.sophe.org/news/sophe-honored-with-asha-2021-whole-school-whole-community-whole-child-wscc-award/

University of Connecticut Collaboratory on School and Child Health. (n.d.). *WSCC: Think about the ink.* https://csch.uconn.edu/wscc-think-about-the-link/

Washington University in St. Louis. (n.d.). *Healthy schools toolkit.* https://healthyschoolstoolkit.wustl.edu/introduction/

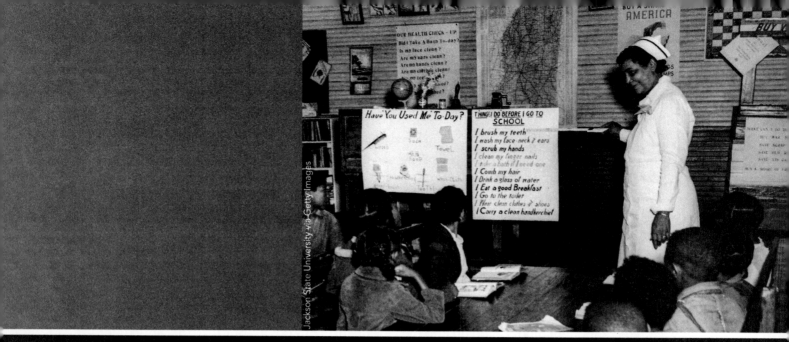

CHAPTER 2

History of WSCC

Diane DeMuth Allensworth • Hannah P. Catalano

LEARNING OBJECTIVES

1. Describe and provide examples of the three stages of health promotion.
2. Compare and contrast various school health models that have evolved over time.
3. Analyze current and historical challenges and barriers to school health programs.

KEY TERMS

Health promotion

School health council

School health team

Social determinants of health

Education and health are inextricably intertwined. Ensuring the maturation of children and youth into productive and contributing members of society is a complex endeavor that requires the collaborative efforts of families, schools, and community agencies as well as the youth themselves. In the United States, approximately 54.6 million young people attend kindergarten through secondary schools (Bauman & Cranney, 2020) for about six hours of classroom time each day for 13 of the most formative years of their lives. Although the primary focus of the education sector is learning and achievement, research has documented the value of addressing the health of students as a means of improving academic achievement (Bradley & Greene, 2013; Bryk et al., 2010; Cabrera et al., 2018; Michael et al., 2015). Students who complete high school live six to nine years longer than those who drop out of school. Students who secure an advanced degree live even longer. At age 25, women with less than a high school degree are estimated to live an average of 50 additional years, whereas women with a graduate degree are estimated to live 62 additional years—a difference of 12 years. For men, the difference in mortality is 16 years (Hummer & Hernandez, 2013). Better educated people are generally healthier and have healthier children (Birch & Auld, 2019; Murray et al., 2006).

In this chapter we explore the evolution of the school health program from its early beginning to its current practices. We describe how a three-component model evolved into the eight-component Coordinated School Health (CSH) model, which has more recently been replaced by the 10-component Whole School, Whole Community, Whole Child (WSCC) model. The context for how the school health program has evolved is placed within the context for health promotion and public health. Finally, we make the case that school health programming is needed today as much as at any time in the past even though the health problems facing students have changed dramatically. The evolution of the school health models is presented in figure 2.1.

Three models have been identified for school health (Birch & Videto, 2015), and there are

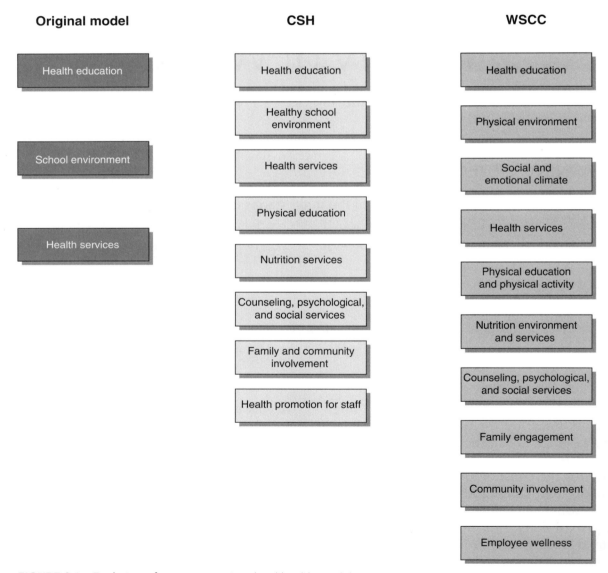

FIGURE 2.1 Evolution of components in school health models.

also three evolutionary stages of **health promotion** (D.D. Allensworth, 2015; Kickbush & Payne, 2003). The history of school health programming closely follows the historical context for health promotion. We may think of this history as having three evolutionary stages in the quest to promote healthy people living in healthy communities (Kickbush & Payne, 2003). The first stage of health promotion, which focused on addressing sanitary conditions and infectious diseases, occurred from the mid-19th century to the mid-20th century. The initiating event occurred in 1854 when John Snow, a physician in London, traced the source of cholera in a community to its water source. By removing the pump handle on the community's water supply, Dr. Snow prevented the cholera bacteria from infecting other community members. This discovery not only led to the development of the modern science of epidemiology but also helped governments around the world recognize the need to address infectious diseases. The second stage of health promotion began approximately 100 years later with the release of the Lalonde report in 1974, when health promotion began to address the behavioral or root causes of diseases and injury. The third and current stage of health promotion began around the beginning of the 21st century as the focus shifted from lifestyle correlates of premature illness and death to the **social determinants of health**.

First Stage of Health Promotion: Addressing Infectious Diseases

Every child should be taught early in life, that, to preserve his own life and his own health and the lives and health of others, is one of the most important and constantly abiding duties.

—*Lemuel Shattuck, Sanitary Commission of Massachusetts, 1850 (Shattuck, 1948, p. 178)*

School health programming in the United States often is traced to the 1850 Shattuck report by the Sanitary Commission of Massachusetts (Shattuck, 1948), which has become a classic in the field of public health and has had a significant influence on school health. Soon after the release of the Shattuck report, the medical and public health sectors recognized that schools could play a major role in controlling communicable disease with their captive audience of children and youth. Medical inspections of children for specific infectious diseases became the forerunner of the current health services component of the WSCC model provided by school nurses. Although medical inspections by school physicians continued into the 1930s, the 1930 White House Conference on Child Health and Protection, which called for the elimination of medical treatments in schools, had the effect of ultimately ensuring that the primary provider of health services in the school would be the school nurse. The school's role was to refer students in need of medical care to their private physicians. It was not until the Robert Wood Johnson Foundation began its work in 1986 to support school-based health clinics that more comprehensive medical services began returning to schools (Institute of Medicine [IOM], 1997).

By the late 1860s New York City had instituted sanitary inspections of schools twice a year because of the poor sanitary conditions in schools (IOM, 1997). This practice became the precursor of the healthy school environment component of CSH. As environmental supports for addressing infectious diseases (e.g., potable water, sanitary latrines) were initiated during the early and mid-20th century, deaths from infectious diseases were dramatically reduced.

World War I marked a turning point in the history of two other current WSCC components: health education and school physical education. Because of the poor physical condition of many draftees, between 1918 and 1921 almost every state enacted laws prescribing health education (hygiene) and physical education (gymnastics). Coursework in health education expanded to include not only hygiene but nutrition, diseases, family health, sex education, and healthy habits as well as the consequences of alcohol and tobacco use. Although Shattuck's 1850 report had also called for physical training as part of his plan for improving the public's health, it was mandated by most states only in the period following World War I (IOM, 1997).

Second Stage of Health Promotion: Addressing Individual Behaviors

Reviews of the leading causes of mortality and morbidity suggest that only six categories of behavior cause most of our major health problems: behaviors that cause unintentional and intentional injuries; drug and alcohol use; sexual behaviors that cause sexually transmitted disease (STD), including HIV infection, and unintended pregnancies; tobacco use; inadequate physical activity; dietary patterns that cause disease. These behaviors usually are established during youth, persist into adulthood and are interrelated. They contribute simultaneously to poor health, education and social outcomes; and they are preventable (Kolbe, 1990; Kann 1993).

—Dr. Lloyd J. Kolbe (1994, p. 58)

By the 1960s, health behaviors linked to physical, mental, social, and emotional problems in children and youth became more prominent than communicable diseases. Of particular concern was the increase in substance abuse, narcotics addiction, homicide, and suicide among adolescents. The timing of this shift in disease causation in youth corresponded with the second stage of health promotion, which began in the 1970s with the release of the Lalonde report (Lalonde, 1974). This report documented that a new perspective was needed to improve the health of the population. The root causes of disease and death could now be traced to four basic causes: biological factors, inadequacies in the health care system, environmental factors, and behavioral or lifestyle factors. This notion directly challenged the prevailing attitude that all improvements in health could be achieved by improving the health care system.

The U.S. Public Health Service (1979) used the Lalonde framework to analyze all deaths in the United States in 1976 (see figure 2.2). It found that the major cause of premature death was lifestyle factors, which were responsible for 50 percent of deaths. Biological factors (i.e., bacteria, viruses, genetics, etc.) were responsible

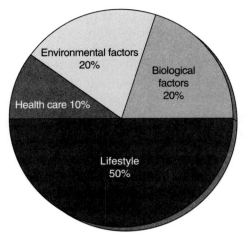

FIGURE 2.2 Root causes of premature deaths.
From U.S. Public Health Service (1979).

for approximately 20 percent of total premature deaths, environmental factors (i.e., toxins, pollutants, safety issues, etc.) for another 20 percent, and health care (e.g., either lack of access to health care or mistakes by health care professionals) for 10 percent. The behaviors that people chose to adopt or not adopt contributed the most to chronic diseases and injury—the leading causes of premature mortality and morbidity by the mid-20th century.

Although the Lalonde framework called attention to the continued need to ensure potable water; effective garbage and sewage disposal; and safe and unpolluted food, medicine, and air, it was the introduction of behavioral factors that shifted the general public's understanding of disease causation. A person's health status became the responsibility of not only the physician, who promotes health with curative treatments, but also the individual, whose choice of lifestyle plays an important role in preventing or promoting disease and injury.

Substituting healthy behaviors for unhealthy behaviors, such as avoiding tobacco use, choosing a healthy diet, and engaging in regular physical activity, could prevent the development of various chronic diseases, including heart disease, type 2 diabetes, and cancer. By adopting many protective behaviors such as wearing seat belts, not riding with someone who has been drinking, and not engaging in fighting, a person could avoid unintentional and intentional injury.

The need to focus more on preventing disease by choosing a health-promoting lifestyle ushered in a focus on health education programs not only for students but also for school staff. School site health promotion for faculty and staff was initiated in 1977 (Drolet & Davis, 1984). Len Tritsch, the Oregon state director for health and physical education, initiated the Seaside Conference, a weeklong statewide summer conference for teams of health educators, administrators, other teachers, school staff, and school board members to develop an action plan for promoting healthy lifestyles in their districts (Girvan, 1987). The purpose was for the teams to develop a plan for how they would apply wellness concepts learned at the conference within their schools. Numerous states replicated the Seaside Conference to promote health education and health promotion for faculty and staff (Davis et al., 1991). An evaluation of this program demonstrated that benefits accrued not only to school staff but also to their students, because as teachers began to focus on their own health, they began to teach more health to students (Girvan, 1987).

Many students engaged in high-risk behaviors at this time. According to Dryfoos (1990), 10 percent of the 28 million students ages 10 to 17 in the United States engaged in a number of high-risk behaviors. Another 4 million students (15 percent) had excessively high prevalence rates for some but not all high-risk behaviors. These figures meant that the future health of 7 million youth in the United States was in jeopardy unless major and immediate changes were made in their lifestyle. Another 25 percent of youth were at moderate risk for negative outcomes associated with their behavior due to school problems, minor delinquencies, light substance abuse, and early intercourse. Only half the nation's youth (14 million) experienced few behavioral problems and were at low risk for negative consequences from their behavior. However, even those students required general preventive services and health promotion programs. Given that approximately 95 percent of children were enrolled in school, a quality school health program was seen as a social necessity for everyone.

To help students choose healthier behaviors, a number of curricula were developed, some with the assistance of federal funding for research and validation of their effectiveness. Examples of curricula developed during the 1980s to encourage the adoption of healthy behaviors included Growing Healthy, Know Your Body, Teenage Health Teaching Modules, and Go for Health. Since the 1980s, the number of evidence-based programs has grown considerably, and information on such programs is now housed in several national and federal clearinghouses, such as the Institute of Education Sciences' What Works Clearinghouse.

Major political developments also contributed to changing the character of school programs. In 1965, a set of domestic programs called the Great Society was enacted by Congress. Two main goals of the Great Society were the elimination of poverty and the elimination of racial injustice. New spending programs that addressed education, medical care, urban problems, and nutrition were launched during this period. Although many of these programs focused on disadvantaged students and students with special needs, one direct effect was to triple the number of school nurses practicing in schools. Relevant legislation included Head Start, Medicaid, the Elementary and Secondary Education Act, the Education for All Handicapped Children Act (Public Law 94-142), and the Child Nutrition Act of 1966 (IOM, 1997).

The Child Nutrition Act established the School Breakfast Program and permanently authorized reimbursements for school lunches served to students in need. In 1946, the U.S. Department of Agriculture began assisting with providing lunch to schoolchildren because of the poor nutrition of many of the draftees into World War II. The Education for All Handicapped Children Act, enacted in 1975, required all public schools that accepted federal funds to provide equal access to education and one free meal a day for children with physical and mental disabilities. Public schools were required to evaluate children with disabilities and create an educational plan in conjunction with parental input that would correspond to, as closely as possible, the educational experience of students without disabilities. Before this law was enacted, many children with disabilities were denied access to education and opportunities to learn because many states had laws excluding children who were "deaf, blind, emotionally disturbed, or had an intellectual disability" (U.S. Department of Education, 2023, para. 2).

Initial Expansion of the School Health Model

During this stage of health promotion, the school health program also changed considerably. From the turn of the 20th century to the late 1980s, the three traditional components articulated for school health programs were health education, health services, and a healthy school environment. Kolbe (1986) suggested that by following an expanded school health model, schools could help students live healthier, longer, more satisfying, and more productive lives. Kolbe proposed that if the three traditional components (health education, health services, and a healthy school environment) were linked with physical education, counseling, school psychology and social services, school nutrition services, family and community involvement, and school site health promotion for faculty and staff, then students' health-related behaviors, health status, and cognitive performance and ultimately their academic achievement would be enhanced.

Kolbe's identification of additional components to expand the CSH model was on target and logical because these services already existed in schools and were contributing to the well-being of students. Counseling services in schools began around the beginning of the 20th century, initially as vocational guidance. However, by the 1930s school counseling started to address personal, social, and emotional problems students were experiencing. Some schools had employed school psychologists since the beginning of the 20th century to provide psychoeducational testing and services to address the diagnosis and treatment of behavioral and learning problems. The passage of the Education for All Handicapped Children Act quadrupled the number of school psychologists from 5,000 in 1970 to 20,000 by 1988 (Fagan, 1990).

In 1986, Lloyd Kolbe's article "Increasing the Impact of School Health Promotion Programs: Emerging Research Perspectives" was published in *Health Education* by the Association for the Advancement of Health Education. At the time, Diane Allensworth was serving as president of the American School Health Association (ASHA) and Kolbe was president-elect. Allensworth suggested that a special issue of ASHA's *Journal of School Health (JOSH)* highlighting the roles and responsibilities of each component might help disseminate the model more quickly. After they started working to secure authors for the special issue, Kolbe's attention was redirected to a new threat to the nation's youth: HIV, which causes AIDS. There was no cure, and the only known treatment at the time was prevention. As the division director for the newly created Division of Adolescent and School Health within the Centers for Disease Control and Prevention (CDC), Kolbe had the responsibility of developing the national plan to reduce the spread of HIV among youth. Although he continued to assist with the development of the special issue of *JOSH*, because of his reduced involvement, he insisted that Allensworth become the lead editor. However, even with the backing of ASHA, the model's adoption faced controversy and challenges from many professionals working within schools.

An initial controversy that surrounded this new model was that physical educators often did not think of themselves as part of the school health program. In addition, school nurses objected in part because the health services component, which had originally been one-third of the school health program, was now reduced to being only one-eighth of the program. In spite of the objections of some professionals and some disciplines, the model endured because ASHA and the CDC continued to support and use it in their various publications. ASHA published a number of articles in *JOSH* focusing on the comprehensive school health model and developed a number

The Landmark Coordinated School Health Issue of the *Journal of School Health*

Many school health professionals and school administrators were first introduced to CSH through a landmark issue of *JOSH* in December 1987. The issue, funded by the Metropolitan Life Foundation, was titled "The Comprehensive School Health Program: Exploring an Expanded Concept." The introductory article, with the same title as the special issue of the journal, was authored by the original visionaries of what is now known as CSH, Lloyd J. Kolbe and Diane D. Allensworth.

Two important concepts were stressed in the introductory article. The first was the importance of coordination among various school programs, the family, and the community. As D.D. Allensworth and Kolbe (1987) emphasized, "These eight components of a Comprehensive School Health Program, if coordinated to address a given health behavior or health problem, could have complementary if not synergistic effects" (p. 409). The second important concept was the connection of the health of students to academic success. In their article, D.D. Allensworth and Kolbe quoted the director of the Office of Disease Prevention and Health Promotion in the U.S. Department of Health and Human Services (USDHHS) at that time, Michael McGinnis, who noted the following:

> What is very clear, is that education and health for children are inextricably intertwined. A student who is not healthy, who suffers from an undetected vision or hearing defect, or who is hungry, or who is impaired by drugs or alcohol, is not a student who will profit from the educational process. Likewise, an individual who has not been provided assistance in the shaping of healthy attitudes, beliefs, and habits early in life, will be more likely to suffer the consequences of reduced productivity in later years. (D.D. Allensworth & Kolbe, p. 409)

Besides the introductory article, the issue included articles that addressed each of the eight components of comprehensive school health. The authors of these articles were asked to address the scope and parameters of the component; specific ways that the component influenced the health and cognitive performance of students, faculty, and staff; results of research that described the effectiveness of the component; and credentials required by practitioners as well as the major national organizations for practitioners related to each component.

Allensworth and Kolbe's intention was that the special issue would influence professionals to function together as a team to have a positive influence on the health and well-being of children and youth. The vision and leadership of Allensworth and Kolbe and the resources developed over the years since the publication of this landmark issue of *JOSH* have certainly made major contributions to maintaining and improving the health and academic achievement of school-age children and youth.

---

of documents for schools explaining how to use the model. D.D. Allensworth et al. (1994) articulated how the model could work at the school level. Strategies included the following:

- Coordinating programming with interdisciplinary and interagency work teams, using the program planning process in a cycle of continuous improvement
- Coordinating the efforts of all faculty, staff, and administrators by focusing on the behaviors that most interfered with learning and well-being
- Replacing a health instruction model with a health promotion model using multiple strategies such as policy, environmental change, direct intervention (screening), role modeling, social support, media, as well as instruction
- Viewing students as resources by soliciting their active involvement in health promotion initiatives

The most dramatic and efficient dissemination of how practitioners at all levels could be organized occurred when Kolbe used the CSH model at the CDC to address HIV prevention nationwide. As the director of a new division at the CDC, the Division of Adolescent and School Health, Kolbe took some bold actions that changed the way the CDC did its work and facilitated the use of the model. Up until this time, the CDC had only funded state departments of health. Yet given the need to address HIV prevention among youth, Kolbe persuaded the CDC to fund state departments of education as well, because education was the only strategy available at that time to prevent the spread of HIV. Kolbe also took the unique and novel position that HIV education should occur within a comprehensive school health model. In addition, the CDC funded approximately 20 national education professional organizations to assist with the dissemination of information about preventing HIV as well as, ultimately, other chronic diseases. This approach diffused resistance to HIV education as exclusively a course in sex education. Furthermore, this approach engaged physical educators, school nurses, counselors, and health education teachers to work collaboratively as they helped school staff understand how to use universal precautions in cases of exposure to blood and bodily fluids in school and how to address the discrimination occurring with students or staff who were HIV positive.

Among the almost 20 national education and school health organizations the CDC funded for HIV and chronic disease prevention, the National Association of State Boards of Education, in cooperation with the National School Boards Association, developed *Fit, Healthy and Ready to Learn*, a policy guide that translated the CDC's school health guidelines into model policy language (Fisher et al., 2003). This document and others developed by the national professional organizations facilitated dissemination of the model. The CDC also developed numerous initiatives and resources that facilitated the use of data to support programming at the state, district, and school levels by identifying students engaged in health-risk and health-promoting behaviors. The Youth Risk Behavior Survey, which has been administered every two years since 1991, monitors six categories of health-related behaviors that contribute to the leading causes of death and disability among youth.

Another major source of controversy and confusion in the early years of CDC funding was the name of the model: the Comprehensive School Health program, which identified the addition of new components to the original three components. Five organizations that received funding from the CDC to work on school health concerns around HIV/AIDS and chronic disease prevention collaborated to conduct market research around the name of the model. Staff from the Council of Chief State School Officers, the National Association of State Boards of Education, the National School Boards Association, ASHA, and the American Cancer Society found that the name "comprehensive" school health programs caused much confusion because health education was at that time also often referred to as "comprehensive health education," and some people would say "comprehensive health education" when they were referring to the comprehensive school health program. Marketing research also discovered that school board members, superintendents, and principals thought that "comprehensive" sounded expensive and complicated. Two major publications of the era, *Schools and Health: Our Nation's Investment* (IOM, 1997) and *Health Is Academic: A Guide to Coordinated School Health Programs* (Marx et al., 1998), were published with the respective editors' full knowledge of the marketing research that had been completed by the five nongovernmental organizations. The editors of both publications agreed to suggest to readers that *coordinated* instead of *comprehensive* was the best word to use when referring to the school health program. The CDC also began using this terminology. By 2006, most state departments of education had adopted the name and components of the CSH program, but adoption at the school level was not as pervasive.

Another issue surrounding the lack of wide-scale adoption by educators at the school level was the lack of easily identified research establishing a link between various components of the model and positive academic achievement. Although the link between health and education was a basic principle of the CSH model

(D.D. Allensworth & Kolbe, 1987), it was not until 2002, nearly 15 years after the model was first proposed that the Association of State and Territorial Health Officials and the Society of State Directors of Health, Physical Education and Recreation (2011) published *Making the Connection: Health and Student Achievement*, a document that presented research on the value of each of the eight components for achieving education goals. This resource included existing research on how each of the components contributed to various education goals, including reducing absenteeism, reducing tardiness, improving comportment, increasing school bonding, decreasing dropout rates, improving achievement, and increasing graduation rates.

In 2010, educational researchers at the University of Chicago identified a safe and nurturing learning environment, family involvement, and linkages with community agencies among the five critical elements needed to improve achievement in elementary grades (Bryk et al., 2010). Although the researchers did not identify these critical elements as components of a comprehensive school health program, their research validated the need for a focus on these three components in an expanded model. A later document presented at the American Educational Research Association in 2018 identified the importance of healthy behaviors to academic performance (Cabrera et al., 2018). Further, while there is value in individual school health components to improve aspects of the health of students, two major reviews noted that cross-cutting programming or multidisciplinary programming of school programs was more effective than individual components working in isolation (Michael et al., 2015; Suto et al., 2021).

Federal Support for Coordinated School Health Programs

A final obstacle for the CSH model was the uncoordinated federal response to school health programming. Federal support for CSH programs began with the CDC, the premier public health agency within the USDHHS. No permanent structure exists linking the U.S. Department of Education and the CDC. Furthermore, in 1992, the Substance Abuse and Mental Health Services Administration was formed within the USDHHS; this helped schools with school health programming, but it was not coordinated with CDC programming.

Unlike other nations, the United States places the responsibility for education at the state level. Therefore, aspects of the curriculum, the amount of funding received per pupil, and the inclusion of school health programming can vary considerably across states. Federal funding for programs such as the Child Nutrition Act and Title I of the Education for All Handicapped Children Act, which are implemented in all schools, provides a mechanism for some continuity in programming across the nation. Funding for demonstration projects as well as resources supporting the various components of school health can be found in most federal offices, including in the U.S. Departments of Education, Health and Human Services, Justice, and Agriculture. The resources and funding for demonstration projects over time can influence programming nationwide. Child Trends completed a major analysis of federal support in 2021 and found that 10 formal interagency groups, 13 formula grant programs, 91 discretionary grant programs, and 67 technical assistance centers and initiatives supported some aspect of school health from 2010 to 2020, although support may vary depending on who applies for federal funding. Unfortunately, existing school health–related interagency collaborations lack representation from all major relevant agencies: the Department of Education, Department of Justice, and USDHHS. For example, although Department of Education and USDHHS agencies are involved in interagency collaboration, the Department of Justice is not currently involved in the two interagency collaborations that are directly focused on school health. Furthermore, few federal school health efforts include a focus on worksite health promotion for schools (Temkin et al., 2021).

One overarching federal initiative that has recognized and promoted school health programming is the Healthy People initiative. This initiative was first released by the Office of Disease Prevention and Health Promotion in 1979. An updated Healthy People document has been published every 10 years (1980 through 2030) by the USDHHS with public health objectives for the ensuing decade. The document is the result of a public–private national initiative that elicits input from a variety of stakeholders, such as national nongovernmental organizations, state health agencies, professional associations, and universities as well as multiple federal agencies. This input provides direction for the identification of national priorities for health promotion at the beginning of each decade. The Healthy People goals and objectives guide and direct the health promotion actions of federal agencies, local and state health departments, health care practitioners, academicians, and health workers at all levels of government. The need to involve practitioners of school health at the school level became critical with the first update of new goals and objectives in 1989. Almost one-third of the objectives published in 1990 for achievement by 2000 could be attained only with the direct participation and support of public schools. The 2020 edition added three new sections: Adolescent Health, Early and Middle Childhood, and Social Determinants (USDHHS, 2010). The number of school health objectives was reduced for the 2030 decade for two basic reasons: (1) The National Center for Health Statistics reduced the number of overall objectives dramatically by almost half so it could better monitor implementation of the remaining objectives; and (2) one of the greatest sources for school health data, the School Health Policies and Practices Study, which provided data at the classroom, school, district, and state levels, had been significantly condensed and was ultimately discontinued. The CDC's last School Health Policies and Practices Study provided district-level data only, not school or classroom data (CDC, 2017).

Third Stage of Health Promotion: Addressing the Social Determinants of Health

That there should be a spread of life expectancy of 48 years among countries and 20 years or more within countries is not inevitable. A burgeoning volume of research identifies social factors at the root of much of these inequalities in health. Social determinants are relevant to communicable and noncommunicable disease alike.

—*Sir Michael Marmot, Lancet, 2005, p. 1099*

By the beginning of the 21st century, it had become apparent that only exhorting people to choose health-enhancing behaviors to improve their health status was insufficient. Individual decisions about behaviors that people could adopt were rooted in the social environments in which they were born, lived, worked, and played. For example, many children lived where they could not play outside because of violence in their neighborhoods. Supermarkets that offered a variety of food and fresh produce were not located in low-income areas. Toxic emissions from industry contaminated the air or water in some communities, and access to medical care was limited. Schools in many low-income communities were often inferior, so students received an inadequate education. The children (as well as the adults who cared for them) had little control over these various social conditions, known as social determinants of health, that precluded their making healthy choices.

Social determinants of health include all societal conditions that affect health—poverty, the economic system, the health care system (including access), the educational system, housing, the transportation system, and the surrounding environment as well as social relationships between community members, such as civic engagement or discrimination and racism. The root causes of premature illness and death have been updated to include social determinants (see figure 2.3).

The United States, one of the richest countries in the world, has one of the highest poverty rates for children of all developed countries and lacks universal health care (Organisation for Economic Co-operation and Development, 2022). Children in poverty experience more of the negative social determinants of health. These children are more likely to experience stressors such as exposure to environmental toxins, food insecurity, housing instability, parent incarceration, household substance abuse, violence, and racial or economic discrimination (Francis et al., 2018). Children living in poverty also experience poorer health and overall well-being and complete less schooling (Balfanz, 2016; Chaudry & Wimer, 2016). The poor health of these students reduces not only their quality of life but also their educational attainment. In fact, educational attainment is the social determinant of health that most strongly correlates with measures of health status, including life expectancy (Hummer & Hernandez, 2013; McGill, 2016). The longer children live in poverty, the slower their general maturation and the lower their educational achievement, not because of innate deficits, but because of the many poverty stressors noted previously, including inequitable educational opportunities (Francis et al., 2018). For many poor students, inequitable educational opportunities and health problems limit their achievement in school, which also limits their productivity as adults. Students who have failed one or more courses in high school are more likely to drop out of school (Farrington, 2014), thus limiting career opportunities that could help them break the cycle of poverty. In summary, there appears to be a reciprocal and causal relationship between (1) academic achievement and educational attainment, (2) familial, economic, social, and physical environment (i.e., poverty), and (3) health (Basch, 2011; Kolbe, 2019).

Healthy People 2020, which was released by the USDHHS in 2010, was the first Healthy People report to include the social determinants of health. The primary health indicator for all social determinant objectives was to increase the proportion of students who graduated with a regular diploma four years after starting ninth grade (USDHHS, 2010). This objective underscored the need for a link between the health and education sectors to ensure educational achievement and health for current students, for the adults they would become, as well as for their future children (see figure 2.4; Birch & Auld, 2019; Murray et al., 2006; Virginia Commonwealth University Center on Society and Health, 2014). Many students continue to have health problems that can reduce their achievement in coursework by limiting their concentration or by increasing their absenteeism. Chronic student absenteeism is related to poor achievement and ultimately dropping out of school (E. Allensworth & Evans, 2016; Garcia & Weiss, 2018; Kearney, 2008). Students who are chronically absent, which is defined as missing at least 10 percent of the school year, can be on a downward spiral of course failure and ultimately failure to graduate (E. Allensworth & Evans, 2016).

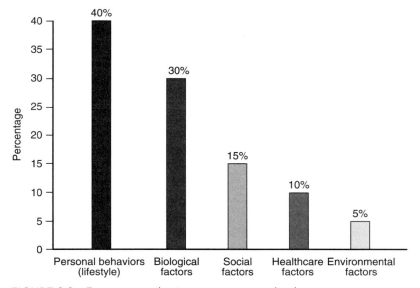

FIGURE 2.3 Factors contributing to premature death.
Data from McGinnis et al. (2002).

The value of addressing health concerns was identified by researchers from the University of Chicago in their work *Organizing Schools for Improvement*. Bryk et al. (2010) demonstrated to principals and superintendents the value of engaging community health organizations to provide for students' health needs if they wanted to see progress in academic achievement. "Community support and linkages" was the phrase used to describe how students' health needs were addressed through linkages to community health and social services agencies to address the social determinants of health—poverty, poor housing, and food insecurity. The educational research team found that students in schools that assembled a first-rate social services support team and accessed external programs and services from community agencies to supplement the health and social services offered by the school system demonstrated improved reading and mathematics scores.

Numerous national organizations have developed and promoted programming that ensures the engagement of community organizations and the services they provide. An umbrella term that describes a variety of national initiatives and organizations is *integrated student services* (ISS). Although the actual strategies may differ by school, most could be described as part of a

> *school-based approach to promoting students' academic success by developing or securing and coordinating supports that target academic and non-academic barriers to achievement. These resources range from traditional tutoring and mentoring to provision of a broader set of supports, such as linking students to physical and mental health care and connecting their families to parent education, family counseling, food banks, or employment assistance. (Moore & Emig, 2014, p. 1)*

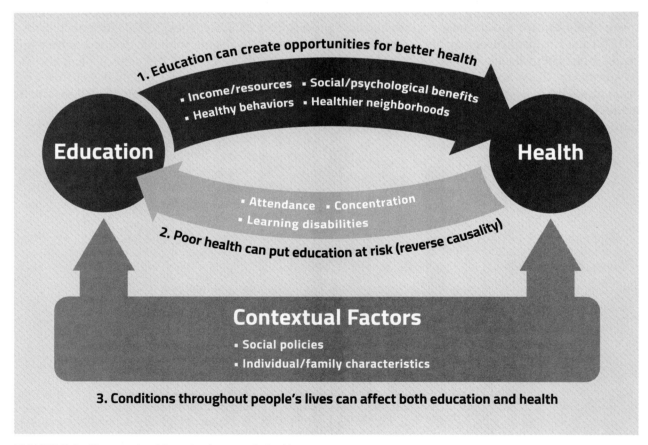

FIGURE 2.4 How are health and education linked?
VCU Center on Society and Health

WSCC IN PRACTICE

Integrated Student Services: A Whole Child Approach With Wraparound Supports

Schools that implement ISS take a Whole Child approach and provide wraparound supports to address students' barriers to learning using a data-driven strategy. Community Schools, Communities in Schools, and City Connects are examples of organizations and models that provide ISS. ISS help schools connect struggling children and their families with housing, medical care, food assistance, tutoring, and other critical supports using programming components similar to those in WSCC (see figure 2.5). Schools that provide ISS are more prevalent among low-income elementary, middle, and high schools. Although the research on these various programs has produced a mix of positive and null (nonsignificant) findings, there are virtually no negative effects across evaluations (Moore et al., 2017). Examples of organizations and programs with particularly strong evaluations include City Connects and Communities in Schools in Chicago (Communities in Schools, 2011, 2022a, 2022b; Pollack et al., 2020). City Connects has demonstrated that its intervention programming reduces absenteeism and promotes retention in elementary schools (City Connects, 2014). In addition, City Connects programming improved postsecondary enrollment and completion of a postsecondary program among predominantly low-income students of color (Pollack et al., 2020). These programs utilize ISS and are compatible with the school health program outlined by the CDC.

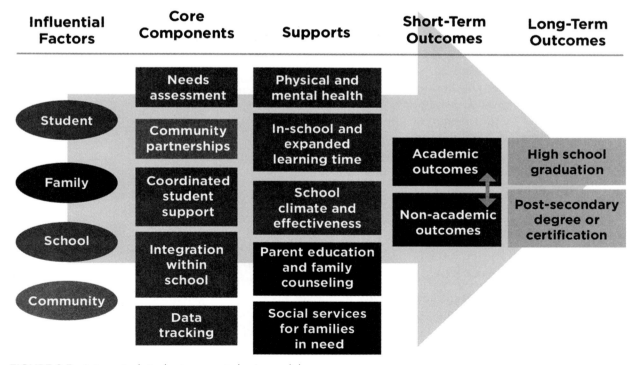

FIGURE 2.5 Integrated student supports logic model.

Reprinted by permission from K.A. Moore, H. Lantos, R. Jones, et al., "Making the Grade: A Progress Report and Next Steps for Integrated Student Supports," *Child Trends* (2017).

Because the federal Every Student Succeeds Act, passed in 2015, encouraged for the first time implementation of ISS, it is assumed that community and family integration by local schools will improve in the coming decades. The need to focus on both community involvement and family engagement as separate but equal components was also demonstrated when the CDC and ASCD combined their two models and the CDC component family and community involvement was separated into two distinct components.

Evolution of the WSCC Model

A model for promoting health and academic success was initiated by ASCD in 2007. The Whole Child initiative focused on ways to ensure that young people's needs were being met both at the higher levels of knowledge and achievement and at the most fundamental levels of health, safety, and belonging. The initiative also challenged schools and communities to work together in new ways as partners, laying aside perennial battles for resources and instead aligning those resources in support of the whole child: "Policy, practice, and resources must be aligned to support not only academic learning for each child, but also the experiences that encourage development of a whole child—one who is knowledgeable, healthy, motivated, and engaged" (ASCD, 2007, p. 5). ASCD's Commission on the Whole Child recommended that local schools work closely with community agencies to address the conditions that affect learning—the social determinants of health. Kolbe was a member of ASCD's commission, an interdisciplinary panel that included leaders in public health, health care, and education. The commission identified the following five elements, known as the Whole Child tenets, as necessary for learning:

- *Each student enters school healthy and learns about and practices a healthy lifestyle.*
- *Each student learns in an intellectually challenging environment that is physically and emotionally safe for students and adults.*
- *Each student is actively engaged in learning and is connected to the school and broader community.*
- *Each student has access to personalized learning and to qualified and caring adults.*
- *Each graduate is prepared for success in college or further study and for employment in a global environment. (ASCD, 2007, p. 20)*

In 2014, ASCD and the CDC merged their respective models into the WSCC model to ensure greater collaboration, integration, and alignment between the health and education sectors. Both Kolbe and Allensworth were among the subject matter experts in health and education who assisted with the development of the WSCC model. To make the original eight-component CDC model more relevant for schools, one panel member suggested separating family and community engagement into two separate components to emphasize the critical role each play. Families are their child's first and primary teachers throughout childhood. Community agencies can provide the physical, mental, and social services needed by students and their families. Furthermore, both family and community agencies have a rich and positive history of improving achievement when they work with schools to improve students' health and learning. Another panel member suggested that a healthy school environment also be separated into two separate components—the physical environment and the social and emotional climate—to highlight the distinct needs of each of these environments. One panel member asked that physical activity be added to the physical education component to emphasize the importance of establishing physical activity for all students outside formal physical education classes. Furthermore, linking the Whole Child model with CSH shifted the focus to students as opposed to the disciplines or services that the components provide, as critical as these services are. It also elevated student voices and the need to view students not just as recipients of programming provided to or for students but also as partners in the process alongside staff, families, and communities. The fact that the CDC and ASCD are so well respected as leaders in their respective sectors bodes well for encouraging both the education sector and the health sector to move simultaneously toward greater collaboration. The structure of the WSCC model is presented in more detail in chapter 3.

Indeed, helping children succeed academically is often predicated on ensuring that their basic health needs are met (IOM, 2015; Michael et al., 2015; Suto et al., 2021). As Kolbe (2019) noted, "Because schools materially influence both health and education outcomes, they substantially determine the future well-being and economic productivity of populations" (p. 443). Research clearly indicates that individuals who attain higher levels of education experience better adult health outcomes resulting in both a longer life expectancy and more quality-adjusted life years (IOM, 2015; Kolbe, 2019; Zimmerman & Woolf, 2014).

The collaborative development of meaningful policies and practices is important in providing direction to the implementation of complementary processes that can guide decisions and actions within both the education and public health sectors as well as coordination between federal, state, district, and local levels (IOM, 2015). When funding became available in the 1990s for both HIV prevention and chronic disease prevention, Kolbe required state departments of education and state departments of health to work collaboratively to address HIV prevention as well as physical inactivity, poor nutrition, and tobacco use—the three major causes of chronic diseases. To receive funding, state education and health departments were asked not only to work collaboratively with each other but also to organize state school health coordinating councils that included representatives from other state agencies responsible for the school-age child along with state professional and voluntary health and education organizations to plan school health programming. This innovative policy decision changed the way states worked. Over the years, more than 20 of the original states, large city school systems, and territories that received this funding set up this collaborative planning between health and education agencies. In addition to being required to set up state coordinating councils, the groups receiving funds were encouraged to develop **school health councils** in each district and **school health teams** at the school level (Fisher et al., 2003). By 2011, secondary schools that had one or more local school health teams ranged from 33.1% to 80.4%, depending on the state (Brenner et al., 2011). The proportion of public health departments working with local schools on school health councils ranged from 17.9 percent to 63.7 percent nationwide, again depending on the state (Brenner et al., 2011). An analysis by the CDC of local school health teams found that schools that had organized such structures had implemented more school health policies and programming (Brenner et al., 2004).

Although coordination and process delineation at the state, district, and school levels has improved overall, it is not in place nationwide. Moreover, coordination between states and federal agencies has remained fragmented (Temkin et al., 2021). Furthermore, no comprehensive federal coordinating body is in place, although there have been several interagency work groups with representation from numerous, but not all, federal agencies (Temkin et al., 2021). The U.S. Departments of Education, Health and Human Services, and Justice all play a central role in federal school health efforts, with each funding significant formula and discretionary grants and technical assistance efforts. However, they need to link with each other as well as with the many other federal agencies with regulatory or funding initiatives to form a comprehensive federal school health interagency collaboration. Doing so would standardize and guide programming across the nation and ensure it addresses health equity issues.

Summary

Over the past century, school health models have evolved from three components to eight components (CSH) to the current WSCC model. Although much progress has been made in improving school health programming since the 1980s, much remains to be done. Many children and youth continue to face threats to their health and well-being. Schools are in a unique position to improve both the education status and the health status of young people. However, the quality and coordination of programming of the various WSCC components in many schools nationwide need to improve because they do not meet the national standards established by respective professional organizations.

To support the whole child, school health programming must continue to evolve. It is recommended that future programs focus on improving the following:

- The 10 components of WSCC to ensure that each component meets the requirements of its respective national professional standards in terms of time, ratio of staff to students, and content
- Youth engagement, voice, and partnership by creating meaningful roles for students as allies, decision-makers, planners, and, foremost, consumers of WSCC
- Health illiteracy and health inequities among youth to further strengthen the implementation of the WSCC model and ultimately to ensure that each child is healthy, safe, engaged, supported, and challenged

These issues are addressed in greater depth throughout the remainder of this book.

LEARNING AIDS

GLOSSARY

health promotion—A planned intervention to improve the health of a target population by changing lifestyle behaviors and environmental conditions through any combination of health education, organizational, economic, or environmental supports.

school health council—A team organized at the district level to facilitate continuous improvement in the school health program as well as collaboration between the school and the community. Ideally, the district school health council includes at least one representative from each of the 10 WSCC components, as well as school administrators, parents, students, and community representatives involved in the health and well-being of students, including a representative from the local health department and the school district's medical consultant.

school health team—A group of teachers, administrators, staff, students, parents, and community members who are focused on implementing work for advancing the WSCC model. The team is often constituted at the individual school level and may inform the work of the school health advisory council. Also known as the *school wellness team*.

social determinants of health—The primary causes of premature illness and death, which are now recognized to be rooted in the social environment in which people are born, live, work, and play. The social determinants of health include all societal conditions that affect health—poverty, the economic system, the health care system (including access), the educational system, housing, the transportation system, and the surrounding environment as well as social relationships between community members, such as civic engagement or discrimination and racism.

APPLICATION ACTIVITIES

1. As a school health professional with a strong background in the WSCC approach, you have been invited by a school administrator to speak to teachers and school staff regarding this approach to school health. You will have 30 minutes for your presentation and 15 minutes for discussion and questions. You are asked to address the three stages of health promotion, the history of the CSH–WSCC approach, and the rationale for promoting school health. Develop a PowerPoint outline for your presentation and a list of questions that may be asked of you by teachers and staff members. Include your responses to the questions.

2. You are invited to write an opinion article (op-ed) for the local online newspaper on WSCC. The purpose of your op-ed is to inform the local community why promoting student health is important for the local district and why WSCC is a logical vehicle for advancing the academic success, health, and wellness of students in the district. Your op-ed cannot be longer than 1,000 words.

3. You are a health educator with a youth health promotion organization that has worked with schools in CSH. Your supervisor has asked you to draft a paper, no longer than two pages, that will be sent to other community organizations that have supported your organization's past CSH efforts. The purpose of the paper is to introduce the WSCC model to these organizations and address potential challenges and barriers that may arise. You have been asked to compare WSCC to the CSH model and to describe both the important elements of WSCC and the benefits of moving from CSH to WSCC. In developing your paper, assume that readers will have limited background on the history of CSH and no background on WSCC.

REFERENCES

Allensworth, D.D. (2015). Historical overview of coordinated school health. In D.A. Birch & D.M. Videto (Eds.), *Promoting health and academic success: The Whole School, Whole Community, Whole Child approach* (pp. 13-28). Human Kinetics.

Allensworth, D.D., & Kolbe, L. (1987). The comprehensive school health program: Exploring an expanded concept. *Journal of School Health, 57*(10), 409-412.

Allensworth, D.D., Symons, C., & Olds, R.S. (1994). *Healthy students 2000: An agenda for continuous improvement in America's schools* [Conference session]. American School Health Association Annual Conference, Kent, OH, United States.

Allensworth, E., & Evans, S. (2016, October). Tackling absenteeism in Chicago: Armed with solid data on student attendance, researchers and practitioners join forces to reduce absenteeism. *Phi Delta Kappan, 98*(2), 16-21.

ASCD. (2007). *The learning compact redefined: A call to action.* https://files.ascd.org/staticfiles/ascd/pdf/Whole%20Child/WCC%20Learning%20Compact.pdf

Association of State and Territorial Health Officials and Society of State Directors of Health, Physical Education and Recreation. (2011). *Making the connection: Health and academic achievement.* Retrieved March 28, 2022, from www.dshs.texas.gov/schoolhealth/tshac/healthand-studentachievement.pdf

Balfanz, R. (2016). Missing school matters. *Phi Delta Kappan, 98*(2), 8-13. https://doi.org/10.1177/0031721716671898

Basch, C.E. (2011). Healthier students are better learners: A missing link in school reforms to close the achievement gap. *Journal of School Health, 81*, 593-598. https://doi.org/10.1111/j.1746-1561.2011.00632.x

Bauman, K., & Cranney, S. (2020). *School enrollment in the United States: 2018 population characteristics—current population report.* U.S. Census Bureau. www.census.gov/content/dam/Census/library/publications/2020/demo/p20-584.pdf

Birch, D.A., & Auld, M.E. (2019). Public health and school health education: Aligning forces for change. *Health Promotion Practice, 20*(6), 818-823. https://doi.org/10.1177/1524839919870184

Birch, D.A., & Videto, D.M. (2015). Whole School, Whole Community, Whole Child: A new model for health and academic success. In D.A. Birch & D.M. Videto (Eds.), *Promoting health and academic success: The Whole School, Whole Community, Whole Child approach* (pp. 3-11). Human Kinetics.

Bradley, B.J., & Greene, A.C. (2013). Do health and education agencies in the United States share responsibility for academic achievement and health? A review of 25 years of evidence about the relationship of adolescents' academic achievement and health behaviors.

Journal of Adolescent Health, 52, 523-532. https://doi.org/10.1016/j.jadohealth.2013.01.008

Brenner, N.D., Kann, L., McManus, T., Stevenson, B., & Wooley, S.F. (2004). The relationship between school health councils and school health policies and programs in U.S. schools. *Journal of School Health, 74*(4), 130-135.

Brenner, N.D., Zewditu, D., Foti, K., McManus, T., Shanklin, S.L., Hawkins, J., & Kann, L. (2011). *School health profiles 2010: Characteristics of health programs among secondary schools in selected U.S. sites*. Centers for Disease Control and Prevention. www.cdc.gov/healthyyouth/profiles/2010/profiles_report.pdf

Bryk, A.S., Sebrig, P.B., Allensworth, E.M., Luppesca, S., & Easton, J.Q. (2010). *Organizing schools for improvement: Lessons from Chicago*. https://press.uchicago.edu/ucp/books/book/chicago/O/bo8212979.html

Cabrera, J.C., Rodriguez, M.C., Karl, S.R., & Chavez, C. (2018, April). *In what ways do health behaviors impact academic performance, educational aspirations, and commitment to learning?* [Paper presentation]. American Educational Research Association Conference, New York, NY, United States. https://conservancy.umn.edu/bitstream/handle/11299/195435/2018-HeathBehaviors-AERA.pdf?sequence=1&isAllowed=y

Centers for Disease Control and Prevention. (2017). *Results from the School Health Policies and Practices Study*. Retrieved July 28, 2022, from www.cdc.gov/healthyyouth/data/shpps/pdf/shpps-results_2016.pdf

Chaudry, A., & Wimer, C. (2016). Poverty is not just an indicator: The relationship between income, poverty, and child well-being. *Academic Pediatrics, 16*(3), S23-S29. https://doi.org/10.1016/j.acap.2015.12.010

City Connects. (2014). *The impact of City Connects: Progress report 2014*. Center for Optimized Student Support, Lynch School of Education, Boston College. www.bc.edu/content/dam/city-connects/Publications/CityConnects_ProgressReport_2014.pdf

Communities in Schools. (2011). *2009-2010 results from the Communities in Schools Network*. www.communitiesinschools.org/media/uploads/attachments/Network_Results_2009-2010.pdf?msclkid=18845daba62211ec-82410ccbd2096463

Communities in Schools. (2022a). *Data*. Retrieved March 28, 2022, from www.communitiesinschools.org/about-us/

Communities in Schools. (2022b). *Our model: Communities in Schools*. www.communitiesinschools.org/our-model/

Davis, T.M., Koch, S., & Ballard, D.J. (1991). The nature of Seaside-style health education conferences. *Journal of Health Education, 22*(2), 73-75. https://doi.org/10.1080/10556699.1991.10628795

Drolet, J.C., & Davis, L.G. (1984). "Seaside"—A model for school health education in-service. *Health Education, 15*(3), 25-32.

Dryfoos, J.G. (1990). *Adolescents at risk: Prevalence and prevention*. Oxford University Press.

Fagan, T. (1990). A brief history of school psychology in the United States. In A. Thomas & J. Grimes (Eds.), *Best practices in school psychology II*, 913-929 National Association of School Psychologists.

Farrington, C.A. (2014). *Failing at school: Lessons for redesigning urban high schools*. Teachers College Press.

Fisher, C., Hunt, P., Kann, L., Kolbe, L., Patterson, B., & Wechsler, H. (2003). *Building a healthier future through school health programs*. Centers for Disease Control and Prevention. www.cdc.gov/healthyyouth/publications/pdf/pp-ch9.pdf

Francis, L., DePriest, K., Wilson, M., & Gross, D. (2018). Child poverty, toxic stress, and social determinants of health: Screening and care coordination. *Online Journal of Issues in Nursing, 23*(3), 1-14. https://doi.org/10.3912/OJIN.Vol23No03Man02

Garcia, E., & Weiss, E. (2018). *Student absenteeism: Who misses school and how missing school matters for performance*. Economic Policy Institute. Retrieved January 20, 2023, from https://files.epi.org/pdf/152438.pdf

Girvan, J.T. (1987, April 13-17). *The impact of the Seaside Health Education Conference on middle school health programs in Oregon* [Paper presentation]. National Convention of the American Alliance for Health, Physical Education, Recreation, and Dance, Las Vegas, NV, United States. https://files.eric.ed.gov/fulltext/ED284850.pdf

Hummer, R.A., & Hernandez, E.M. (2013). The effect of educational attainment on adult mortality in the United States. *Population Bulletin, 68*(1), 1-16.

Institute of Medicine. (1997). *Schools and health: Our nation's investment*. National Academy of Sciences. https://doi.org/10.17226/5153

Institute of Medicine. (2015). Why educational attainment is crucial to improving population health. In Institute of Medicine (Ed.), *Exploring opportunities for collaboration between health and education to improve population health: Workshop summary*. National Academies Press, 13-24. https://doi.org/10.17226/18979

Kann, L. (Ed.). (1993). *Measuring adolescent health behaviors: The Youth Risk Behavior Surveillance System (YRBSS) and recent research reports on reaching high-risk adolescents*. Public Health Reports.

Kearney, C.A. (2008). An interdisciplinary model of school absenteeism in youth to inform professional practice and public policy. *Educational Psychology Review, 20*, 257-282. https://doi.org/10.1007/s10648-008-9078-3

Kickbush, I., & Payne, L. (2003). Twenty-first century health promotion: The public health revolution meets the wellness revolution. *Health Promotion International, 18*(4), 275-278. https://doi.org/10.1093/heapro/dag418

Kolbe, L.J. (1986). Increasing the impact of school health promotion programs: Emerging research perspectives. *Journal of Health Education, 17*(5), 47-52.

Kolbe, L.J. (1990). An epidemiological surveillance system to monitor youth behaviors that most affect health. *Health Education, 22*, 252-255.

Kolbe, L.J. (1994). An essential strategy to improve the health and education of Americans. In P. Cortese and K. Middleton (Eds.), *The comprehensive school health challenge* (Vol. 1; pp. 55-80). ETR Associates.

Kolbe, L.J. (2019). School health as a strategy to improve both public health and education. *Annual Review of Public Health, 40*, 443-463. https://doi.org/10.1146/annurev-publhealth-040218-043727

Lalonde, M. (1974). *A new perspective on the health of Canadians: A working document.* Government of Canada.

Marmot, M. (2005). Social determinants of health inequalities. *Lancet, 365*, 1099-1104. https://doi.org/10.1016/S0140-6736(05)71146-6

Marx, E., Wooley, S.F., & Northrop, D. (1998). *Health is academic: A guide to coordinated school health programs.* Teachers College Press.

McGill, N. (2016). Education attainment linked to health throughout lifespan: Exploring social determinants of health. *The Nation's Health, 46*(6), 1-19. www.thenationshealth.org/content/46/6/1.3

McGinnis, J.M. (1981). Health problems of children and youth: A challenge for schools. *Health Education Quarterly, 8*(1), 11-14. https://doi.org/10.1177/109019818100800103

Michael, S.L., Merlo, C., Basch, C., Hoe, R.M., Wentzel, K.R., & Wechsler, H. (2015). Critical connections: Health and academics. *Journal of School Health, 85*(11), 740-758. https://doi.org/10.1111/josh.12309

Moore, K.A., & Emig, C. (2014). *Integrated student supports: A summary of the evidence base for policymakers.* Child Trends. https://cms.childtrends.org/wp-content/uploads/2014/02/2014-05ISSWhitePaper3.pdf

Moore, K.A., Lantos, H., Jones, R., Schindler, A., Belford, J., & Sacks, V. (2017). *Making the grade: A progress report and next steps for integrated student supports.* Child Trends. www.childtrends.org/wp-content/uploads/2017/12/ISS_ChildTrends_February2018.pdf

Murray, N., Franzini, L., Marko, D., Lupo, P., Garza, J., & Linder, S. (2006). *Code red: The critical condition of health in Texas: Appendix E: Education and health: A review and assessment.* www.utsystem.edu/sites/default/files/documents/Code%20Red%3A%20The%20Critical%20Condition%20of%20Health%20in%20Texas/report.pdf

Organisation for Economic Co-operation and Development. (2022). *Poverty rate.* https://data.oecd.org/inequality/poverty-rate.htm#indicator-chart

Pollack, C., Lawson, J.L., Raczek, A.E., Dearing, E., Walsh, M.E., & Kaufman, G. (2020, January 21). *Long-term effects of integrated student support: An evaluation of an elementary school intervention on postsecondary enrollment and completion.* https://doi.org/10.35542/osf.io/byadw

Shattuck, L. (1948). *Report of the Sanitary Commission of Massachusetts, 1850.* Harvard University Press.

Suto, M., Miyazaki, C., Yanagawa, Y., Takehara, K., Kato, T., Gai, R., Ota, E., & Mori, R. (2021). Overview of evidence concerning school-based interventions for improving the health of school-aged children and adolescents. *Journal of School Health, 91*(6), 499-517. https://doi.org/10.1111/josh.13021

Temkin, D., Steed, H., Her, S., & Guros, C. (2021). *The landscape of federal K-12 school health efforts, 2010-2020.* Child Trends. www.childtrends.org/wp-content/uploads/2021/08/KaiserSchoolHealthReport_ChildTrends_August2021-1.pdf

U.S. Department of Education. (2023, January 11). *A history of the Individuals with Disabilities Act.* https://sites.ed.gov/idea/IDEA-History

U.S. Department of Health and Human Services. (2010). *Healthy People 2020.* Office of Disease Prevention and Health Promotion. www.healthypeople.gov/2020/topics-objectives

U.S. Public Health Service. (1979). *Healthy People: The U.S. Surgeon General's report on health promotion and disease prevention.* U.S. Department of Health, Education and Welfare.

Virginia Commonwealth University Center on Society and Health. (2014). *Why education matters to health: Exploring the causes* (Issue brief). www.rwjf.org/en/library/research/2014/04/why-education-matters-to-health.html

Zimmerman, E., & Woolf, S.H. (2014). *Understanding the relationship between education and health.* https://nam.edu/wp-content/uploads/2015/06/BPH-UnderstandingTheRelationship1.pdf

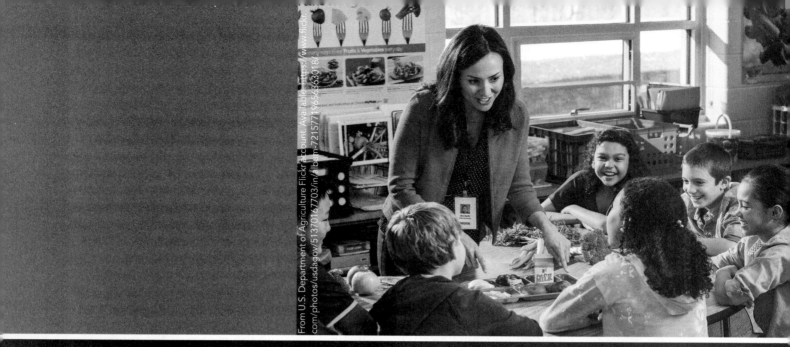

CHAPTER 3

Overview of the WSCC Model

Hannah P. Catalano • David A. Birch • Donna M. Videto

LEARNING OBJECTIVES

1. Describe how the Whole School, Whole Community, Whole Child (WSCC) framework integrates and expands on the Whole Child initiative and the Coordinated School Health model.
2. Analyze the essential elements of the WSCC model, including the five Whole Child tenets, 10 components, and community-focused orientation.
3. Identify potential interrelationships among and between the various components of the WSCC model.

KEY TERMS

Comprehensive school health education
Maslow's hierarchy of needs
National Health Education Standards (3rd ed.)
National School Lunch Program
School-based health center (SBHC)
WSCC components

Since the early 1900s school health models have evolved from a three-component framework (health education, health services, school environment) to the eight-component Coordinated School Health (CSH) framework. Key leaders from the school health, public health, and education sectors have called for increased collaboration and alignment between leaders and professionals in these sectors to support each child's physical, emotional, social, and intellectual development (Centers for Disease Control and Prevention [CDC], 2022f). Consequently, for the benefit of all school-age children, in 2014 ASCD and the CDC combined their respective models into a more unified and collaborative approach: the Whole School, Whole Community, Whole Child (WSCC) model. The WSCC model aims to engage the whole school and whole community in the promotion of health and academic success through its policies, processes, practices, and programs. As Sean Slade, a key leader in the development of the model, explained, "WSCC is not a model that calls for health for education's sake. Nor does it call for education for health's sake. Rather, it is a call for health and education for each child's sake" (ASCD, 2016, p. 2).

As presented in chapter 2, WSCC combines and expands on the Whole Child approach and the CSH model. Coordination among **WSCC components** has been stressed as an essential aspect of both CSH and WSCC. Even with coordination, however, quality in each of the components is essential for maximum effect on both health and learning. Although these components often exist in schools, the mere presence of a program does not mean that the program is implemented in a quality manner that aligns with WSCC.

The purpose of this chapter is to present an overview of the WSCC model, including its Whole Child tenets and community-focused orientation, and highlight background knowledge related to program quality for each of the 10 components of the WSCC approach. Essential information related to program quality is presented for each component. This information includes appropriate national guidelines or standards, faculty or staff qualifications, and best practices related to implementation.

WSCC Model Overview

The WSCC model is a framework that aims to improve learning and health for every child through greater alignment and integration of education and health (Society for Public Health Education [SOPHE], n.d.c). WSCC emphasizes school- and community-wide engagement to support each child's development through a coordinated, multicomponent approach. A visual depiction of the model is presented in figure 3.1. At the center of the model is a child engaged in physical activity. The placement of the child at the center of the model is intentional and symbolizes that children's well-being should be at the forefront of all school-based policies, processes, programs, and practices (Birch, 2023). Furthermore, children and youth are the primary recipients of services in the WSCC model (SOPHE, n.d.c); therefore, the central placement underscores the importance of children and youth being recognized as full partners in school and community decision-making. In the diagrammatic representation of the WSCC model, the child is surrounded by the five Whole Child tenets. The Whole Child tenets, or key principles of WSCC, "are the desired outcomes for every student and are critical for supporting academic achievement and student health" (SOPHE, n.d.c, p. 4). The placement of the tenets around the child in the model illuminates their importance as strategic goals or outcomes to guide curriculum or school-related policies and processes (Birch, 2023).

Whole Child Tenets

The Whole Child tenets are as follows:

- Healthy. *Each student enters school healthy and learns about and practices a healthy lifestyle.*
- Safe. *Each student learns in an environment that is physically and emotionally safe for students and adults.*

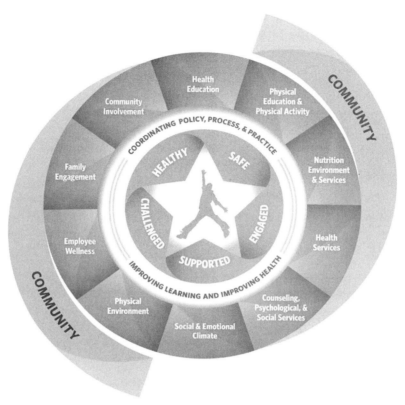

FIGURE 3.1 Whole School, Whole Community, Whole Child model.
Reprinted from ASCD, *Whole School, Whole Community, Whole Child: A Collaborative Approach to Learning and Health* (2014).

- Engaged. *Each student is actively engaged in learning and is connected to the school and broader community.*
- Supported. *Each student has access to personalized learning and is supported by qualified, caring adults.*
- Challenged. *Each student is challenged academically and prepared for success in college or further study and for employment and participation in a global environment. (ASCD, 2015)*

The premise behind the Whole Child tenets is that children cannot learn unless they are healthy and safe. The tenets are derived from Abraham **Maslow's hierarchy of needs**, in which children's physiological needs (e.g., physical health, sense of belonging, safety) provide the foundation for human development and must be met before children can be engaged, supported, and challenged (Slade, 2015). Maslow's hierarchy of needs was initially presented in the paper "A Theory of Human Motivation" (Maslow, 1943). In this original hierarchy, physiological needs were deemed foundational, placed at the base of a pyramid, and listed subsequently in top-up order: safety, belonging, esteem, and self-actualization. The pyramid structure of the hierarchy illustrated that some needs were achievable only after others had been met. Building on this structure, the Whole Child tenets were organized to illustrate that health, followed by safety, is fundamental in creating environments in which children can then be engaged, supported, and challenged (figure 3.2; Slade, 2015, p. 54).

Each of the five tenets has a unique set of 10 indicators. The indicators provide a scaffold that outlines in greater detail what each tenet encompasses (Scharberg, 2013). The indicators offer direction for schools and districts to assess and analyze needs and assets and support planning for improved alignment between education and health (Slade, 2015).

Coordinating Policy, Process, and Practice and Improving Learning and Improving Health

The intent of the WSCC model is to "permeate all school programs, policies, processes, and practices" (Birch, 2023, p. 191). In figure 3.1, the text "Coordinating Policy, Process, and Practice" and "Improving Learning and Improving Health" is in the white inner ring that circles the image of the child and the tenets. This part of the model signifies the collaborative work of the school health team in coordinating school policy, processes, and practices and ensuring that each child is given the opportunity to be healthy, safe, engaged, supported, and challenged (SOPHE, n.d.c).

To maximize the potential of WSCC and maintain its presence, coordination is essential and must be planned in a prudent manner. Coordination should originate from two groups: school health teams and a school health advisory council (Allensworth, 2015; S.D. Murray et al., 2015). School health teams offer leadership at the individual school level, and school health advisory councils do the same at the district level. School health advisory councils select policies, processes, and practices for districtwide WSCC implementation; school health teams translate district-level guidance for individual school-level implementation while accounting for the school's mission and values, resources, facilities, and grade levels and characteristics of the local community. Both groups must have a designated coordinator. The role of the coordinator is to plan and facilitate team or council meetings, maintain the team's vision and commitment, provide leadership related to the group's work, and offer coordination among the range of interests and activities. It is essential for the school health team and district-level group to communicate effectively.

The 10 components of the WSCC model are listed on the following page in clockwise order based on their placement in the visual model. Each component is discussed in greater detail later in the chapter.

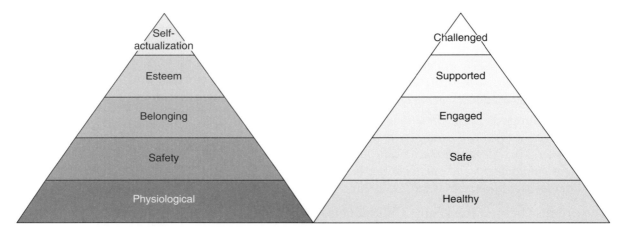

FIGURE 3.2 "Maslow's hierarchy of needs (left) and the five Whole Child tenets (right) are both built on a structure that presumes that the body's physiological needs must be met before other human needs (such as emotional and social needs) may be addressed" (Slade, 2015, p. 55)

- Health education
- Physical education and physical activity
- Nutrition environment and services
- Health services
- Counseling, psychological, and social services
- Social and emotional climate
- Physical environment
- Employee wellness
- Family engagement
- Community involvement

The 10 WSCC Components

The 10 components of the WSCC model offer a framework for integrating and coordinating the WSCC approach (Birch, 2023). The components represent the professional workforce and school-based services available to support the health, safety, and well-being of students and staff (SOPHE, n.d.c, p. 5). This section of the chapter includes a description of each component as well as recommendations and best practices for effective implementation of the WSCC model.

WSCC IN PRACTICE
Journal of School Health: 2020 Special Issue on WSCC

An important feature of *Promoting Health and Academic Success: The WSCC Approach* is the inclusion of WSCC knowledge and experience that have been gained since the publication of the first edition of the book in 2015. One excellent source for this information is the December 2020 special issue of the *Journal of School Health (JOSH)*. This special issue includes two commentaries that present an overview of 14 articles that showcase various aspects of WSCC implementation and research. The articles address important issues related to WSCC, including the presence of and potential for the integration of equity in education and health within the WSCC approach, and the interconnectedness and coordination of multiple elements within the model. This issue of *JOSH* represents an incredibly valuable resource for administrators and professionals who work, or should work, within the WSCC model and for researchers and thought leaders who consider the model an important focus of their work.

The following are examples of the 14 excellent articles included in the special issue:

- "State Laws Matter When It Comes to District Policymaking Relative to the Whole School, Whole Community, Whole Child Framework" (Chriqui et al., 2020)
- "Development of a Comprehensive Tool for School Health Policy Evaluation: The WellSAT WSCC" (Koriakin et al., 2020)
- "Research to Translation: The Healthy Schools Toolkit and New Approaches to the Whole School, Whole Community, Whole Child Model" (Purnell et al., 2020)
- "Community-Based System Dynamics for Mobilizing Communities to Advance School Health" (Ballard et al., 2020)
- "Every School Healthy: Creating Local Impact Through National Efforts" (Pufall Jones et al., 2020)
- "Unusual Suspects: The People Inside and Outside of School Who Matter in Whole School, Whole Community, Whole Child Efforts" (Pittman et al., 2020)
- "Every School Healthy: An Urban School Case Study" (Baldwin & Ventresca, 2020)

Health Education

Quality school health education is based on sequential, grade level–appropriate, culturally inclusive content taught by qualified, professionally prepared teachers. The health education curriculum should be based on relevant health behavior theories; focus on the emotional, intellectual, physical, and social dimensions of health; provide students with exposure to diverse instructional techniques; and evaluate student achievement through a variety of assessment strategies (National Consensus for School Health Education [NCSHE], 2022). The learning experiences within the curriculum should be developed to help students acquire functional health information; identify personal values that support healthy behaviors; analyze the influence of family, peers, media, technology, and social justice on personal and community health; and develop the skills necessary to adopt, practice, and maintain behaviors that enhance individual health and the health of others (NCSHE, 2022). A **comprehensive school health education** curriculum addresses a variety of topics, such as the use and abuse of alcohol and other drugs, healthy eating and nutrition, mental and emotional health, physical activity, safety and injury prevention, sexual health, tobacco use, and violence prevention (CDC, 2021).

Specific direction for curriculum development and health instruction is presented in the third edition of the national school health education standards, titled *National Health Education Standards: Model Guidance for Curriculum and Instruction* (NCSHE, 2022). This 2022 edition of the standards was developed by NCSHE, a group of six leading national health education organizations in the United States: the American School Health Association, Eta Sigma Gamma (the national health education honor society), the Foundation for the Advancement of Health Education, the National Commission for Health Education Credentialing, the Society of State Leaders of Health and Physical Education, and SOPHE. In the development of the standards, the national consensus involved health education leaders from throughout the United States. These leaders included kindergarten through grade 12 (K-12) health teachers, local school district curriculum directors, health education directors in state education agencies, leaders of national nongovernmental organizations, curriculum developers, academicians in health education (including teacher educators and members of higher education management), and other experts in education and public health. In addition, a draft of the standards was made available for public comment. This step generated input from more than 500 stakeholders in school health education (NCSHE, 2022).

The standards provide a resource for the development of state standards and health education curricula in local school districts. For each of the eight standards (figure 3.3), suggestions are presented for how teachers

---

FIGURE 3.3   NATIONAL HEALTH EDUCATION STANDARDS

Standard 1: Students comprehend functional health knowledge to enhance health.

Standard 2: Students analyze the influence of family, peers, culture, social media, technology, and other determinants on health behaviors.

Standard 3: Students demonstrate health literacy by accessing valid and reliable health information, products, and services to enhance health.

Standard 4: Students demonstrate effective interpersonal communication skills to enhance health.

Standard 5: Students demonstrate effective decision-making skills to enhance health.

Standard 6: Students demonstrate effective goal-setting skills to enhance health.

Standard 7: Students demonstrate observable health and safety practices.

Standard 8: Students advocate for behaviors that support personal, family, peer, school, and community health.

Reprinted from National Consensus for School Health Education, *National Health Education Standards: Model Guidance for Curriculum and Instruction*, 3rd ed. (2022). www.schoolhealtheducation.org.

can address the standard through instruction, and indicators are given for grade-level–appropriate attainment of the standard by students at the end of 2nd, 5th, 8th, and 12th grades. Access to the standards is available at no charge through the NCSHE website (NCSHE, 2022).

Beyond the **National Health Education Standards (3rd ed.)**, other considerations are important in the development and implementation of quality school health education. The following list is an adaptation and expansion of CDC recommendations for school health education (Birch et al., 2015; CDC, 2019a). Quality school health education

- involves stakeholders in the planning and curriculum development processes,
- focuses on clear health goals and related behavioral outcomes,
- is research based and theory driven,
- incorporates issues related to health equity and health-related social justice,
- is based on the National Health Education Standards,
- is taught by professionally prepared teachers passionate about teaching health education,
- addresses individual values, attitudes, and beliefs,
- addresses individual and group norms that support health-enhancing behaviors,
- focuses on reinforcing protective factors and increasing perceptions of personal risk and the harmfulness of engaging in specific unhealthy practices and behaviors,
- addresses social pressures and influences,
- addresses the influence of social injustices, including systemic racism and other systemic discrimination, on health disparities and overall well-being,
- builds personal competence, social competence, and self-efficacy through skill development,
- provides functional health knowledge that is basic, is accurate, and contributes directly to health-promoting decisions and behaviors,
- uses strategies designed to personalize information and engage students,
- addresses content sequentially from elementary school through middle school and high school,
- involves age-appropriate and developmentally appropriate information, learning strategies, teaching methods, and materials,
- incorporates learning strategies, teaching methods, and materials that actively engage students in learning and are culturally inclusive,
- provides adequate time for instruction and learning,
- provides opportunities to reinforce skills and positive health behaviors,
- provides opportunities to make positive connections with influential others,
- evaluates learning through authentic assessment techniques,
- includes teacher information and plans for professional development and training that enhance the effectiveness of instruction and student learning, and
- is a component of an active WSCC model.

Physical Education and Physical Activity

Schools can play an important role in providing opportunities for regular physical activity for students. These opportunities can occur through quality physical education programs and other physical activities during and beyond the school day that can lead to the attainment of knowledge and skills and engagement in lifelong physical activity. The CDC views physical education as the foundation for a comprehensive school physical activity program that includes five components: physical education, physical activity during school, physical activity before and after school, staff involvement, and family and community engagement (CDC, 2013).

The Society of Health and Physical Educators (SHAPE America) defines physical education as an academic subject that provides a planned, sequential, K-12 standards-based program of curriculum and instruction designed to develop motor skills, knowledge, and behaviors for healthy and active living, physical fitness, sporting conduct, self-efficacy, and emotional intelligence (SHAPE America, 2015). SHAPE America describes the goal of physical education as developing physically literate individuals who have the knowledge, skills, and dispositions to enjoy a lifetime of healthy and meaningful physical activity (SHAPE America, in press).

The physical education profession has developed national standards to provide direction to school districts and schools relative to curriculum development and instruction (figure 3.4). Each of the standards relates to the knowledge, skills, and attitudes of a physically literate person. Each standard has grade-span learning indicators and learning progressions that delineate the knowledge and skills students should learn from prekindergarten through grade 12 (preK-12), including a trajectory for those learning experiences (SHAPE America, in press). The grade-span learning indicators are grouped by preK to 2, 3 to 5, 6 to 8, and 9 to 12 rather than individual grades.

FIGURE 3.4 NATIONAL STANDARDS FOR PHYSICAL EDUCATION

Standard 1: Develops a variety of motor skills.

Standard 2: Applies knowledge related to movement and fitness concepts.

Standard 3: Develops social skills through movement.

Standard 4: Develops personal skills, identifies personal benefits of movement, and chooses to engage in physical activity.

Reprinted by permission from SHAPE America, *National Physical Education Standards*, 2nd ed. (Champaign, IL: Human Kinetics, in press).

In addition to national standards, other considerations are important in the development and implementation of quality physical education programs. SHAPE America has identified four essential components: policy and environment, curriculum, appropriate instruction, and student assessment. The organization has presented considerations for each of these four components in a document titled *The Essential Components of Physical Education* (SHAPE America, 2015).

Although quality physical education serves as the foundation for a comprehensive school physical activity program, in most cases such a program by itself is not able to provide the 60 minutes per day of moderate to vigorous physical activity recommended for school-age children and youth (CDC, 2018). Numerous opportunities exist for schools to offer additional opportunities for physical activities for students. Especially at the elementary school level, recess has long presented an opportunity for physical activity during the school day. Beyond physical activity, recess provides students with an opportunity to develop life skills related to communication, conflict resolution, cooperation, creativity, decision-making, problem-solving, taking turns, and sharing (Kohl & Cook, 2013). Research suggests that recess promotes positive emotional health, social development, school behavior, and cognitive performance among students (Massey et al., 2021). Numerous organizations have developed policy statements supporting the importance of recess, including the American Academy of Pediatrics, National Association of Early Childhood Specialists in State Departments of Education, National Association of Elementary School Principals, National Association for the Education of Young Children, and National Parent Teacher Association (Kohl & Cook, 2013; Murray et al., 2013). The Great Recess Framework–Observational Tool provides direction for schools to assess the quality of their recess offerings through an examination of the size of the playground, its location, and any hazards on it; access to equipment, boundaries, and the availability of organized games and play; the number, spacing, and various engagement levels of adults; and various factors related to play, conflict, and communication among students (Massey et al., 2018).

Since the turn of the 21st century, interest has increased in the use of classroom-based physical activities with students (van Sluijs et al., 2021). These activities may take place within the context of classroom instruction or occur during breaks from instruction (CDC, 2022b).

Research indicates that classroom-based physical activity can improve on-task classroom behaviors, reduce negative off-task behaviors, and have a positive impact on academic outcomes (Watson et al., 2017).

Physically active travel to and from school, or active transport, presents an opportunity for students to engage in daily physical activity. This form of physical activity can include walking, biking, skateboarding, or some other type of travel to and from school. Active transport might involve walking the entire distance to and from school or being transported by auto, school bus, or public transportation to a certain point and then walking the remainder of the way (Kohl & Cook, 2013). School staff members or parents and family members often serve as supervisors for these activities. Factors that may affect the feasibility of active transport can include the location of schools; the existence of sidewalks, walking and bike paths, pedestrian crossings, and traffic lights; neighborhood safety; weather conditions; and the possible need for adult supervision.

One structured method of active transport for students is the walking school bus. The walking school bus involves a group of children walking together to and from school with adult supervision. The group of children and the adult supervisor or supervisors walk along a predetermined route and may pick up other children at designated stops along the way. On the way to school, the adult supervision starts at the beginning of the route; after school, the adult meets the children at school and reverses the route to lead them all home (County Health Rankings and Roadmaps, 2019). In addition to increasing students' physical activity, the walking school bus may have other benefits, including increased social interaction among

WSCC IN PRACTICE
Society for Public Health Education WSCC Team Training Modules

SOPHE, in collaboration with CDC Healthy Schools, has developed 10 WSCC Team Training Modules for use by local schools, districts, or states to facilitate planning and implementing the WSCC model. These ready-made professional development modules are free and publicly accessible from the SOPHE website. The trainings are intended to be conducted face to face. Each training module stands alone and is approximately one hour in length, though individual training sessions can be broken up into smaller chunks. None of the training modules is dependent on any other; therefore, an individualized professional development plan can be constructed based on the needs and interests of local schools or districts. Each training session includes a detailed script, a PowerPoint slide deck, and handouts, including directions for facilitators. Step-by-step instructions are available on the SOPHE website to support effective facilitation of trainings.

The modules include the following:

- Whole School, Whole Community, Whole Child (WSCC) Overview
- Making the Case: Building and Sustaining Administrative Support
- Organizing for Success: Establishing Your WSCC Team
- Creating Engaging and Productive Meetings
- Assessing School Health Needs
- Transforming the School Environment: Policy, Systems, and Environmental Change
- Using Data to Create a Whole School, Whole Community, Whole Child (WSCC) Improvement Plan
- Communicating School Health Results and Improvements
- Engaging Youth
- Health Equity in Schools (SOPHE, n.d.b)

students and with adults, increased parent and community member engagement with schools, reduced traffic to and from schools, an enhanced sense of community among student walkers and adult supervisors, and increased knowledge and skills around traffic safety among students (Blue Zones, n.d.; National Center for Safe Routes to School, n.d.). Step by Step: How to Start a Walking School Bus at Your School (Moening et al., 2016), a collaborative project of the California Department of Public Health and Safe Routes to School National Partnership, presents detailed directions for developing, maintaining, and evaluating walking school bus programs along with a list of additional resources.

Interscholastic and intramural sports also provide students with opportunities for physical activity. Though research suggests academic benefits from participating in high school sports, most students do not participate. Research by the Aspen Institute indicates that only 39 percent of high school students are engaged in school sports and that engagement is lower in urban (32 percent) and high-poverty (27 percent) schools (Farrey, 2020). To increase participation in both interscholastic and intramural programs, schools need policies and practices in place that support the involvement of students.

Nutrition Environment and Services

Schools play an important role in the eating habits of children and youth. For some students, school meals may be the primary or only daily source of nutritious foods. Components of the school nutrition environment include school lunch and breakfast programs, foods sold outside school meal programs (e.g., in vending machines, in school stores, at grab-and-go kiosks, at school fundraisers, at concession stands), food provided at classroom or school celebrations, and nutrition education and messages about food presented in the school cafeteria and other areas of the school campus (CDC, 2021).

All students in schools that participate in the federal **National School Lunch Program** can purchase lunch through this program. Eligible students in these schools can receive free or reduced-price lunches (U.S. Department of Agriculture [USDA], Economic Research Service, 2022). The 2020 USDA standards require schools to offer fruits and vegetables with every lunch and weekly vegetable offerings that include legumes and dark green and red or orange vegetables. Students are required to take at least one half-cup serving of fruits or vegetables with every school breakfast and lunch. At least half of the grains offered with school meals must be rich in whole grains (at least 51 percent whole grain). Age-appropriate calorie minimums and maximums, which are determined by the USDA, must be met in all meals. In addition, meals cannot contain added trans fat, and no more than 10 percent of calories can come from saturated fat. Meals must also offer one cup of fat-free or 1 percent milk. Free drinking water must also be available in the cafeteria during lunch and breakfast (CDC, 2022e). Schools must also meet USDA Smart Snacks nutrition standards, which were mandated by the Healthy, Hunger-Free Kids Act beginning in July 2014 (CDC, 2022d). These snack standards apply to beverages and foods sold in competition with reimbursable meals through vending machines, snack bars, school stores, and a la carte lines (USDA, Food and Nutrition Service, 2022). Furthermore, the standards require competitive foods to be rich in whole grains or to have a vegetable, fruit, dairy product, or protein food as its first ingredient or a combination of food that includes at least a quarter cup of vegetable or fruit. In addition, the standards place restrictions on the total amounts of calories, dietary fats, sugars, and sodium in snacks and entrees served onsite. They also restrict the types of drinks that can be sold. The standards do not apply to beverages and food brought from home or sold during nonschool hours, at off-campus events, or on weekends. Detailed information on these standards is presented in *A Guide to Smart Snacks in School* (USDA, Food and Nutrition Service, 2022).

Keys to Excellence: Standards of Practice for Nutrition Integrity, a resource of the School Nutrition Association, is intended to assist schools in achieving nutrition integrity goals at the administrative, management, and operational levels. It includes 10 best practices in relation to a school's services and environment. Multiple indicators are presented for each of the practices. Best practices are also presented for physical activity, operations, administration, and marketing and communication. The 10 best practices are as follows:

1. *School meals and snacks are planned and prepared to improve and sustain the health and well-being of all students and to contribute to the development of healthy eating habits.*
2. *Competitive foods are planned and served to encourage healthy choices and comply with federal guidelines.*
3. *The school nutrition program (SNP) addresses competitive food issues to reflect the best interest of student health.*
4. *The SNP participates in national, state, or local initiatives to encourage students to consume healthy foods.*
5. *The SNP participates in the Farm to School program.*
6. *The SNP encourages and supports nutrition education.*
7. *The school dining area serves as a dynamic nutrition learning center where students are engaged in healthy eating.*
8. *The SNP ensures that school nutrition personnel receive training that [meets] USDA's professional standards for SNP personnel.*
9. *The SNP provides opportunities for the community to learn how school meals are a model for healthy eating.*
10. *The SNP is engaged in wellness activities in schools and communities. (School Nutrition Association, 2019)*

Health Services

Health services include first aid, emergency care, assessment and planning for the management of chronic conditions such as asthma or diabetes, and, when needed, coordination between the school and family members and students' medical home (CDC, 2021). School nurses often serve as coordinators of school health services. Beyond the direct provision of health care to students, the school nurse's responsibilities can include leadership in the development of policies, programs, and procedures at the school and district levels; the development, implementation, and evaluation of students' individualized health care plans; communication with teachers, administrators, parents, and, in some cases, the community in regard to students' health issues and needs; case management for students' health care in the context of the school, family, and medical home; the establishment of relationships and referral procedures with medical partners and social agencies; the elicitation of program support; and the development of school safety emergency management plans (McClanahan & Weismuller, 2015; National Association of School Nurses, 2016). Other professionals, such as nurse practitioners, dentists, health educators, physicians, physician assistants, and allied health personnel, may also provide health care within the context of the school health program (CDC, 2022c).

The National Association of School Nurses (2020) recommends that every school have one full-time registered professional nurse. Each day, all students should have access to the school nurse throughout the entire school day. In large schools, providing this level of access may require having more than one nurse. Decisions related to the staffing of school nurses should consider not only the number of students in the school but also the special health, education, and safety needs of students (National Association of School Nurses, 2020). Research indicates that the presence of a school nurse is associated with decreased student absenteeism and less missed class time (Yoder, 2020). Beyond having an impact on academic factors, research indicates that school nursing also is a cost-saving investment, based on a reduction in emergency room visits and a decrease in parents' time away from work to care for sick children (Wang et al., 2014).

Physicians can serve as key members of the health services team. The American Academy of Pediatrics Council on School Health recommends that every school district have a school physician. In the 2013 American Academy of Pediatrics Policy Statement *Role of the School Physician*, it is recommended that school physicians have expertise in pediatrics or be nationally board-certified pediatricians (Devore et al., 2013). School physicians should possess knowledge related to public health, adolescent health, infectious disease, immunizations, medical-legal issues, health and learning, social services resources, environmental and occupational health, emergency preparedness, sports medicine, and coordinated school health (Devore et al., 2013).

Some schools offer an expanded health services program through **school-based health centers (SBHCs)**. The overall goal of SBHCs is to promote and support students' health and academic performance. SBHCs supplement the work of the school nurse by providing primary health care, mental health care, social services, dental care, and health education (Knopf et al., 2016). In addition, SBHCs can provide an accessible referral site for students who are without a medical home or in need of more comprehensive services, such as primary, mental, oral, or vision health care (School-Based Health Alliance, n.d.). SBHCs are housed in the school or, in some cases, outside the school grounds (the latter are referred to as "school-linked centers"; Knopf et al., 2016). In some cases, SBHCs provide services to school staff, students' family members, and others within the surrounding community. The American Academy of Pediatrics recommends that SBHCs serve as health care resources for children who are uninsured, are underinsured, or have limited access to health care (Council on School Health, 2012). Given evidence that indicates effectiveness in improving both health and education outcomes, the CDC recommends that SBHCs be implemented and maintained in low-income communities (Community Preventive Services Task Force, 2016). Extensive research indicates that SBHCs can have positive effects on both students' health and their academic outcomes (Arenson et al., 2019; Soleimanpour & Geierstanger, 2014). Research also indicates that the economic benefits of SBHCs exceed the intervention cost (Ran et al., 2016).

Counseling, Psychological, and Social Services

Certified school counselors, school psychologists, and school social workers are essential in schools to promote and support students' mental, behavioral, and social-emotional health; academic success; career development; and progress toward a productive and fulfilling adulthood. Research supports the impacts of these three disciplines on these outcomes (American School Counselor Association [ASCA], n.d.; National Association of School Psychologists [NASP], 2020; National Association of Social Workers [NASW], 2012). These professionals provide services that include psychological, psychoeducational, and psychosocial assessments; interventions such as individual or group counseling and consultation to address barriers to learning; and, when needed, referrals to school and community support services. Beyond these services, school mental health professionals can also provide assessment, prevention, intervention, and programs that address overall school environment and engage in consultation with other school staff and community resources and providers. These actions are intended to contribute to the health and educational needs of all students.

School counselors should have a presence at the elementary, middle, and high school levels (ASCA, 2023). ASCA recommends that, at a minimum, school counselors have a master's degree in school counseling, meet certification and licensure standards, and uphold ASCA ethical and professional standards. Specific responsibilities of school counselors include providing individual student academic planning and goal setting, school counseling classroom lessons, short-term counseling to students, and referrals for long-term support; collaborating with families, teachers, administrators, and community members for student success; advocating for students at individualized education plan meetings and other student-focused meetings; and conducting data analysis to identify student issues, needs, and challenges. ASCA (2023) recommends 250 to 1 as the ideal student-to-counselor caseload. Research supports the importance of an appropriate student-to-counselor ratio for services to have a positive impact on students (Kearney et al., 2021; Lapan et al., 2012; Parzych et al., 2019).

School psychologists work with students, families, educators, and community members to resolve students' chronic mental health problems and issues through engagement with students; consultation with teachers, school administrators, families, and other mental health professionals employed by the school (i.e., school counselors, school social workers); and collaborative efforts with community providers. These efforts focus on improving academic achievement, promoting positive behavior and mental health, supporting diverse learning, creating safe and positive school climates, strengthening family–school partnerships, providing direct support, improving schoolwide assessment and accountability, and monitoring individual student progress in academics and behavior. NASP (2020) recommends one school psychologist for every 500-700 students.

Regarding professional preparation, school psychologists complete a specialist-level degree (at least 60 graduate semester hours) or a doctoral degree (at least 90 graduate semester hours; NASP, 2020). As a result of this graduate study, school psychologists develop knowledge and skills related to topics such as schoolwide practices to promote learning; resilience and risk factors; consultation and collaboration; academic learning interventions; mental health interventions; behavioral interventions; instructional support; special education services; and crisis preparedness, response, and recovery. School psychologists must be credentialed by the state in which they work and may also be certified nationally by the National School Psychology Certification Board (NASP, 2020).

School social workers provide services and coordinate efforts with students, parents, teachers, administrators, and other school staff to promote students' academic achievement; educational equity; social, emotional, and behavioral competence; and life adjustment to school and society (NASW, 2012). Specifically, these actions include the following:

- Addressing students' mental health concerns and behavioral issues
- Providing academic and classroom support
- Consulting with teachers, parents, administrators, and other staff members
- Providing individual and group counseling or therapy
- Assisting in special education planning and assessment
- Mobilizing family, school, and community resources to support individual students
- Developing and conducting professional development sessions
- Advocating for community services to meet the needs of students and families (MSW@USC, 2019; School Social Work Association of America, n.d.a, n.d.b)

School social workers must have a graduate degree in social work from a program accredited by the Council on Social Work Education (NASW, 2012). The recommended entry-level requirement is a master's in social work. A focus on the school setting should be an important part of school social workers' professional preparation or should be attained through professional development. School social workers should understand education issues and be knowledgeable about evidence-informed approaches to teaching and learning. School social workers are licensed by state boards of social work and, in some states, certified through state departments of education. An appropriate ratio of school social workers to students is 1 to 250 for a full-time social worker; when a school social worker is providing services to students with intensive needs, a lower ratio, such as 1 to 50, is suggested (NASW, 2012). This ratio may vary within school districts, depending on factors such as the experience and expertise of the school social worker, percentage of high-risk students, and availability of other services within the school and around the community (Frey et al., 2012, p. 2).

Social and Emotional Climate

The school social and emotional climate can be described as the quality of life in school for students, teachers, and all stakeholders. Characteristics of a positive social and emotional climate include equity and inclusivity; physical, social, and psychological safety; meaningful, respectful relationships among teachers, administrators, staff members, family members, and students; a safe and supportive learning environment that provides academic challenges and opportunities for engagement in learning for all students; a commitment to social-emotional learning (SEL); opportunities for student involvement in school decision-making; and a student-centered disciplinary policy (CDC, 2017; Osher & Berg, 2017). It is important to note that school activities and interactions that influence the social and emotional climate occur in hallways, playgrounds, cafeterias, and classrooms and during travel to and from school. Community support and professional development for teachers and all staff members are important in initiating and developing these characteristics (CDC, 2017).

SEL has received considerable attention since 2016. Birch (2023) presented SEL as an element of the social-emotional component of the WSCC model. SEL is usually based on two components: classroom-based instruction and a safe and supportive total school environment (Durlak et al., 2011). Through these two components, SEL provides students with the opportunity to learn and apply social, emotional, behavioral, and character skills that are important in academic endeavors, work, relationships, and citizenship (Jones et al., 2019).

Perceptions of the school climate can vary by student. School leaders must be aware of these varying perceptions and be cognizant of the factors that affect students' school experiences. Osher and Berg (2017) reported that students of color and students who are economically disadvantaged are more likely to report worse perceptions of the school climate than their peers. Simmons (2019) suggested that SEL can provide a venue for initiating conversations that enable students to confront injustice, hate, and inequity related to racism, poverty, violence, sexism, homophobia, transphobia, and other forms of marginalization. As a result of addressing these issues, students can develop an understanding of power and privilege, examine their own personal positions and actions, and consider their roles as community members in addressing social justice. Policies and practices that promote a positive, inclusive approach to the school climate can not only be supportive to marginalized students but also present opportunities for engaging parents and family members of students from marginalized groups (Osher & Berg, 2017).

Research supports the contribution of a positive school climate to improved social and education outcomes for students. These outcomes include increased bonding with teachers and peers, greater respect for school rules, reduced aggression and violence, better classroom behavior, improved grades, increased satisfaction with school, reduced absenteeism, decreased suspension rates, and a higher level of school connectedness (Daily et al., 2020; Michael et al., 2015). Research findings from two meta-analyses identified positive outcomes for SEL including enhanced social and emotional skills, positive attitudes toward self and others, positive social behaviors, fewer conduct problems, reduced emotional distress, and improved academic performance (Durlak et al., 2011; Taylor et al., 2017).

All stakeholders in the school community should recognize and feel the message transmitted from a positive social climate. The message should clearly indicate that all students, family members, staff and teachers, and community members are important to the success and well-being of schools; that all cultures represented in the school community are recognized, appreciated, and celebrated; that social injustices that may be present in the school community are recognized and addressed; that there is a commitment to the academic success of all students; and that stakeholders recognize that students learn and demonstrate their learning in different ways.

Physical Environment

The physical environment of a school has an important impact on students' academic success, their enjoyment of the school experience, and their safety and overall well-being. An accessible, healthy, safe, learning-centered, and physically attractive school environment will not only benefit students but also enhance the instructional environment for teachers; improve the work environment for school staff members; and provide a welcoming environment for visitors, including family and community members.

The physical environment includes the school building and everything within the building, such as classrooms, hallways, restrooms, teaching and learning resources, furniture, and instructional and safety equipment. In addition, ventilation, moisture, temperature, noise level, and natural and artificial lighting within the building are all factors that influence the physical environment. A healthy school environment also provides protection for school staff, students, and visitors from crime, violence, and injuries and prevents exposure to mold, hazardous materials, pesticides, cleaning agents, and biological and chemical agents. Safe school grounds, including playgrounds and athletic fields, are also an important component of the physical environment (CDC, 2021). Student transportation is another factor. School buses and other vehicles used for transportation must be maintained for safety and compliance with environmental regulations and should provide an attractive, comfortable travel environment for passengers. The flow of pedestrian, bicycle, and motor vehicle traffic outside the school should be efficient and safe (ASCD, 2014).

Two resources can provide direction for schools in the assessment of important factors within the school physical environment. The first resource, the report *Schools for Health: Foundations for Student Success—How School Buildings Influence Student Health, Thinking and Performance*, was developed by the Healthy Buildings Program at the Harvard T.H. Chan School of Public Health, under the direction of Dr. Joseph Allen. Based on extensive research, the report presents the evidence-based impact of nine fundamental building factors on student health, thinking, and performance (Eitland et al., 2017). The nine foundational building factors are air quality, thermal health, moisture, dust and pests, safety and security, water quality, noise, lighting and views, and ventilation. The second resource, the *School Health Index (SHI) Self-Assessment and Planning Guide*, is a guide developed by the CDC to help schools identify strengths and weaknesses in all components of the WSCC model, including the school physical environment, to develop an action plan for improving student health (CDC, 2019b).

Further details on the SHI are presented later in the School Health Index section. Both the SHI and *Schools for Health: Foundations for Student Success—How School Buildings Influence Student Health, Thinking and Performance* are available at no cost online.

The health and safety of students and school staff can be threatened by episodic events such as natural disasters, disease outbreaks, crime, and violence. To be as prepared as possible for these types of events, schools should develop an emergency operations plan to ensure a coordinated response in case of any health or safety emergency. Schools should engage community partners, government agencies, various public health and safety representatives, and other stakeholders in the development process. The U.S. Department of Education has developed two complementary resources related to emergency operations plans, one for school districts (*The Role of Districts in Developing High-Quality School Emergency Operations Plans*; Office of Elementary and Secondary Education, 2019) and the other for schools (*Guide for Developing High-Quality School Emergency Operations Plans*; U.S. Department of Education et al., 2013). The school guides frame preparedness within five areas: prevention, protection, mitigation, response, and recovery. Both resources are free and available online.

Employee Wellness

Promoting the physical and mental health of school employees can not only benefit school staff but also support students' health and academic success. A variety of positive health behaviors and outcomes have been identified for school employees who participate in wellness programs. These benefits include improved behaviors and outcomes such as increased physical activity, improved diet, reduced hypertension, weight loss, better stress management, and improvements in overall well-being (Kolbe, 2019). Regarding benefits to students, when teachers and other staff members are absent from school, students' learning can be disrupted. School employees—including teachers, administrators, bus drivers, cafeteria and custodial staff, and contractors—who experience positive health are more productive and less likely to be absent from work. Through their behaviors, these employees can serve as powerful health role models for students. In addition, employees who pay more attention to their own health may increase their support for efforts to improve students' health and support initiatives such as the WSCC model (Birch, 2023; CDC, 2021). Collectively, school employee wellness programs have the potential to have a national impact on health. As one of the largest employers in the United States, school programs can make an important contribution to improving the health status of the overall population (Herbert et al., 2017).

Other benefits from participating in school employee wellness programs have been identified. Research indicates a difference in absenteeism between teachers who participate in programs (less absenteeism) and those who do not participate in programs (Birch, 2023; Herbert et al., 2017). These differences result in reduced costs through decreased payments for substitute teachers (Herbert et al., 2017; Miller, 2008). Employee wellness programs can also contribute to the attractiveness of a school as a work setting to current and prospective teachers. Employees' perceptions of the benefits of school wellness programs can contribute to a school district's retention of quality teachers and valuable staff members and enhance a district's ability to recruit new teachers (Kolbe, 2019).

With regard to implementation, in comparison to non-school worksites, schools have advantages in terms of onsite resources for employee wellness activities. These resources often include gyms, walking and running tracks, and other sites for physical activity; equipment for physical activity; health educators, physical educators, school nurses, and other professionals who can serve as content specialists and program instructors; instructional materials; and classroom and conference room space. Potential programs include employee assistance programs; health-risk appraisals; health screening (blood pressure, diabetes, serum cholesterol); physical activity programs, such as walking, running, resistance activities, aerobics, swimming, and yoga; health education addressing topics such as nutrition, injury prevention, mindfulness, and stress management; ongoing information from program websites, social media communication, newsletters, and bulletin boards; and healthy social events.

Ideally, employee wellness programs should be a component of a school or school district's WSCC program. School employee wellness programs are more likely to attain school- or school district–level support, implement meaningful activities, experience high levels of participation, and be sustained over time when a systematic planning, implementation, and evaluation process is in place. The following steps in sequence are recommended for inclusion in this process: gain administrative support; form an employee wellness committee or team (this could be a subgroup of a WSCC team); identify employee health needs, interests, and assets; identify administrative goals and objectives; identify program activities; market activities; implement activities; evaluate activities; and maintain interest and involvement by showcasing positive evaluation data and testimonials, providing ongoing health information, and gathering input for possible new activities.

Family Engagement

Well-planned, meaningful family engagement efforts can support teaching and learning and enhance not only academic success but also the overall well-being of students, families, and all school staff members. Research indicates that teachers and administrators value school partnerships with families and that the majority of parents want to be engaged with schools to support their children's education. Improving the school climate, strengthening school and classroom programs, providing family service programs, enhancing parents' skills, connecting families with others in the school and community, and supporting teachers are all possible outcomes of school partnerships with families (Epstein et al., 2018). These outcomes can contribute to students' academic and social success in schools.

For important reasons, the terminology related to the interaction between families and schools has shifted from *parent involvement* to *family engagement*. Students' life situations vary, and some may not have parents who are able or available to engage in a partnership with their school. Other family members, such as grandparents, foster parents, guardians, siblings, and other influential adults, may serve as students' primary caregivers and important sources of support. Thus, the term *family* is more appropriate for many students than *parent*. Shifting the terminology from *involvement* to *engagement* signifies a movement from schools having power over (whether intentionally or unintentionally) to schools sharing power with family members (Marchand et al., 2019). Ferlazzo (2011) suggested that engagement is "doing with" rather than "doing to" and is highlighted by communication that goes two ways rather than one way. Examples of involvement activities include school-identified activities such as orientations for parents at the beginning of the school year, parent–teacher conferences, attendance at student performances, and parent volunteer opportunities. Parents are often invited through communication from the school to attend these activities. Although these involvement activities are important, family engagement is based on the recognition that schools and families are essential partners in students' academic success and well-being. In an engaged partnership, schools clearly welcome all family members, and engagement activities are collaboratively identified, planned, and evaluated through active participation among family members, teachers, administrators, and other school staff members. Engagement includes family input into school decision-making through membership on committees and decision-making bodies, the use of focus groups, and family surveys.

The positive impact of family engagement on students' academic achievement at all grade levels and across a diverse range of students is supported by an extensive body of research. Although *family engagement* is the suggested term, the term *parent involvement* is still commonly used in both research and practice and is reflected in the following research findings. Multiple meta-analyses have been conducted to systematically examine the relationship between parent involvement and academic achievement for students at the preK-12 levels. Smith et al. (2020) based on a meta-analysis of 77 parent involvement studies, Castro et al. (2015) based on 37 studies, Higgins and Katsipataki (2015) based on 13 studies, and Hill and Tyson (2009) based on 50 studies all found positive associations through their analyses between parent involvement and academic achievement. The 50 studies in the Hill and Tyson meta-analysis focused on the middle school grades, whereas the other three meta-analyses focused on studies at multiple preK-12 grade levels. Three separate meta-analyses conducted by Jeynes (2012, 2016, 2017) investigated the relationship between parent involvement and academic achievement among African American students (42 studies), Latino students (28 studies), and urban students (51 studies) in preK-12. In each of the three analyses, Jeynes concluded that a positive association existed between parent involvement and academic achievement.

Additional research has identified benefits of family engagement for students' school behavior. On the basis of an analysis of a national database, Domina (2005) concluded that parent involvement contributes to the prevention of school behavior problems. Sheldon (2018), linking parent involvement to academic achievement, identified several studies of large data sets that demonstrate linkages between parent involvement and improvements in students' school behavior (Beyers et al., 2003; El Nokali et al., 2010; Hill et al., 2004). Sheldon and Epstein (2002) found that an improvement from one year to the next in schools' family and community involvement efforts resulted in a decrease in student referrals to the principal, detention, and in-school suspensions. Research has also linked parent involvement with improved school attendance (Michael et al., 2015; Sheldon, 2018).

Epstein et al. (2018) suggested that family engagement should promote both family-like schools and school-like families. Family-like schools welcome all families, recognize the uniqueness of families (including differences in resources and availability), and include all students and families. School-like families emphasize the importance of education to their children, promote regular school attendance, and support students' involvement in activities that help them develop academic and life skills. Epstein et al. (2002) developed a research-based framework for family engagement that has been widely used by schools since the turn of the 21st century. The framework features six types of engagement that provide direction for the development of comprehensive programs for school, family, and community engagement. Comprehensive programs should include activities for each of the following six components:

1. *Parenting:* providing supportive home environments and helping school personnel gain an awareness and understanding of students' families
2. *Communicating:* engaging in two-way communication using a variety of methods, including technology
3. *Volunteering:* recruiting family members to provide assistance at school, at home, and in other locations
4. *Learning at home:* providing education programs and activities for parents
5. *Decision-making:* inviting parents to serve as leaders in decision-making situations in the school
6. *Collaborating with the community:* identifying resources and services in the community that support and engage families and students (Epstein et al., 2018)

Several considerations are of importance in maximizing the impact of parent engagement. These considerations include using multiple methods to promote ongoing, two-way communication between schools and families; demonstrating cultural responsiveness on the part of school administrators, teachers, and other school staff members that is highlighted by an understanding of the various assets, challenges, and needs of the cultures represented in the school community; and addressing barriers to engagement that may result from parents and family members speaking multiple languages, not being able to leave work during school hours, and lacking transportation.

Community Involvement

School partnerships with community members, businesses, and various organizations can provide education and health benefits to students, families, administrators, teachers, other school staff members, and the community itself. Potential partners for schools include service and volunteer organizations such as the Rotary, Lions, and Kiwanis clubs; the YMCA and YWCA; Boys and Girls Clubs; faith-based organizations; the United Way; local businesses; libraries and museums; local colleges and universities; voluntary health agencies; hospitals and clinics; the local recreation department; the fire and police departments; media; and sports franchises (Sanders, 2018).

Community partnerships can provide schools with volunteers, external expertise, unique sites for teaching and learning, and financial and material resources. For example, individual community members, businesses, and organizations can provide funding for instructional resources and facilities. Partners can also provide expertise for teaching and learning that is not available from teachers and staff and provide sites for student field trips. School and community decision-making presents an important opportunity for engagement. Community members can bring outside perspectives to school decision-making bodies, and staff members and students can bring a school perspective to community policy and decision-making entities. Other school–community activities and interactions can demonstrate the idea of schools being a part of the community rather than a separate institution. School staff members and students can engage with community members by exhibiting at community art or health fairs or participating in community–school book clubs in which school staff, students, and individual community members read the same book and discuss it. Schools can also share facilities with community members. School physical activity facilities can be used for programs for community members, and school classrooms can be used for community education classes.

Local colleges and universities can also present opportunities for mutually beneficial partnerships with schools. Colleges and universities can provide schools with access to faculty members with expertise related to specific areas in education, school health, and research and evaluation. In addition, colleges and universities can provide opportunities for school-age students to observe classes and visit campus centers, museums, and other facilities. Conversely, school administrators and teachers can provide perspectives based on experiences from early childhood, elementary, middle, and high school settings. Another partnership activity between schools and universities is offering dual enrollment courses for both high school and college credit. These courses are often offered for free or at a lesser cost than regular college courses and provide students with an introduction to college-level instruction.

A specific approach to partnerships is the Community Schools model. This model, often described as "wraparound services," represents an integrated approach to academics, services, supports, and opportunities. It is intended to promote student learning, stronger families, and healthier communities (California School Boards Association, n.d.). The services and supports are coordinated and provided by the school, community health and social services agencies, civil rights organizations, faith-based organizations, food banks, colleges and universities, the business sector, and other community agencies and organizations. Examples of these services include expanded learning activities for students, family, and community members; health and social services sometimes through school-based clinics; legal assistance; and programs to support college admission, career preparation, and the attainment of citizenship (Blank & Villarreal, 2015; Weingarten, 2015). Evaluations of the Community Schools model found improvements in math and reading standardized test scores in schools in Boston, Chicago, and Tulsa (Adams, 2019; Bryk et al., 2010; Walsh et al., 2014) and improved attendance rates and a decrease in chronic absenteeism in Baltimore and Chicago schools (Bryk et al., 2010; Olson, 2014). A structured examination of 143 research studies indicated that the Community Schools model had a positive impact on school attendance, academic achievement, and high school graduation rates and reduced racial and economic achievement gaps (Maier et al., 2017).

For community–school partnerships to thrive, it is important to keep in mind the following considerations regarding planning, implementation, and evaluation:

- Promote an understanding among all partners that the education of children and youth is a shared responsibility of families, schools, and the community. All representatives should have an awareness of the potential benefits of the partnership and examples of possible activities.
- Help community partners understand the school's mission, vision, philosophy, and core values and the lifelong recipro-

cal relationship between education and health.
- Create an awareness of the impact of social injustices on children's health and school success.
- Ensure that community partners represent all segments of the community and that the individuals involved reflect the population of the community.
- Demonstrate collaborative decision-making, transparency, and two-way communication in all partnership activities.
- Conduct ongoing evaluation of the processes and impact of the partnership (Birch, 2023).

School Health Index

The *School Health Index (SHI) Self-Assessment and Planning Guide* is a CDC resource developed in partnership with school administrators and staff, school health experts, parents, and nongovernmental health agencies. This guide provides schools with a tool to examine health and safety policies and programs to provide direction for the development of an action plan for addressing student health. The SHI uses the 10 WSCC components as a framework for reviewing policies, programs, and services related to seven health topic areas: physical activity and physical education, nutrition, tobacco use prevention, alcohol and other drug use prevention, chronic health conditions, unintentional injury and violence prevention (safety), and sexual health (including sexually transmitted disease and HIV education and pregnancy prevention). The SHI provides direction for a self-assessment process that engages members of the school community to identify the strengths and weaknesses of the school's health-related policies and practices. The self-assessment assists in the identification of actions that can be taken to improve areas of weakness. The WSCC in Practice sidebar on page 51 provides an example of priority school districts in Washington that have used the SHI to review and improve their wellness policies.

Community as an Overarching WSCC Concept

The communities in which children live have an impact on their health and access to high-quality schools. How a community supports its schools is indicative of how the community supports its children (Birch, 2023). Furthermore, schools are reflective of their local communities. As shown in figure 3.1, the full WSCC model is enclosed within the outer community ring, which demonstrates the prominent role of the community as a critical partner in supporting schools and children. Within the WSCC model diagram, the space between the school and the community represents an open two-way passage with continuous traffic, which indicates ongoing communication and a mutually beneficial partnership. As presented earlier in the chapter, the center and focal point of the WSCC model is the child. To maximize the WSCC model's potential in positively affecting children's health and academic success, schools and their communities must have strong partnerships: Communities must support their schools and vice versa.

Communities and schools that work together effectively share values and interests, utilize an inclusive decision-making process, and assist community members in engaging with children and schools in a meaningful manner (SOPHE, n.d.a). Moreover, developing and sustaining a strong school–community partnership requires an acknowledgment of the essential nature of the partnership, ongoing communication and transparency, an understanding of the needs and assets that the partners bring to the relationship, and, finally, an enduring commitment to address the barriers and issues within both sectors (Birch, 2023). The WSCC model presents an opportunity to engage school staff and community members in decision-making and action. In return, this results in communities and schools that support and implement coordinated policies and activities that improve students' academic success and health and reciprocally benefit school staff and community members.

WSCC IN PRACTICE
Priority School Districts in Washington State Use the School Health Index to Improve Wellness Policies

In Washington, 82.5 percent of 10th-grade students do not eat the recommended servings of fruits and vegetables per day and only 57.9 percent reported being physically active for at least 60 minutes on most days (Healthy Youth Survey, 2018). As a result, the Healthy Schools Washington (HSW) Program took action.

The HSW Program works to improve student health and academic achievement by improving opportunities for healthy eating, physical activity, and chronic disease management. Before the COVID-19 pandemic, Washington's priority school districts had planned to complete the School Health Index (SHI) and WellSAT 3.0 to assess school environment and policies that affect student health, such as those pertaining to fruit and vegetable consumption and physical activity. However, in-person meetings and trainings transitioned into virtual formats. In May and June 2020, the HSW Program developed a four-step process to complete the assessments virtually to address the issues identified in the Healthy Youth Survey:

1. Identified and assembled a team of content experts to be responsible for completing the SHI.
2. Used a skilled group facilitator to navigate each SHI team through SHI modules to enable schools to identify strengths and weaknesses of health and safety policies and programs.
3. Convened a two-hour professional development (PD) session to review SHI results.
4. Completed the WellSAT 3.0 in another two-hour PD session.

Impact: The COVID-19 pandemic limited the ability of the HSW Program and Washington's priority school districts to take measurable actions based on these assessments. However, the school districts that participated in the four-step process trainings submitted health improvement action plans describing the policies and procedures they intended to address once COVID-19 restrictions were lifted. Among other actions, districts intend to:

- Incorporate physical activity breaks in the classroom and provide teachers with resources to take this action.
- Improve marketing of school meals and grab-and-go bags.
- Provide and promote locally grown foods to students.
- Provide enough time for all students to eat breakfast and lunch.
- Provide recommendations to all schools, parents, and the community on foods offered to students for parties and rewards, in school stores, and a la carte items.
- Hire a nurse's aide for the elementary school to manage injuries, health concerns, and chronic health conditions.
- Improve the social and emotional climate by creating a professional development plan for staff that addresses the following:
  – How discussions with students during discipline can lead to healthier student behavior.
  – How to engage students to ensure they feel heard and valued.
  – How to teach coping skills during interactions and conversations with students.
  – How to use student surveys to understand student social and emotional needs.
  (CDC, 2022a, pp. 1-2)

Community partners can help:

- *Arrange for schools to serve as hubs to organize and deliver a range of services beyond their traditional core offerings;*
- *Build individual and institutional networks, assets, and resources—like facilities, materials, skills, and economic power—to promote school and community health;*
- *Provide wraparound services that students need to be successful, such as health care and social services;*
- *Offer learning and enrichment activities to strengthen student outcomes and skills. (SOPHE, n.d.a, p. 2)*

Summary

This chapter presented an overview of the WSCC model and highlighted background information related to program quality for each of the 10 components. The goal of WSCC is for every child to be healthy, safe, engaged, supported, and challenged for maximum well-being and academic success. Ensuring quality in the WSCC approach is essential for communities and schools to maximize health and academic success for students. Overall support and coordination among the various components of WSCC are essential, but the efficacy of that support and coordination can be negated if there are issues related to the overall quality of the individual components of WSCC. Weakness in one or more of the individual components could diminish the effect of the total WSCC approach. To move forward and address such gaps, schools and communities must make efforts to strengthen their commitment to quality across the WSCC components, adhere to national guidelines and standards, have well-prepared professionals and staff, and implement best practices for all WSCC components. Beyond the individual components, schools and communities must collaborate; coordinate school policies, practices, and processes; and commit to a school-wide continuous improvement approach to maximally support each child's well-being and educational success.

LEARNING AIDS

GLOSSARY

comprehensive school health education—Defined by the CDC as a course of study for students in preK-12 that addresses a variety of topics, such as the use and abuse of alcohol and other drugs, healthy eating and nutrition, mental and emotional health, personal health and wellness, physical activity, safety and injury prevention, sexual health, tobacco use, and violence prevention.

Maslow's hierarchy of needs—Abraham Maslow's presentation of the needs for human development. The hierarchy of needs is frequently displayed as a pyramid with the foundational needs at the base and self-actualization at the top.

National Health Education Standards (3rd ed.)—Eight instructional standards and related performance expectations that provide direction for the development of state health education standards, local school district curricula, and related instruction. The standards reflect the functional health knowledge, beliefs, and skills necessary for students to adopt and maintain healthy behaviors, achieve health literacy, and enhance health and academic outcomes.

National School Lunch Program—A federally assisted meal program operating in public and nonprofit private schools and residential child care institutions. It provides nutritionally balanced low-cost or free lunches to children each school day. The program was established under the National School Lunch Act, which was signed by President Harry Truman in 1946.

school-based health center (SBHC)—A health center located in a school or on school grounds that provides, at a minimum, on-site primary and preventive health care, mental health counseling, health promotion referral, and follow-up services for young people enrolled. The center may be staffed by physicians, physician assistants, school nurses, or mental health professionals. Services are provided without consideration for a student's financial circumstances.

WSCC components—The 10 WSCC components represent the professional workforce and school-based services available to support the health, safety, and well-being of students and staff (SOPHE, n.d.c, p. 5).

APPLICATION ACTIVITIES

1. Create a one-hour professional development training presentation intended for colleagues in the school district in which you work (real or imagined). In the training presentation, be sure to (1) present a rationale for the WSCC model and (2) describe the WSCC model (five tenets, 10 components, and community emphasis). Next, develop a PowerPoint presentation to highlight the key points of the training.

2. Interview at least three college students regarding their memories of their experiences related to nine of the WSCC components (health education; physical education and physical activity; health services; nutrition environment and services; counseling, psychological, and social services; the physical environment; family engagement; community involvement; and the social and emotional climate). Request that the students describe the extent to which they felt healthy, safe, engaged, supported, and challenged as students. For the activity, develop a list of interview questions related to the nine WSCC components. Then, following the interviews, develop a summary of the interviews and a written reflection.

3. The WSCC model is going to be presented at a school health conference in your region of the state. The rationale, components, and important considerations related to the model will be included in the presentation. You have been asked to be a member of a respondent panel to provide your thoughts on the presentation of the WSCC model. You will have 15 minutes to provide your response. It should include your thoughts of the model and your perception of its applicability for students, schools, parents and family members, and the community. Perhaps you might have other ideas for the model; if so, identify anything you think should be added to or eliminated from the WSCC model. Develop a detailed outline for your 15-minute response.

REFERENCES

Adams, C.M. (2019). Sustaining full-service community schools: Lessons from the Tulsa area community schools initiative. *Journal of Education for Students Placed at Risk*, 24(3), 288-313. https://doi.org/10.1080/10824669.2019.1615924

Allensworth, D. (2015). Historical overview of coordinated school health. In D.A. Birch & D.M. Videto (Eds.), *Promoting health and academic success: The Whole School, Whole Community, Whole Child approach* (pp. 13-28). Human Kinetics.

American School Counselor Association [ASCA]. (2023). *The role of the school counselor*. https://www.schoolcounselor.org/getmedia/ee8b2e1b-d021-4575-982c-c84402cb2cd2/Role-Statement.pdf

American School Counselor Association [ASCA]. (n.d.). *Empirical research studies supporting the value of school counseling*. https://www.schoolcounselor.org/getmedia/7d00dcff-40a6-4316-ab6c-8f3ffd7941c2/Effectiveness.pdf

Arenson, M., Hudson, P.J., Lee, N., & Lai, B. (2019). The evidence on school-based health centers: A review. *Global Pediatric Health*, 6, 1-10. https://doi.org/10.1177%2F1942602X19852749

ASCD. (2014). *Whole School, Whole Community, Whole Child: A collaborative approach to learning and health*. https://files.ascd.org/staticfiles/ascd/pdf/siteASCD/publications/wholechild/wscc-a-collaborative-approach.pdf

ASCD. (2015). *About—Whole child education*. www.wholechildeducation.org/about/

ASCD. (2016). *The Whole School, Whole Community, Whole Child model: Ideas for implementation*. https://files.ascd.org/staticfiles/ascd/pdf/siteASCD/wholechild/WSCC_Examples_Publication.pdf

Baldwin, S., & Ventresca, A. R. C. (2020). Every school healthy: An urban school case study. *Journal of School Health, 90*(12), 1045–1055. https://doi.org/10.1111/josh.12965

Ballard, E., Farrell, A. & Long, M. (2020). Community-based system dynamics for mobilizing communities to advance school health. Journal of School Health, *90(12)*, 964-975. https://doi.org/10.1111/josh.12961

Beyers, J.M., Bates, J.E., Pettit, G.S., & Dodge, K.A. (2003). Neighborhood structure, parent processes, and the development of externalizing behaviors: A multilevel analysis. *American Journal of Community Psychology, 31*, 35-53. https://doi.org/10.1023/A:1023018502759

Birch, D.A. (2023). *Leveraging the education-health connection: How educators, physicians, and public health professionals can improve education and health outcomes throughout the lifespan*. Johns Hopkins University Press.

Birch, D.A., Priest, H.M., & Mitchell, Q.P. (2015). Advocacy for quality school health education: The role of public health educators as professionals and community members. *The Health Educator, 47*(1), 38-44.

Blank, M.J., & Villarreal, L. (2015). Where it all comes together: How partnerships connect communities and schools. *American Educator, 39*(3), 4-9, 43. https://files.eric.ed.gov/fulltext/EJ1076382.pdf

Blue Zones. (n.d.). *Walking school buses get kids moving, alert, and ready to learn*. www.bluezones.com/2017/09/walking-school-buses-get-kids-moving-alert-and-ready-to-learn/#

Bryk, A.S., Bender Sebring, P., Allensworth, E., Luppescu, S., & Easton, J.Q. (2010). *Organizing schools for improvement: Lessons from Chicago*. University of Chicago Press.

California School Boards Association. (n.d.). *Community schools*. www.csba.org/en/GovernanceAndPolicyResources/ConditionsOfChildren/ParentFamComEngageandCollab/CommunitySchools

Castro, M., Expósito-Casas, E., López-Martín, E., Lizasoain, L., Navarro-Asencio, E., & Gaviria, J.L. (2015). Parental involvement on student academic achievement: A meta-analysis. *Educational Research Review, 14*, 33-46. https://doi.org/10.1016/j.edurev.2015.01.002

Centers for Disease Control and Prevention. (2013). *Comprehensive school physical activity programs: A guide for schools*. www.cdc.gov/healthyschools/physicalactivity/pdf/13_242620-A_CSPAP_SchoolPhysActivityPrograms_Final_508_12192013.pdf

Centers for Disease Control and Prevention. (2017). *2017 School Health Index (SHI) elementary version*. www.cdc.gov/healthyschools/shi/pdf/Elementary-Total-2017.pdf

Centers for Disease Control and Prevention. (2018). *Strategies for classroom physical activity in schools*. www.cdc.gov/healthyschools/physicalactivity/pdf/2019_04_25_Strategies-for-CPA_508tagged.pdf

Centers for Disease Control and Prevention. (2019a). *Characteristics of an effective health education curriculum*. www.cdc.gov/healthyschools/sher/characteristics/

Centers for Disease Control and Prevention. (2019b). *School Health Index*. www.cdc.gov/healthyschools/shi/index.htm

Centers for Disease Control and Prevention. (2021). *Components of the Whole School, Whole Community, Whole Child (WSCC)*. www.cdc.gov/healthyschools/wscc/components.htm

Centers for Disease Control and Prevention. (2022a). *CDC Healthy Schools stories of achievement: Healthy students, ready to learn: Washington*. www.cdc.gov/healthyschools/achievement_stories/documents/Stories-of-Achievement-Washington_final-508.pdf

Centers for Disease Control and Prevention. (2022b). *Classroom physical activity*. www.cdc.gov/healthyschools/physicalactivity/classroom-pa.htm

Centers for Disease Control and Prevention. (2022c). *School health services*. www.cdc.gov/healthyschools/schoolhealthservices.htm

Centers for Disease Control and Prevention. (2022d). *Smart snacks and school vending machines*. www.cdc.gov/healthyschools/nutrition/smartsnacks.htm

Centers for Disease Control and Prevention. (2022e). *Water access in schools*. www.cdc.gov/healthyschools/nutrition/wateraccess.htm

Centers for Disease Control and Prevention. (2022f). *Whole School, Whole Community, Whole Child (WSCC)*. https://www.cdc.gov/healthyschools/wscc/index.htm

Chriqui, J.F., Leider, J., Temkin, D., Piekarz-Porter, E., Schermbeck, R.M. and Stuart-Cassel, V. (2020). State laws matter when it comes to district policymaking relative to the whole school, whole community, whole child framework. *Journal of School Health, 90*, 907-917. https://doi.org/10.1111/josh.12959

Community Preventive Services Task Force. (2016). School-based health centers to promote health equity: Recommendation of the Community Preventive Services Task Force. *American Journal of Preventive Medicine, 51*(1), 127-128. https://doi.org/10.1016/j.amepre.2016.01.008

Council on School Health. (2012). School-based health centers and pediatric practice. *Pediatrics, 129*(1), 387-393. www.pediatrics.org/cgi/doi/10.1542/peds.2011-3443

County Health Rankings and Roadmaps. (2019, November 4). *Walking school buses*. www.countyhealthrankings.org/take-action-to-improve-health/what-works-for-health/strategies/walking-school-buses

Daily, S.M., Mann, M.J., Lilly, C.L., Dyer, A.M., Smith, M.L., & Kristjansson, A.L. (2020). School climate as an intervention to reduce academic failure and educate the whole child: A longitudinal study. *Journal of School Health, 90*(3), 182-193. https://doi.org/10.1111/josh.12863

Devore, C.D., Wheeler, L.S.M., & American Academy of Pediatrics Council on School Health. (2013). Role of the school physician. *Pediatrics, 131*(1), 178-182. https://doi.org/10.1542/peds.2012-2995

Domina, T. (2005). Leveling the home advantage: Assessing the effectiveness of parental involvement in elementary school. *Sociology of Education, 78*(3), 233-249. https://doi.org/10.1177%2F003804070507800303

Durlak, J.A., Weissberg, R.P., Dymnicki, A.B., Taylor, R.D., & Schellinger, K.B. (2011). The impact of enhancing students' social and emotional learning: A meta-analysis of school-based universal interventions. *Child Development, 82*, 405-432. https://doi.org/10.1111/j.1467-8624.2010.01564.x

Eitland, E., MacNaughton, P., Cedeno Laurent, M., Spengler, J., Bernstein, A., & Allen, J. (2017, October 5). *School buildings and student success*. Harvard T.H. Chan School of Public Health. www.hsph.harvard.edu/c-change/news/school-buildings-and-student-success/

El Nokali, N.E., Bachman, H.J., & Votruba-Drzal, E. (2010). Parent involvement and children's academic and social development in elementary school. *Child Development, 81*, 988-1005. https://doi.org/10.1111/j.1467-8624.2010.01447.x

Epstein, J.L., Sanders, M.G., Sheldon, S.B., Simon, B.S., Salinas, K.C., Jansorn, N.R., Van Voorhis, F.L., Martin, C.S., Thomas, B.G., Greenfield, M.D., Hutchins, D.J., & Williams, K.J. (Eds). (2018). *School, family, and community partnerships: Your handbook for action* (4th ed.). Corwin Press.

Epstein, J. L., Sanders, M. G., Simon, B. S., Salinas, K. C., Jansorn, N. R., & Van Voorhis, F. L. (2002). *School, family, and community partnerships: Your handbook for action* (2nd ed.). Corwin Press.

Farrey, T. (2020, June 22). *Why we're reimagining school sports in America*. Aspen Institute. www.aspeninstitute.org/blog-posts/why-were-reimagining-school-sports-in-america/

Ferlazzo, L. (2011). Involvement or engagement? *Educational Leadership, 68*(8), 10-14.

Frey, A. J., Alvarez, M. E., Sabatino, C. A., Lindsey, B. C., Dupper, D. R., Raines, J. C., Streeck, F., McInerney, A., & Norris, M. P. (2012). The development of a national school social work practice model. *Children and Schools, 34*(3), 131-134. https://doi.org/10.1093/cs/cds025

Herbert, P.C., Lohrmann, D.K., & Hall, C. (2017). Targeting obesity through health promotion programs for school staff. *Strategies, 30*(1), 28-34. https://doi.org/10.1080/08924562.2016.1251867

Higgins, S., & Katsipataki, M. (2015). Evidence from meta-analysis about parental involvement in education which supports their children's learning. *Journal of Children's Services, 10*(3), 280-290. https://doi.org/10.1108/JCS-02-2015-0009

Hill, N.E., Castellino, D.R., Lansford, J.E., Nowlin, P., Dodge, K.A., Bates, J.E., & Pettit, G.S. (2004). Parent academic involvement as related to school behavior, achievement, and aspirations: Demographic variations across adolescence. *Child Development, 75*(5), 1491-1509. https://doi.org/10.1111/j.1467-8624.2004.00753.x

Hill, N.E., & Tyson, D.F. (2009). Parental involvement in middle school: A meta-analytic assessment of the strategies that promote achievement. *Developmental Psychology, 45*(3), 740-763. https://psycnet.apa.org/doi/10.1037/a0015362

Jeynes, W. (2012). A meta-analysis of the efficacy of different types of parental involvement programs for urban students. *Urban Education, 47*(4), 706-742. https://doi.org/10.1177%2F0042085912445643

Jeynes, W.H. (2016). A meta-analysis: The relationship between parental involvement and African American school outcomes. *Journal of Black Studies, 47*(3), 195-216. https://doi.org/10.1177%2F0021934715623522

Jeynes, W.H. (2017). A meta-analysis: The relationship between parental involvement and Latino student outcomes. *Education and Urban Society, 49*(1), 4-28. https://doi.org/10.1177%2F0013124516630596

Jones, S.M., McGarrah, M.W., & Kahn, J. (2019). Social and emotional learning: A principled science of human development in context. *Educational Psychologist, 54*(3), 129-143. https://doi.org/10.1080/00461520.2019.1625776

Healthy Youth Survey. (2019). *Healthy Youth Survey 2018 | report of results | statewide results grades 6, 8, 10 and 12*. https://doh.wa.gov/sites/default/files/legacy/Documents/8350/HYSStateMultiGradeReport.pdf

Kearney, C., Akos, P., Domina, T., & Young, Z. (2021). Student-to-school counselor ratios: A meta-analytic review of the evidence. *Journal of Counseling & Development, 99*(4), 418-428. https://doi.org/10.1002/jcad.12394

Knopf, J.A., Finnie, R.K., Peng, Y., Hahn, R.A., Truman, B.I., Vernon-Smiley, M., Johnson, V.C., Johnson, R.L., Fielding, J.E., Muntaner, C., Hunt, P.C., Jones, C.P., Fullilove, M.T., & Community Preventive Services Task Force. (2016). School-based health centers to advance health equity: A community guide systematic review. *American Journal of Preventive Medicine, 51*(1), 114-126. https://doi.org/10.1016/j.amepre.2016.01.009

Kohl, H.W., III, & Cook, H.D. (Eds.). (2013). *Educating the student body: Taking physical activity and physical education to school*. National Academies Press.

Kolbe, L. J. (2019). School health as a strategy to improve both public health and education. *Annual Review of Public Health, 40*, 443–463. https://doi.org/10.1146/annurev-publhealth-040218-043727

Koriakin, T.A., McKee, S.L., Schwartz, M.B., & Chafouleas, S.M. (2020). Development of a comprehensive tool for school health policy evaluation: The WellSAT WSCC. *Journal of School Health, 90*(12), 923-939. https://doi.org/10.1111/josh.12956

Lapan, R.T., Gysbers, N.C., Stanley, B., & Pierce, M.E. (2012). Missouri professional school counselors: Ratios matter, especially in high-poverty schools. *Professional School Counseling, 16*(2). https://doi.org/10.1177/2156759X0001600207

Maier, A., Daniel, J., Oakes, J., & Lam, L. (2017, December). *Community schools as an effective school improvement strategy: A review of the evidence*. Learning Policy Institute. https://learningpolicyinstitute.org/media/137/download?inline&file=Community_Schools_Effective_REPORT.pdf

Marchand, A.D., Vassar, R.R., Diemer, M.A., & Rowley, S.J. (2019). Integrating race, racism, and critical consciousness in Black parents' engagement with schools. *Journal of Family Therapy and Review, 11*(3), 367-384. https://doi.org/10.1111/jftr.12344

Maslow, A.H. 1943. A theory of human motivation. *Psychological Review, 50*(4), 370–96. http://psychclassics.yorku.ca/Maslow/motivation.htm

Massey, W.V., Stellino, M.B., Mullen, S.P., Claassen, J., & Wilkison, M. (2018). Development of the Great Recess Framework–Observational Tool to measure contextual and behavioral components of elementary school recess. *BMC Public Health, 18*(1), 1-11. https://doi.org/10.1186/s12889-018-5295-y

Massey, W.V., Thalken, J., Szarabajko, A., Neilson, L., & Geldhof, J. (2021). Recess quality and social and behavioral health in elementary school students. *Journal of School Health, 91*(9), 730-740. https://doi.org/10.1111/josh.13065

McClanahan, R., & Weismuller, P.C. (2015). School nurses and care coordination for children with complex needs: An integrative review. *Journal of School Nursing, 31*(1), 34-43. https://doi.org/10.11772F1059840514550484

Michael, S.L., Merlo, C.L., Basch, C.E., Wentzel, K.R., & Wechsler, H. (2015). Critical connections: Health and academics. *Journal of School Health, 85*(11), 740-758. https://doi.org/10.1111/josh.12309

Miller, R. (2008). *Tales of teacher absence: New research yields patterns that speak to policymakers*. Center for American Progress.

Moening, K., Lieberman, M., & Zimmerman, S. (2016). *Step by step: How to start a walking school bus at your school*. California Department of Public Health. www.saferoutespartnership.org/sites/default/files/resource_files/step-by-step-walking-school-bus-2017.pdf

MSW@USC. (2019, February 4). *Role of school social workers*. University of Southern California. https://msw.usc.edu/mswusc-blog/what-is-a-school-social-worker/

Murray, R., Ramstetter, C., & American Academy of Pediatrics Council on School Health. (2013). The crucial role of recess in school. *Pediatrics, 131*(1), 183-188. https://doi.org/10.1542/peds.2012-2993

Murray, S.D., Hurley, J., & Ahmed, S.R. (2015). Supporting the whole child through coordinated policies, processes, and practices. *Journal of School Health, 85*(11), 795-801. https://doi.org/10.1111/josh.12306

National Association of School Nurses. (2016). The role of the 21st century school nurse. *NASN School Nurse, 32*(1), 56-58.

National Association of School Nurses. (2020). *School nurse workload: Staffing for safe care*. www.nasn.org/advocacy/professional-practice-documents/position-statements/ps-workload#:~:text=of%20School%20Nurses.,(2020).,Nurse%20Workload%20(Position%20Statement).&text=%E2%80%9CTo%20optimize%20student%20health%2C%20safety,all%20day%2C%20every%20day.%E2%80%9D

National Association of School Psychologists. (2020). *Who are school psychologists*. www.nasponline.org/about-school-psychology/who-are-school-psychologists

National Association of Social Workers. (2012). *NASW standards for school social work services*. www.socialworkers.org/LinkClick.aspx?fileticket=5qpx4B6Csr0%3d&portalid=0

National Center for Safe Routes to School (n.d.). *Deciding if a walking school bus is the right fit*. http://guide.saferoutesinfo.org/walking_school_bus/deciding_if_a_walking_school_bus_is_the_right_fit.cfm

National Consensus for School Health Education. (2022). *National Health Education Standards: Model guidance for curriculum and instruction* (3rd ed.). www.schoolhealtheducation.org/

Office of Elementary and Secondary Education, Office of Safe and Supportive Schools. (2019). *The role of districts in developing high-quality school emergency operations plans*. https://rems.ed.gov/docs/District_Guide_508C.pdf

Olson, L. S. (2014). *A first look at community schools in Baltimore*. Baltimore Education Research Consortium.

Osher, D., & Berg, J. (2017). *School climate and social and emotional learning: The integration of two approaches*. Edna Bennet Pierce Prevention Research Center, Pennsylvania State University.

Parzych, J.L., Donohue, P., Gaesser, A., & Chiu, M.M. (2019, February 1). *Measuring the impact of school counselor ratios on student outcomes* (ASCA Research Report). www.schoolcounselor.org/getmedia/5157ef82-d2e8-4b4d-8659-a957f14b7875/Ratios-Student-Outcomes-Research-Report.pdf

Pittman, K., Moroney, D. A., Irby, M., & Young, J. (2020). Unusual suspects: The people inside and outside of school who matter in whole school, whole community, whole child efforts. *Journal of School Health, 90*(12), 1038–1044. https://doi.org/10.1111/josh.12966

Pufall Jones, E., Hatfield, D. P., & Connolly, N. (2020). Every school healthy: Creating local impact through national efforts. *Journal of School Health, 90*(12), 995–1003. https://doi.org/10.1111/josh.12963

Purnell, J.Q., Lobb Dougherty, N., Kryzer, E.K., Bajracharya, S., Chaitan, V.L., Combs, T., Ballard, E., Simpson, A., Caburnay, C., Poor, T.J., Pearson, C.J., Reiter, C., Adams, K.R., & Brown, M. (2020). Research to translation: The Healthy Schools Toolkit and new approaches to the whole school, whole community, whole child model. *Journal of School Health, 90*(12), 948-963. https://doi.org/10.1111/josh.12958

Ran, T., Chattopadhyay, S.K., Hahn, R.A., & Community Preventive Services Task Force. (2016). Economic evaluation of school-based health centers: A community guide systematic review. *American Journal of Preventive Medicine, 51*(1), 129-138. https://doi.org/10.1016/j.amepre.2016.01.017

Sanders, M.G. (2018). School-community partnerships: The little extra that makes a big difference. In J.L. Epstein, M.G. Sanders, S.B. Sheldon, B.S. Simon, K.C. Salinas, N.R. Jansorn, F.L. Van Voorhis, C.S. Martin, B.G. Thomas, M.D. Greenfield, D.J. Hutchins, & K.J. Williams, *School, family, and community partnerships: Your handbook for action* (4th ed., pp. 33-42). Corwin Press.

Scharberg, K. (2013). Understanding the Whole Child approach with tenets, indicators, and components—Whole child education. *The Whole Child Blog.* www.wholechildeducation.org/blog/understanding-the-whole-child-approach-with-tenets-indicators-and-component.html

School-Based Health Alliance. (n.d.). *About school-based health care.* www.sbh4all.org/what-we-do/school-based-health-care/aboutsbhcs/

School Nutrition Association. (2019). *Keys to excellence: Standards of practice for nutrition integrity.* https://schoolnutrition.org/wp-content/uploads/2022/09/Keys-to-Excellence-Standards.pdf

School Social Work Association of America. (n.d.a). *Role of school social work.* www.sswaa.org/school-social-work

School Social Work Association of America. (n.d.b). *Role of school social work* [Infographic]. https://aab82939-3e7b-497d-8f30a85373757e29.filesusr.com/ugd/426a18_003ab15a5e9246248dff98506e46654b.pdf

SHAPE America. (in press). *National physical education standards.* (2nd ed.). Human Kinetics.

SHAPE America. (2015). *The essential components of physical education.* https://www.shapeamerica.org//Common/Uploaded%20files/uploads/pdfs/TheEssentialComponentsOfPhysicalEducation.pdf

Sheldon, S.B. (2018). Improving student outcomes with school, family, and community partnerships: A research review. In J. L. Epstein, M.G. Sanders, S.B. Sheldon, B.S. Simon, K.C. Salinas, N.R. Jansorn, F.L. Van Voorhis, C. S. Martin, B.G. Thomas, M.D. Greenfield, D. J. Hutchins, & K. J. Williams (Eds.), *School, family, and community partnerships: Your handbook for action* (4th ed., pp. 43-62). Corwin Press.

Sheldon, S.B., & Epstein, J.L. (2002). Improving student behavior and school discipline with family and community involvement. *Education and Urban Society, 35*(1), 4-26. https://doi.org/10.1177%2F001ASCD312402237212

Simmons, D. (2019). How to be an antiracist educator. *ASCD Education Update, 61*(10). https://eastsideforall.org/wp-content/uploads/2020/01/How-to-Be-an-Antiracist-Educator.pdf

Slade, S. (2015). The whole child initiative. In D.A. Birch & D.M. Videto (Eds.), *Promoting health and academic success: The Whole School, Whole Community, Whole Child approach* (pp. 53-63). Human Kinetics.

Smith, T.E., Sheridan, S.M., Kim, E.M., Park, S., & Beretvas, S.N. (2020). The effects of family-school partnership interventions on academic and social-emotional functioning: A meta-analysis exploring what works for whom. *Educational Psychology Review, 32,* 511-544. https://doi.org/10.1007/s10648-019-09509-w

Society for Public Health Education. (n.d.a). *Creating school and community partnerships.* https://83d1c0c27a041a7d5507-d5b2ab4b603312217b3d4630a3b284aa.ssl.cf2.rackcdn.com/sophelms_d662359f4017bc922d-70b2ada3b6e998.pdf

Society for Public Health Education. (n.d.b). *SOPHE learning: SOPHE WSCC team training modules.* https://elearn.sophe.org/wscc-training-modules

Society for Public Health Education. (n.d.c). *SOPHE WSCC script overview.* www.sophe.org/wp-content/uploads/2020/03/SOPHE-WSCC-Script-Overview.pdf

Soleimanpour, S., & Geierstanger, S. (2014). *Documenting the link between school-based health centers and academic success: A guide for the field.* California School-Based Health Alliance. www.schoolhealthcenters.org/wp-content/uploads/2014/07/SBHCs-Academic-Success-CA-Alliance-2014.pdf

Taylor, R.D., Oberle, E., Durlak, J.A., & Weissberg, R.P. (2017). Promoting positive youth development through school-based social and emotional learning interventions: A meta-analysis of follow-up effects. *Child Development, 88*(4), 1156-1171. https://doi.org/10.1111/cdev.12864

U.S. Department of Agriculture, Economic Research Service. (2022, August 3). *National School Lunch Program.* www.ers.usda.gov/topics/food-nutrition-assistance/child-nutrition-programs/national-school-lunch-program.aspx

U.S. Department of Agriculture, Food and Nutrition Service. (2022, May). *A guide to smart snacks in school.* https://fns-prod.azureedge.us/sites/default/files/resource-files/smartsnacks.pdf

U.S. Department of Education, U.S. Department of Health and Human Services, U.S. Department of Homeland Security, U.S. Department of Justice, Federal Bureau of Investigation, & Federal Emergency Management Agency. (2013). *Guide for developing high-quality school emergency operations plans.* https://rems.ed.gov/docs/School_Guide_508C.pdf

van Sluijs, E.M.F., Ekelund, U., Crochemore-Silva, I., Guthold, R., Ha, A., Lubans, D., Oyeyemi, A.L., Ding, D., & Katzmarzyk, P.T. (2021). Physical activity behaviours in adolescence: Current evidence and opportunities for intervention. *The Lancet, 398*(10298), 429-442. https://doi.org/10.1016/S0140-6736(21)01259-9

Walsh, M.E., Madaus, G.F., Raczek, A.E., Dearing, E., Foley, C., An, C., Lee-St. John, T.J., & Beaton, A. (2014). A new model for student support in high-poverty urban elementary schools: Effects on elementary and middle school academic outcomes. *American Educational Research Journal, 51*(4), 704-737. https://doi.org/10.3102/0002831214541669

Wang, L.Y., Vernon-Smiley, M., Gapinski, M.A., Desisto, M., Maughan, E., & Sheetz, A. (2014). Cost-benefit study of school nursing services. *JAMA Pediatrics, 168*(7), 642-648. https://doi.org/10.1001/jamapediatrics.2013.5441

Watson, A., Timperio, A., Brown, H., Best, K., & Hesketh, K.D. (2017). Effect of classroom-based physical activity interventions on academic and physical activity outcomes: A systematic review and meta-analysis. *International Journal of Behavioral Nutrition and Physical Activity, 14*(1), Article 114. https://doi.org/10.1186/s12966-017-0569-9

Weingarten, R. (2015). Schools at the center of communities. *American Educator, 39*(3), 14, 1.

Yoder, C.M. (2020). School nurses and student academic outcomes: An integrative review. *Journal of School Nursing, 36*(1), 49-60. https://doi.org/10.1177/1059840518824397

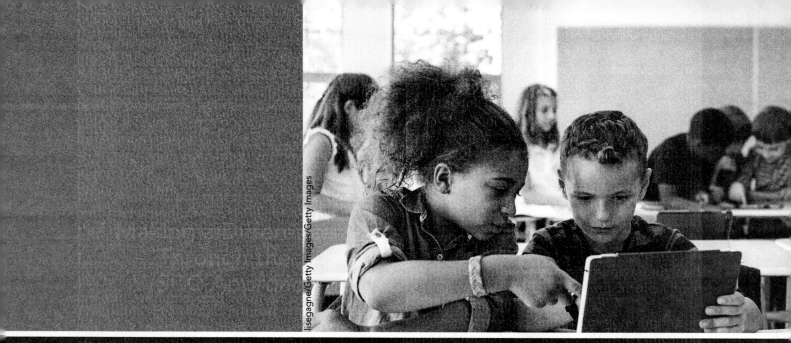

CHAPTER 4

Health and Academic Success

Michele Wallen

LEARNING OBJECTIVES

1. Examine the relationship between students' health and academic success.
2. Describe the relationship between educational attainment and adult health outcomes.
3. Analyze factors that promote and support students' health and academic success.

KEY TERMS

Academic achievement
Adverse childhood experiences
Cognitive skills
Educational attainment
Health
Health-risk behavior

Longitudinal study
Meta-analysis
Randomized controlled trial
School climate
School connectedness

Students' **health** and their **academic achievement** are inextricably linked. Learning can be impeded by hunger, illness, and emotional and physical trauma (Michael et al., 2015). Statistical analyses reflect a negative association between high school students' **health-risk behaviors** and their academic performance (Rasberry et al., 2017). Students who engage in health-risk behaviors are more likely to have lower grades than those who do not.

Improvement in even one risk factor may help improve academic performance, which is significant, because **educational attainment** is a strong predictor of health and health outcomes (Birch, 2023; Lawrence et al., 2016; Raghupathi & Raghupathi, 2020; Roy et al., 2020). Education affects a variety of skills that are associated with employment and health later in life. Education has the potential to enhance individuals' literacy skills, problem-solving ability, self-control, self-efficacy, and self-directedness. These skills assist individuals in navigating health care decisions, adhering to treatment protocols, and accessing health care services when needed (Azkan et al., 2022; Hickey et al., 2018; Lee et al., 2020). As educational attainment increases, students further develop and practice **cognitive skills** and traits that offer economic and health advantages (Zimmerman & Woolf, 2014). Enhanced cognitive skills can lead to more competitive employment opportunities and a higher socioeconomic status with access to health-promoting resources and preventive care. Educational attainment is also associated with improved social support. Social networks can provide financial, psychological, and emotional support and are associated with positive health behaviors and outcomes (Hunter et al., 2019).

Empirical studies that have used data from nationally representative samples have reported education-related disparities in life expectancy from 1980 to 2010 and increases in these disparities through the 2000s and 2010s (Crimmins & Saito, 2001; Meara et al., 2008; Olshansky et al., 2012; Roy et al., 2020). In the United States, adults who do not complete high school face the greatest social, economic, and health challenges. People who do not graduate from high school are more likely than college graduates to be in poor or fair health. The age-adjusted mortality rate for high school dropouts (ages 25-64) is twice that for adults who have some college education. One in four households headed by people without a high school education face food insecurity. People who do not finish high school are more likely to experience acute and chronic illnesses and conditions, such as heart disease, hypertension, stroke, high cholesterol, emphysema, diabetes, asthma attacks, and ulcers. This is compounded by the fact that people with less than a high school education experience substantial barriers to health care and are nearly three times as likely as college graduates to be uninsured. College graduates live on average five years longer than people who do not complete high school (Arendt, 2005; United Health Foundation, 2022).

Health is an essential component of educational attainment, and education is a significant contributing factor to limiting premature morbidity and mortality (Roy et al., 2020). Therefore, educators and public health professionals benefit from working together to implement the Whole School, Whole Community, Whole Child (WSCC) approach and improve integration and collaboration between the health and education sectors. This chapter explores the relationship between health and academic achievement in schools and examines strategies for advancing these important outcomes.

Health-Risk Behaviors

The Centers for Disease Control and Prevention (CDC) oversees the collection of data from middle and high school students every other year through the Youth Risk Behavior Survey. This surveillance effort allows researchers to follow trends and identify relationships associated with adolescent health-risk behaviors. One relationship important to educators and health professionals is the link between academic achievement and engagement in health-risk behaviors. Researchers investigating the correlation between health and academics use measures such as grade point averages (GPAs) and standardized test scores to quantify academic performance. Students who follow public health recommendations for lifestyle choices achieve higher GPAs (Hershner, 2020; Raley et al., 2016; Reuter & Forster, 2021; Wald et al., 2014). Evidence suggests that optimal nutrition, physical activity, and sleep are important for academic achievement (Burrows et al., 2017; Fedewa & Ahn, 2011; Hershner, 2020; Schmidt & Van der Linden, 2015).

Longitudinal studies have concluded that less engagement in health-risk behaviors among youth ages 10 to 18 corresponds with higher academic achievement during high school, higher education attainment, and engagement in fewer health-risk behaviors in adulthood (Bradley & Greene, 2013). After researchers control for sex, race, ethnicity, and grade level, data for high school students from the 2019 Youth Risk Behavior Survey suggest a negative association between health-risk behaviors and academic achievement. Additional analysis of academic grades and positive health behaviors, individually and collectively among U.S. high school students, suggests that higher academic grades are associated with more positive individual and cumulative health behaviors (Hawkins et al., 2022). As reflected in table 4.1, students with higher grades are less likely than students

TABLE 4.1 Percentage of High School Students Who Engaged in Health-Risk Behaviors by Type of Grades Earned—United States, Youth Risk Behavior Survey, 2019

Health-risk behavior	A's	B's	C's	D's or F's
ALCOHOL USE				
Drank alcohol before age 13	12	15	19	26
Currently drink alcohol	27	30	33	40
Currently binge drink	13	13	15	23
TOBACCO PRODUCT USE				
Currently use an electronic cigarette or other electronic vapor product	26	34	41	52
Currently smoke cigarettes	4	5	8	19
Currently smoke cigars	4	5	8	16
Currently use smokeless tobacco	2	3	5	12
DIETARY BEHAVIORS				
Ate breakfast on all 7 days	42	31	23	20
Ate fruit or drank 100% fruit juice one or more times per day	62	58	56	54
Ate vegetables one or more times per day	66	58	53	52
Drank one or more glasses of milk per day	30	28	27	26
Did not drink a can, bottle, or glass of soda or pop	41	28	22	21
PHYSICAL ACTIVITY AND SEDENTARY BEHAVIORS				
Was physically active at least 60 minutes per day on all 7 days	24	25	21	20
Played on at least one sports team	66	57	41	42
Attended physical education classes on all 5 days	26	26	27	23
Watched television for 3 hours or more per day	15	21	24	28
Played video or computer games or used a computer for 3 hours or more per day	41	47	54	54
OTHER HEALTH BEHAVIORS				
Got 8 hours or more of sleep	25	21	18	14
Never saw a dentist	1	2	2	5
Been told by a doctor or nurse that they have asthma	22	21	23	25

Adapted from Centers for Disease Control and Prevention (2020).

with lower grades to use alcohol and tobacco products. Health-promoting behaviors are positive predictors of GPA (Hershner, 2020; Wald et al., 2014). Compared to students with lower grades, students with higher grades are more likely to engage in healthy dietary behaviors and physical activity and less likely to engage in sedentary behaviors. Students with higher grades are less likely than their peers with lower grades to experience certain health conditions and are more likely to receive preventive care.

As research continues to demonstrate the connections between education and health, it is essential to prioritize WSCC policies and practices and to prioritize programs that address the root causes of health and educational inequities so children can reach their academic potential and limit their risk for poor health outcomes (CDC, 2020).

Health and Education in Early Childhood

High-quality early childhood education can increase parental involvement, lead to the identification of learning delays in children and the use of relevant resources, contribute to improved education outcomes, increase future earning potential, and lead to healthier and longer lives. Researchers investigated the relationship between child health and academic achievement during the formative years by using a large database of former Head Start children. Child health status was found to be an independent risk factor for lower academic achievement. Longitudinal analyses showed that poor general health status in kindergarten independently predicted lower reading and math scores in third grade (Spernak et al., 2006). National early childhood education programs such as Head Start emphasize both the health and educational needs of children and demonstrate benefits in language and literacy development, social-emotional skills, and parent–child closeness (Puma et al., 2012). More recent studies have found that participating in Head Start and other model programs reduces depression and disability rates in adolescence and early adulthood. In **randomized controlled trials**, both model early childhood and model prekindergarten programs have benefits for health and health behaviors in adolescence and adulthood, specifically reduced smoking and improved cardiovascular and metabolic health (Morrissey, 2019). Health and educational priorities do not recede after kindergarten for children and should therefore be a central focus of policymakers and educators. Resources and priority should be given to both educational and health outcomes in all grades because students' engagement in health-risk behaviors increases with age (CDC, 2020).

The National Education Goals Panel, a bipartisan intergovernmental body of federal and state officials, was created to assess and report progress toward national education goals. The panel identified five distinct yet connected domains of school readiness that serve as developmental building blocks within the Head Start child development and early learning framework:

- Language and literacy
- Approaches to learning
- Cognitive and general knowledge
- Physical development and health
- Social and emotional development

Note that two of the five domains of early learning, physical development and health and social and emotional learning, can be specifically addressed with the WSCC approach. Given the critical role that health and physical development play in early learning and school readiness, it is understandable that longitudinal studies have found that children who experience poor health at a young age have lower academic achievement while in school, attain lower levels of post-secondary educational attainment, and experience lower social status and poorer health as adults (Arpin et al., 2023; Case et al., 2005).

Adverse Childhood Experiences

Barriers to advanced educational attainment need to be identified and addressed early in schools to improve economic and health outcomes later in life. An increasing body of literature suggests that chronic exposure to stressors and trauma in childhood from birth to age 17, described as **adverse childhood experiences**, can affect brain development and is linked to chronic health problems, mental illness, substance use problems in adolescence and adulthood, and poor performance in school. Adverse childhood experiences can include exposure to violence, abuse, neglect, or household conditions such as substance use problems, mental health issues, and instability due to parental separation (Larson et al., 2017; Merrick et al., 2019). Preventing adverse childhood experiences by using the best available evidence to create safe, stable, nurturing relationships and environments in early childhood programs could potentially prevent chronic conditions, mental health problems, and health-risk behaviors later in life. Investing in high-quality early childhood education programs, in particular those with health components, may provide lasting health benefits (Morrissey, 2019). Several states have regulations that require screening for adverse childhood experiences. The WSCC approach to mental, physical, and social health provides a framework to guide schools in addressing trauma through services, trainings, policies, and practices that support the whole child. Schools can use the WSCC approach to integrate support services and instructional practices that create safe and welcoming spaces for all students in which their basic needs are met. Recognizing that action steps must be customized for schools and communities, Temkin et al. (2020) recommended inviting stakeholder groups to review current legislation, policies, funding streams, organizational capacities, data collection, and reporting practices to identify gaps in integration, support, and processes. Addressing these gaps will help school communities create healthier learning environments. It is important that these stakeholder groups represent a cross-section of school community members and reflect the demographic diversity of the region. Intentional efforts should be made to include underrepresented and marginalized communities. Policies should leverage the direct support of state education and health agencies to include technical assistance and guidance for local school districts, reduce barriers to accessing health and safety resources, and clarify how state and federal funding streams can be used to support coordinated health services through schools and communities. As state policymakers acknowledge that adverse childhood experiences and trauma negatively affect teaching and learning, schools and communities should be funded and incentivized to integrate trauma-informed approaches and training into their programs and practices (Temkin et al., 2020).

Chronic Absenteeism

Having two or more adverse childhood experiences, especially neighborhood violence or family substance abuse, is associated with chronic absenteeism (Stempel et al., 2017). "Chronic absenteeism" refers to missing too much school; it is commonly defined as missing 10 percent or more of school days in a school year for any reason. It can begin as early as preschool or kindergarten. Chronic absenteeism puts children at risk for poor school performance and school dropout, which puts them at risk for unhealthy behaviors as adolescents and young adults, which in turn can result in poor long-term health outcomes (Allison et al., 2019). Absenteeism due to physical health conditions can be exacerbated by the presence of mental or behavioral health conditions (Stempel et al., 2017). Declining health throughout childhood due to either the accumulation of health problems or the progression of a chronic condition has a detrimental impact on academic achievement (Jackson, 2015). Students with treatable conditions miss a combined 14 million days of school each year in the United States (Robert Wood Johnson Foundation, 2016). Food insecurity, unstable housing or transportation, bullying, fear of violence, and other social factors cause students to be chronically absent from school (Robert Wood Johnson Foundation, 2016). Other physical and behavioral factors associated with absenteeism include cyberbullying risk behaviors and the **school climate**. Students who are chronically absent between grades 8 and 12 are seven times more likely than students who are not chronically absent to drop out of school (Robert Wood Johnson

WSCC IN PRACTICE
The Education Attainment–Adult Health Connection

Education is the single most modifiable social determinant of health.
Anthony Iton, Senior Vice President for Healthy
Communities, California Endowment (McGill, 2016)

Education and health represent a reciprocal relationship. Health affects education, and education affects health. Students dealing with physical, emotional, social, or family health issues often face challenges in being successful academically. Thus, health is an education issue. High school graduates who move on to attain higher levels of postsecondary education are more likely to have better adult health outcomes, including longer life, a higher quality of life, and lower levels of chronic disease than those without higher levels of education. Thus, education is a health issue. It is important to note that the WSCC model can have a positive impact on both education and health.

National attention has been focused on the impact of education attainment on adult health outcomes. One example of this attention is a one-day workshop held by the National Academies of Sciences, Engineering, and Medicine's Roundtable on Population Health Improvement. The workshop titled "School Success: An Opportunity for Population Health" held in Oakland, California, on June 14, 2018, was designed to explore how health sector capabilities can assist and support schools to improve educational outcomes from prekindergarten through grade 12. The proceedings of the workshop were published in a report, *School Success: An Opportunity for Population Health* (National Academies of Sciences, Engineering, and Medicine, 2020). The workshop proceedings include the following chapters:

- The Relationship Between Education and Health
- Exploring the Role of the Health Sector in Supporting Educational Success and Improving Outcomes
- Case Examples of Health–Education Collaboration to Improve Specific Educational Outcomes
- Exploring Policy Issues and Opportunities
- Reflections on the Day (pp. xi-xii)

Based on the workshop presentations and discussion, participants identified the following perspectives:

- "Educational outcomes are health outcomes. . . . Mutual and shared outcomes are essential to the health–education partnership" (pp. 67-68).
- "School health initiatives are not about 'fixing' the child," but instead the goal should be meeting the needs of children and families (p. 67).
- "There is synergy of interventions" that help children succeed in schools. "For example, breakfast in school meets a child's need for nourishment, but it also makes the child feel connected and cared for, which might help that child perform better and stay in school" (p. 67).
- Health professionals need to understand and "speak the language of educators" (p. 67). This understanding of language is important in promoting interdisciplinary collaboration.
- The presentation of data should accompany stories and stories should accompany the presentation of data (p. 68).
- The WSCC model should be embraced by both professions as an approach for meeting the needs of the whole child (p. 68).

The workshop proceedings provide important background information on the education attainment–health relationship. The document provides an open-access resource that can serve as an important tool for professional practice, interdisciplinary collaboration, and advocacy related to WSCC planning and implementation.

Foundation, 2016). Because of the linkage between health and academic success and educational attainment, reducing school absenteeism should be a priority for both public health and education professionals. Interventions to reduce school absences can mitigate lifelong negative academic, social, and health outcomes associated with missing school (Allen et al., 2018). The WSCC approach provides a framework for integrating services and resources to efficiently provide prevention and care strategies and effectively address the complex and interrelated causes of absenteeism. Examples of school and community interventions to reduce school absences and improve academic success include access to medical care, center-based preschool programs, collaboration between schools and medical professionals, parental education campaigns, school-based mental health programs, school-based support for vulnerable and at-risk populations, and school nurse interventions (Allen et al., 2018). These strategies and other interventions grounded in the WSCC model are discussed in detail in the next section.

Making a Difference Through the WSCC Approach

The public health and education professions can work together to implement effective and efficient school health programs and policies to improve students' cognitive, physical, social, and emotional development. Through the coordination and planning of policies, programs, and services, schools can reduce violence and aggression, address mental health problems, provide health services, promote family and community involvement and parental engagement, provide a healthy breakfast and offer other balanced nutritional services, and provide quality physical education and additional opportunities for physical activity. All these efforts are addressed in following subsections. Focused efforts to promote WSCC provide students with a healthy, safe, engaging, supportive, and challenging environment and improve school connectedness.

Create School Connectedness

Studies show that students who experience positive school connectedness are less likely to experience mental health problems, less likely to engage in health-risk behaviors, and more likely to have positive education outcomes (Forrest et al., 2013; Raniti et al., 2022; Wilkins et al., 2023). **School connectedness** emerges when students feel as though they are a part of the school and perceive an attachment between themselves and the adults and other students at school. Connectedness occurs when students feel as though adults care about their success in learning and their well-being as people. Increased school connectedness is related to educational motivation, classroom engagement, and better attendance. School connectedness is also related to lower rates of poor mental health, marijuana use, prescription opioid use, unprotected sex, sexual intercourse, experiencing forced sex, and missing school because of feeling unsafe (Wilkins et al., 2023). Family and school connectedness may have lasting protective effects that continue through adulthood across multiple health outcomes related to mental health, violence, sexual behavior, and substance use (see figure 4.1). Schools have the potential to promote overall health in adulthood by improving family and school connectedness during adolescence (Steiner et al., 2019).

Research reviews and discussions among an interdisciplinary group of leaders in education distilled the following key factors related to school connectedness:

- Student success can be improved through strengthened bonds with the school, increasing connectedness.
- Students must experience high expectations for academic success and feel supported by staff.
- Students need to feel as though they belong to a positive peer group.
- Students need to feel safe and supported in a positive school environment (Blum & Libbey, 2004; Wilkins et al., 2023; Wingspread, 2004).

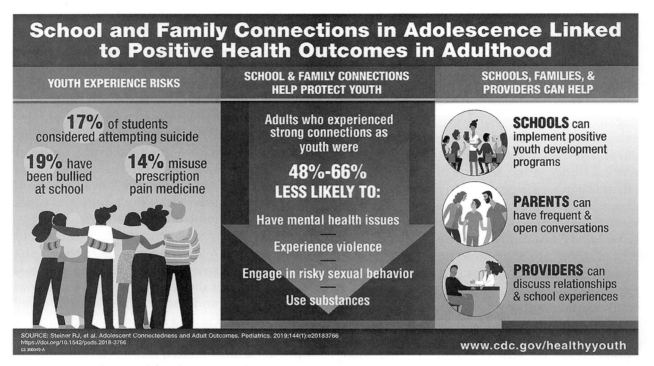

FIGURE 4.1 School and family connectedness provides immediate and long-term benefits to individuals, schools, and communities.
Reprinted from Centers for Disease Control and Prevention (2023).

The WSCC approach, which involves families, schools, and communities and emphasizes the need for a healthy social and emotional school climate, can help build school connectedness. Regular communication and collaboration between school staff members, school counselors, school social workers, and school psychologists allow professionals to provide varying levels of assistance and care to students. By coordinating existing resources and services, school staff can effectively and efficiently meet the needs of students without working outside their areas of expertise and while avoiding the duplication of services (ASCD & CDC, 2014).

The CDC (2022b) outlined the following science-based strategies for building school connectedness:

1. Promote the use of effective classroom management strategies that foster a positive learning environment.
2. Build strong, supportive, trusting relationships with students.
3. Maintain high expectations for students.
4. Create opportunities for students to collaborate with and actively engage with their peers.
5. Provide clear and consistent expectations for behavior in the classroom, and take actions to promote positive, prosocial behaviors.
6. Use instructional approaches that monitor the needs of students and explicitly focus on increasing students' interest and engagement.
7. Provide professional development and support for teachers and other school staff to enable them to meet the diverse cognitive, emotional, and social needs of their students.

Safe classrooms and a positive school climate can also contribute to school connectedness. An assessment of school climate and school connectedness should be part of a school's accountability measures. A poor school climate can dramatically affect connectedness and engagement levels and lead to absenteeism, dropping out, and subsequently poor educational and health outcomes. Examples of specific strategies for developing a safe school climate include engaging in planned supervision, especially during noninstructional periods (e.g., during class changes, before and after school, during lunch periods); making intentional efforts to greet each student by name; and using physical education classes to develop collaboration skills and promote fair play and conflict resolution (CDC, 2023b).

School health educators also have a role in helping students develop connectedness and creating a safe learning environment. The National Health Education Standards serve as a framework for curriculum, instruction, and assessment in health education. Reviews of effective health education curricula indicate that students should be given the opportunity to practice and refine key skills reflected in the standards, such as interpersonal communication skills, refusal skills, and decision-making and conflict resolution skills, in a safe environment while receiving constructive feedback for improvement (National Consensus for School Health Education, 2022). These skills are critical for building effective relationships, creating a safe social and emotional climate, and developing school connectedness (Li et al., 2022).

Enhancing School Climate and Culture and Promoting Emotional and Mental Health

A study of key stakeholders focused on identifying policy opportunities to promote the WSCC framework. Stakeholder groups identified emotional and mental health and school climate and culture as high-priority areas (Solomon et al., 2018). Teachers of all disciplines must make efforts to monitor student behavior in classrooms, in hallways, and on school grounds to correct inappropriate actions that could be perceived as hurtful or disrespectful by others. School staff must actively create a culture of intolerance for violence by addressing all acts of bullying and by enforcing all policies promptly, fairly, and consistently (Brewer et al., 2018). These policies should also establish a climate of high academic standards and zero tolerance for weapons, hate-related words or symbols, and name-calling (CDC, 2022b). Teachers, staff, and administrators should receive professional development in the social, mental, and emotional health of youth (Brewer et al., 2018). Bullying, violence, and aggression in schools threaten students' academic performance, engagement, and sense of connectedness (Johansson et al., 2022). Cyberbullying often occurs outside school hours, which makes it difficult to address within schools; however, the victimization that occurs has implications for students' sense of safety, mental and emotional health, attendance, and academic performance and for the campus culture as well (Grinshteyn & Yang, 2017). Therefore, the health education curriculum should also include activities that define cyberbullying as well as the social, emotional, and legal ramifications that cyberbullies and their victims face. Administrators, faculty, and staff—specifically school counselors, social workers, and school psychologists—must work together to identify, intervene in, and prevent violent and aggressive behaviors among students. A comprehensive health education program that helps students build effective skills in the areas of collaboration, negotiation, conflict resolution, respect for others' consent or nonconsent, empathy, compassion, listening, decision-making, self-management, and goal setting is a logical setting for creating a culture of intolerance for violence in the school and community. Building these health assets may buffer adolescents from the negative effects on academic performance that are often linked to the social and emotional challenges associated with puberty and transitions from elementary to middle school and from middle to high school (Forrest et al., 2013).

Professional preparation programs for educators and administrators can benefit students by emphasizing the relationship between school climate, student health, and academic achievement. These three factors are intricately linked and key to success in schools. Educators can better serve students when they know how to build relationships with students, can demonstrate a level of cultural competency in their thoughts and actions, and know how to use support services to help students who are facing challenges and crises. Academic and safety concerns support the need for focused mental health resources in schools. In one study, Lipson and Eisenberg (2018) identified depression among college students, independent of other factors, as a significant predictor of academic dissatisfaction and dropout intentions; in contrast, positive mental health served as a significant predictor of satisfaction and persistence. Another study measuring the effect of poor health on academic achievement found that depression could lead to a 0.45 decrease in GPA (Ding et al., 2009). Depression is also associated with an increased probability of dropping out of school. Depression and anxiety are the two most common mental health conditions among adolescents. The co-occurrence of these health problems serves as a significant predictor of a lower GPA (Kilgore et al., 2023). Abundant evidence supports the need for early identification and appropriate intervention for students' health, future academic performance, and educational attainment. Coordinated assistance from guidance counselors, school psychologists, social workers, parents, faculty, and administrators can drastically alter the personal, academic, and economic trajectories of a student with a mental health disorder.

Provide Health Services and School-Based Health Centers

The health problems experienced by adolescents can be complex and may require the services of multiple health providers for prevention, intervention, and crisis services. The WSCC approach promotes coordination of the provision of health services through schools. In some schools, these services are provided through a school-based health center (SBHC). In other schools, students' health care is the primary responsibility of the school nurse. The American Academy of Pediatrics and the National Association of School Nurses recommend a minimum of a full-time registered nurse for every school to help keep students safe and healthy (Maughn et al., 2018). In schools with SBHCs, school nurses act in partnership with SBHC staff members in leadership and care coordination to protect and advance the health of students (National Association of School Nurses & School-Based Health Alliance, n.d.).

SBHCs are intended to create access to a variety of services, especially for children and adolescents in underserved communities. SBHCs typically provide a combination of medical and preventive care and mental health services to students at school. These services are provided without consideration for a student's financial circumstances. Previous studies have documented the cost-effectiveness of SBHCs, which includes reducing emergency room visits, improving health outcomes, and increasing school attendance and graduation rates (Allison et al., 2007; Wade & Guo, 2010; Westbrook et al., 2020). When students can seek medical treatment or preventive services without having to leave campus, the positive effect for students and schools can be observed through improvements not only in the health and well-being of students but also in attendance rates and GPA over time (Lintz et al., 2019; Walker et al., 2010). SBHCs can help to reduce the unmet mental health needs of adolescents, which can have compounding effects on academic achievement and educational attainment (Larson et al., 2017). The prevalence of major depressive episodes in youth is estimated to be 17 percent, and it is estimated that less than half of these adolescents receive treatment (National Institute of Mental Health, 2022). For those who receive treatment, follow-up care for mental health services is critical and is linked to reduced suicidal ideation and suicide attempts; reduced substance abuse; reduced emergency department use; and better identification and treatment of behavioral, mental, and physical health issues. Students who access mental health services at SBHCs return for follow-up visits at higher rates than students who only see primary care providers (Stempel et al., 2019). A systematic review found that SBHCs improve educational and health-related outcomes among disadvantaged students and can be effective at advancing health equity (Knopf et al., 2016).

School nursing is a specialized nursing practice that not only protects and promotes student health but also eliminates or reduces barriers to learning (National Association of

School Nurses, 2017). School nurses serve as coordinators of a school's health services, and their responsibilities can include leadership in the development of policies, programs, and procedures at the school and district level; the development, implementation, and evaluation of students' individualized health care plans; communication in regard to students' health issues and needs with teachers, administrators, parents, and, in some cases, the community; case management for students' health care in the context of the school, family, and medical home; the establishment of relationships and referral procedures with the medical partners and social agencies; elicitation of program support; and the development of school safety emergency management plans (McClanahan & Weismuller, 2015; National Association of School Nurses, 2016). Beyond coordination, specific school services provided in schools can include primary health care, including emergency care for illness or injury; referral to specialized medical care; daily care of students with chronic conditions, such as asthma and diabetes; preventive care, such as flu shots and hearing and vision screening; and health education for students and parents (CDC, 2022b).

Financial support is critical to the provision of school health services. Policymakers have acknowledged the positive return on educational attainment gained by investing in school health services. The Every Student Succeeds Act authorizes the use of funds to support school nursing services for Title I schools (i.e., schools in which 40 percent of children come from lower socioeconomic households; Blackborow et al., 2017). Multiple funding sources should be explored to support and provide health care services in schools, including partnerships with local health care systems or hospitals, public health departments, and community-based agencies.

Promote Family and Parental Engagement

Family engagement is a critical element of the WSCC approach. Schools cannot effectively address the learning, emotional, social, and developmental needs of students without communication and collaboration with the families of the students they serve. Studies have shown a positive relationship between parental engagement in a child's education and academic achievement. Students with engaged parents are more likely than students whose parents are not engaged to earn higher grades and have higher test scores, attend school regularly, and demonstrate positive social skills and behaviors (Al-Alwan, 2014; El Nokali et al., 2010). The greater the degree of involvement by parents in all types of learning and at all levels, the greater the academic gains and benefits (Boonk et al., 2018; Dotterer & Wehrspann, 2015). The WSCC approach promotes early family engagement in the education process. The early involvement of parents and active involvement by parents (e.g., working with children at home on school assignments and projects, volunteering in the classroom and school building, communicating with teachers and school staff about learning progress) significantly increase students' academic gains (El Nokali et al., 2010). Programs can effectively connect with families and communities when they welcome parental involvement, listen to and address parent and community concerns, and develop trusting relationships (Al-Alwan, 2014; El Nokali et al., 2010). The WSCC approach fosters respecting the needs of the family, which is of great value when connecting with parents. Examples of recognizing the needs of families include providing child care during meetings and events at school, identifying alternative locations and times for meetings with parents outside the school building, sending educational kits and resources home with students, creating discussion groups with other families, and encouraging family members to send a representative for the family to meetings or trainings when necessary.

Provide Both a Healthy Breakfast and Balanced Nutritional Services

Schools and families often need to work together to provide students with one of life's most basic needs: healthy food options. The nutrition environment and services component of the WSCC approach describes the critical intersection of schools, families, and communities working together to address the nutritional needs of students, which can improve their physical, cognitive, social, and emotional well-being. Research has shed light on the educational challenges associated with skipping breakfast. Eating breakfast enhances cognitive performance, especially on complex tasks that require extensive processing and visual learning (Peña-Jorquera et al., 2021). A systematic review found that tasks that require attention, executive function, and memory are executed more reliably when breakfast is consumed (Adolphus et al., 2016). Inadequate or no breakfast consumption is associated with depression, lower happiness, posttraumatic stress disorder, loneliness, and sleep problems (Pengpid & Peltzer, 2020). Some studies suggest that eating breakfast at school results in less student tardiness, decreased absences, improved attention and behavior, and increased math grades and test scores (Bartfeld et al., 2019; Murphy, 2007). Children and adolescents skip breakfast more than they do any other meal (Sincovich et al., 2022). When students are hungry or have not eaten a nutritious meal, they may have trouble concentrating and experience short-term memory lapses. Schools should try to serve breakfast to all students each day. Creative programs such as breakfast bags at the school entrance, breakfast carts to serve students in classrooms, and breakfast periods in the school day help students access the nutrients they need to focus, process, and retain new learning each day (GENYOUth Foundation, 2020).

Although breakfast is not the only nutritional factor that affects cognitive performance and health, it is one that is frequently monitored and measured in the literature because of its importance to educational attainment and its availability at school sites. Associations between unhealthy eating patterns and unfavorable school performance in children are well documented (Chan et al., 2017). Poor overall school performance is positively associated with unhealthy eating patterns, which include low consumption of nutrient-dense foods and dairy products and high consumption of nonnutritive sources of food (Burrows et al., 2017). Given that students eat two of the three traditional meals at school, school nutrition services can partner with school health specialists to create nutrition education programs that teach students to plan a balanced approach to meal selection that meets dietary recommendations without ignoring their personal taste preferences. Schools can empower students in their meal selections by providing for a student voice in the meal planning and food options with comment cards and advisory committee meetings.

Besides considering student interests and cultural influences, school districts should comply with federal standards for school breakfast, lunch, and competitive food sales. Using locally grown and raised foods can promote sustainability and lower costs for schools. School and community gardens offer opportunities for parental and community involvement, nutrition education, analyses of the scientific origins and processing of foods, and healthy taste testing for students and families. The Community Eligibility Provision is a federal provision available for school districts that serve areas with high poverty rates. This program allows schools to offer breakfast and lunch at no cost to students regardless of income, which has resulted in higher student participation rates in these meals. Schools can also offer summer meal programs to make food available and accessible for children and families during the summer months (GENYOUth Foundation, 2020).

Provide Quality Physical Education and Physical Activity

Schools can provide a healthy and inviting environment for food choices and physical activity. Physical activity in public schools has declined since the 1980s. Administrators and school officials are keenly aware of the importance of using instructional time wisely to increase students' academic proficiency. Some school administrators fear that dedicating time to nontested disciplines such as physical education may take time away from tested subject areas and subsequently lower standardized test scores used for assessment and accountability purposes. Yet research suggests a positive correlation between the amount of time spent being physically active during school and on weekends and higher standardized test scores in reading, math, and spelling. Time dedicated to physical activity during instructional hours did not negatively affect students' test scores (Donnelly et al., 2009, 2016). Studies continually show that more participation in physical education is associated with better grades, higher standardized test scores, and more positive classroom behavior. Time spent in recess is positively associated with cognitive performance and positive classroom behaviors (Michael et al., 2015). Educators should recognize the benefits of physical activity and feel confident that providing opportunities such as recess to students on a regular basis can benefit academic behaviors and at the same time facilitate fundamental social skills (Stapp & Karr, 2018).

Even short bouts of physical activity can have positive effects. Researchers have studied the association between physical activity and academic achievement over several decades, and reviews using **meta-analysis** techniques found a significant positive association between students' cognitive functioning and physical activity (Álvarez-Bueno et al., 2017; Michael et al., 2015). Improved cognition among students has been attributed to physical activity during the school day, and research shows that teachers observe additional positive effects on focus and memory (Hillman et al., 2009). Unexpected improvements in attention to task and task performance in preadolescent children have been documented following brief bouts of exercise in school (Hillman et al., 2009; Mahar, 2011). Classroom teachers can collaborate with physical education teachers to plan integrated lessons and units, structured recess, and options for physical activity before, during, and after school. Donnelly et al. (2017) studied the effect of classroom activities that integrate movement and physical activity with academic lessons. These lessons did not require extensive teacher preparation, were enjoyable for teachers and students, and resulted in improved academic scores. Figure 4.2 includes tips for using classroom activity breaks to provide short bouts of physical activity throughout the school day.

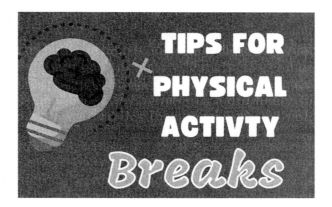

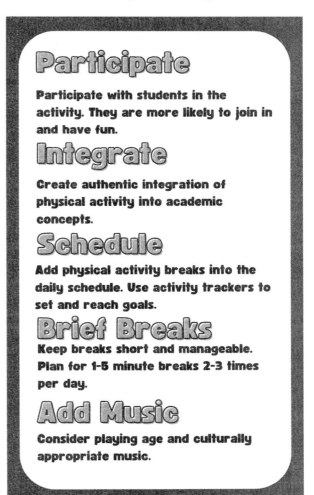

FIGURE 4.2 Tips for physical activity breaks.

Schools can promote learning and help students develop skills and behaviors that have a lasting effect. Because children and youth spend the majority of their time in school, schools can have a positive impact on the foods they eat and the quality and quantity of physical activity they engage in. The WSCC approach can contribute to increased physical activity and healthy diets for students that are positively associated with children's weight, health outcomes, and academic and behavioral problems at school (Shi et al., 2013). Figure 4.3 highlights improvements in academic performance as a result of eating healthy and getting physical activity as recommended by the CDC. More information can be found at www.cdc.gov and https://genyouthnow.org.

HEALTHY EATING AND PHYSICAL ACTIVITY YIELD IMPROVED ACADEMIC PERFORMANCE

Students who regularly eat breakfast
- earn better grades and have higher standardized test scores,
- miss fewer days of school, and
- demonstrate better concentration and memory.

Students who skip breakfast
- exhibit poor memory and inattentiveness and
- miss more school than students who usually eat breakfast.

Students who are physically active (e.g., during physical education, recess, or classroom activities)
- experience improved academic performance, concentration, and attention;
- have fewer disciplinary problems; and
- are less likely to drop out of school.

FIGURE 4.3 The effects of healthy eating and physical activity on students and learning.

Summary

A common mission among schools is to prepare students to be successful and productive citizens in the world in which they live. An evolving body of literature supporting the academic benefits of health promotion can be used to encourage the coordination of school health programs through WSCC. With careful attention to school climate and strategies to create connectedness for students and their families, schools can improve educational attainment for their students. Administrators and policymakers must focus on health and education outcomes through all grade levels beginning in early childhood. Schools can provide mental, emotional, and physical health education and services; daily opportunities for a balanced and accessible breakfast and nutritious food choices; and dedicated time for physical education and planned integration of physical activity into the school day. Coordinating these programs and services can benefit students' academic performance, attention to task, cognition, and educational and economic outcomes. By coordinating efforts to promote the health and well-being of students, schools and communities are investing in a better future for all.

LEARNING AIDS

GLOSSARY

academic achievement—Often considered the outcome of an educational endeavor (the end of a kindergarten through grade 12 education). The extent to which students, teachers, or institutions have achieved their education goals. Academic achievement is commonly measured by examinations or continuous assessment.

adverse childhood experiences—Chronic exposure to stressors and trauma in childhood from birth to age 17, including violence, abuse, neglect, or conditions in the home such as substance use problems among family members, mental health issues, and instability due to parental separation. These experiences can affect brain development and are linked to chronic health problems, mental illness, substance use problems in adolescence and adulthood, and poor performance in school.

cognitive skills—Skills individuals use to learn. Examples of these skills include remembering, understanding, applying, analyzing, evaluating, and creating.

educational attainment—The highest level of education attained by an individual, such as a high school degree, bachelor's degree, master's degree, or doctoral degree.

health—The World Health Organization defines health as a state of complete physical, mental, and social well-being, not merely the absence of disease or infirmity. Another definition is physical, mental, and social wellness or a state of well-being.

health-risk behaviors—Actions taken by an individual that increase the likelihood of diminished health status or safety. The CDC has identified six categories of priority health-risk behaviors for youth in the United States: behaviors that contribute to unintentional injuries and violence; tobacco use; alcohol and other drug use; sexual behaviors that contribute to unintended pregnancy and sexually transmitted diseases, including HIV infection; unhealthy eating; and physical inactivity.

longitudinal study—A study in which the behaviors or outcomes of individuals or groups are monitored or tracked on a continual basis over a period of time.

meta-analysis—A systematic statistical procedure in which data from multiple studies are combined and analyzed to synthesize and summarize research findings.

randomized controlled trial—A study that measures the impact of a program or treatment. In a randomized controlled trial, one group of participants receives the program or treatment, and another group does not. The results can be compared between the two groups.

school climate—The educational and social atmosphere of a school. The quality of life experienced in the school by students and school staff.

school connectedness—Students' belief that adults and peers in their school care about their learning as well as about them as individuals; the comfort and satisfaction students feel related to their school experience.

APPLICATION ACTIVITIES

1. You are responsible for developing a presentation to the local school board on improving academic performance. The board has invited education professionals from various disciplines to address this topic. Your 20-minute presentation should focus on the relationship between students' health and their academic success. You should also include in your presentation the role that WSCC can play as a method for promoting academic success. Develop a detailed outline for your presentation.

2. Select one of the following influences on students' health and academic success: early childhood education, adverse childhood experiences, school connectedness, or school climate. Find five sources related to the influence you choose as well as to health and academic success. These sources can be articles in professional journals, organization websites, blogs, documentaries, interviews with professionals who work in the area you selected, or other resources you identify. For each of your five sources, write a two- or three-paragraph summary of the important information. In addition, write a two- or three-paragraph reaction to the totality of the readings. Be prepared to present an informal 5-minute summary of your paper.

3. Either through individual discussions or in several small-group discussions, ask other students to describe a time when their physical, mental, or emotional health affected their academic performance or the academic performance of a friend or family member. As part of the discussion, ask them to provide recommendations for how schools can help promote health and academic success. Write a paper that includes a summary of selected issues described in the discussion, the students' recommendations, and your overall reaction to your findings.

REFERENCES

Adolphus, K., Lawton, C.L., Champ, C.L., & Dye, L. (2016). The effects of breakfast and breakfast consumption on cognition in children and adolescents: A systematic review. *Advances in Nutrition, 7*(3), 590S-612S. https://doi.org/10.3945/an.115.010256

Al-Alwan, A.F. (2014). Modeling the relations among parental involvement, school engagement and academic performance of high school students. *International Education Studies, 7*(4), 47-56. https://doi.org/10.5539/ies.v7n4p47

Allen, C.W., Diamon-Myrsten, S., & Rollins, L. (2018). School absenteeism in children and adolescents. *American Family Physician, 98*(12), 738-744.

Allison, M.A., Attisha, E., & Council on School Health. (2019). The link between school attendance and good health. *Pediatrics, 143*(2), e20183648. https://doi.org/10.1542/peds.2018-3648

Allison, M.A., Crane, L.A., Beaty, B.L., Davidson, A.J., Melinkovich, P., & Kempe, A. (2007). School-based health centers: Improving access and quality of care for low-income adolescents. *Pediatrics, 120*(4), e887-e894. https://doi.org/10.1542/peds.2006-2314

Álvarez-Bueno, C., Pesce, C., Cavero-Redondo, I., Sánchez-López, M., Garrido-Miguel, M., & Martínez-Vizcaíno, V. (2017). Academic achievement and physical activity: A meta-analysis. *Pediatrics, 140*(6), e20171498. https://doi.org/10.1542/peds.2017-1498

Arendt, J.N. (2005). Does education cause better health? A panel data analysis using school reforms for identification. *Economics of Education Review, 24*(2), 149-160.

Arpin, E., de Oliveira, C., Siddiqi, A., & Laporte, A. (2023). Beyond the mean: Distributional differences in earnings and mental health in young adulthood by childhood health histories. *SSM—Population Health, 23*, Article 101451. https://doi.org/10.1016/j.ssmph.2023.101451

ASCD & Centers for Disease Control and Prevention. (2014). *Whole School, Whole Community, Whole Child: A collaborative approach to learning and health.* The ASCD Whole Child Initiative.

Azkan, T.D., Bhattacharya, S., Demirci, H., & Yildiz, T. (2022). Health literacy and health outcomes in chronic obstructive pulmonary disease patients: An explorative study. *Frontiers in Public Health, 10.* https://doi.org/10.3389/fpubh.2022.846768

Bartfeld, J.S., Berger, L., Men, F., & Chen, Y. (2019). Access to the school breakfast program is associated with higher attendance and test scores among elementary school students. *Journal of Nutrition, 149*(2), 336-343. https://doi.org/10.1093/jn/nxy267

Birch, D.A. (2023). *Leveraging the education-health connection*. Johns Hopkins University Press.

Blackborow, M., Clark, E., Combe, L., Morgitan, J., & Tupe, A. (2017). There's a new alphabet in town: ESSA and its implications for students, schools, and school nurses. *NASN School Nurse, 33*(2). https://doi.org/10.1177/1942602X17747207

Blum, R., & Libbey, H.P. (2004). Executive summary: Healthier students are better learners. *Journal of School Health, 74*(7), 231-232.

Boonk, L., Gijselears, H.J.M., Ritzen, H., & Brand-Gruwel, S. (2018). A review of the relationship between parental involvement indicators and academic achievement. *Educational Research Review, 24*(1), 10-30.

Bradley, B.J., & Greene, A.C. (2013). Do health and education agencies in the United States share responsibility for academic achievement and health? A review of 25 years of evidence about the relationship of adolescents' academic achievement and health behaviors. *Journal of Adolescent Health, 52*(5), 523-532. https://doi.org/10.1016/j.jadohealth.2013.01.008

Brewer, S.L., Jr., Brewer, H.J., & Kulik, K.S. (2018). Bullying victimization in schools: Why the Whole School, Whole Community, Whole Child model is essential. *Journal of School Health, 88*(11), 794-802. https://doi.org/10.1111/josh.12686

Burrows, T., Goldman, S., Pursey, K., & Lim, R. (2017). Is there an association between dietary intake and academic achievement: A systematic review. *Journal of Human Nutrition and Dietetics, 30*(2), 117-140. https://doi.org/10.1111/jhn.12407

Case, A., Fertig, A., & Paxson, C. (2005). The lasting impact of childhood health and circumstance. *Journal of Health Economics, 24*(2), 365-389. https://doi.org/10.1016/j.jhealeco.2004.09.008

Centers for Disease Control and Prevention. (2020). Youth risk behavior surveillance—United States, 2019. *MMWR Supplement, 69*(1), 1-88. www.cdc.gov/healthyyouth/data/yrbs/pdf/2019/su6901-H.pdf

Centers for Disease Control and Prevention. (2022a). *Making the connection: Research on health and academics. Youth Risk Behavior Survey data*. Retrieved December 26, 2022, from www.cdc.gov/healthyschools/health_and_academics/index.htm

Centers for Disease Control and Prevention. (2022b). *What can schools do? School connectedness*. www.cdc.gov/healthyyouth/protective/school-connectedness/connectedness_schools.htm

Centers for Disease Control and Prevention. (2023a). *Infographics*. www.cdc.gov/healthyyouth/multimedia/infographics_posters/infographics.htm

Centers for Disease Control and Prevention. (2023b). *What works in schools: Health services*. https://www.cdc.gov/healthyyouth/whatworks/what-works-health-services.htm

Chan, H.S.K., Knight, C., & Nicholson, M. (2017). Association between dietary intake and "school-valued" outcomes: A scoping review. *Health Education Research, 32*(1), 48-57. https://doi.org/10.1093/her/cyw057

Crimmins, E.M., & Saito, Y. (2001). Trends in healthy life expectancy in the United States, 1970-1990: Gender, racial, and educational differences. *Social Science & Medicine, 52*(11), 1629-1641. https://doi.org/10.1016/s0277-9536(00)00273-2

Ding, W., Lehrer, S. F., Rosenquist, J. N., & Audrain-McGovern, J. (2009). The impact of poor health on academic performance: New evidence using genetic markers. *Journal of Health Economics, 28*(3), 578–597. https://doi.org/10.1016/j.jhealeco.2008.11.006

Donnelly, J.E., Greene, J.L., Gibson, C.A., Smith, B.K., Washburn, R.A., Sullivan, D.K., DuBose, K., Mayo, M.S., Schmelzle, K.H., Ryan, J.J., Jacobsen, D.J., & Williams, S.L. (2009). Physical Activity Across the Curriculum (PAAC): A randomized controlled trial to promote physical activity and diminish overweight and obesity in elementary school children. *Preventive Medicine, 49*(4), 336-341. https://doi.org/10.1016/j.ypmed.2009.07.022

Donnelly, J.E., Hillman, C.H., Castelli, D., Etnier, J.L., Lee, S., Tomporowski, P., Lambourne, K., & Szabo-Reed, A.N. (2016). Physical activity, fitness, cognitive function, and academic achievement in children: A systematic review. *Medicine and Science in Sports and Exercise, 48*(6), 1197-1222. https://doi.org/10.1249/MSS.0000000000000901

Donnelly, J.E., Hillman, C.H., Greene, J.L., Hansen, D.M., Gibson, C.A., Sullivan, D.K., Poggio, J., Mayo, M.S., Lambourne, K., Szabo-Reed, A.N., Herrmann, S.D., Honas, J.J., Scudder, M.R., Betts, J.L., Henley, K., Hunt, S.L., & Washburn, R.A. (2017). Physical activity and academic achievement across the curriculum: Results from a 3-year cluster-randomized trial. *Preventive Medicine, 99*, 140-145. https://doi.org/10.1016/j.ypmed.2017.02.006

Dotterer, A.M., & Wehrspann, E. (2015). Parent involvement and academic outcomes among urban adolescents: Examining the role of school engagement. *Educational Psychology, 36*(4), 812-830. https://doi.org/10.1080/01443410.2015.1099617

El Nokali, N.E., Bachman, H.J., & Votruba-Drzal, E. (2010). Parent involvement and children's academic and social development in elementary school. *Child Development, 81*(3), 988-1005. https://doi.org/10.1111/j.1467-8624.2010.01447.x

Fedewa, A.L., & Ahn, S. (2011). The effects of physical activity and physical fitness on children's achievement and cognitive outcomes: A meta-analysis. *Research Quarterly for Exercise and Sport, 82*(3), 521-535. https://doi.org/10.1080/02701367.2011.10599785

Forrest, C.B., Bevans, K.B., Riley, A.W., Crespo, R., & Louis, T.A. (2013). Health and school outcomes during children's transition into adolescence. *Journal of Adolescent Health, 52*(2), 186-194. https://doi.org/10.1016/j.jadohealth.2012.06.019

GENYOUth Foundation. (2020). *Healthier school communities: What's at stake now and what we can do about it.* Retrieved December 27, 2022, from https://genyouthnow.org/reports/healthier-school-communities-what-is-at-stake-now/

Grinshteyn, E., & Yang, Y.T. (2017). The association between electronic bullying and school absenteeism among high school students in the United States. *Journal of School Health, 87*(2), 142-149. https://doi.org/10.1111/josh.12476https://doi.org/10.1177/0020731415585986

Hawkins, G.T., Lee, S.H., Michael, S.L., Merlo, C.L., Lee, S.M., King, B.A., Rasberry, C.N., & Underwood, J.M. (2022). Individual and collective positive health behaviors and academic achievement among U.S. high school students, Youth Risk Behavior Survey 2017. *American Journal of Health Promotion, 36*(4), 651-661. https://doi.org/10.1177/08901171211064496

Hershner, S. (2020). Sleep and academic performance: Measuring the impact of sleep. *Current Opinion in Behavioral Sciences, 33,* 51-56.

Hickey, K., Masternon Creber, R., Reading, M., Sciacca, R., Riga, R., Frulla, A., & Casida, J. (2018). Low health literacy: Implications for managing cardia patients in practice. *Nurse Practitioner, 43*(8), 49-55. https://doi.org/10.1097/01.NPR.0000541468.54290.49

Hillman, C.H., Pontifex, M.B., Raine, L.B., Castelli, D.M., Hall, E.E., & Kramer, A.F. (2009). The effect of acute treadmill walking on cognitive control and academic achievement in preadolescent children. *Neuroscience, 159*(3), 1044-1054. https://doi.org/10.1016/j.neuroscience.2009.01.057

Hunter, R.F., de la Haye, K., Murray, J.M., Badham, J., Valente, T.W., Clarke, M., & Kee, F. (2019). Social network interventions for health behaviours and outcomes: A systematic review and meta-analysis. *PLOS Medicine, 16*(9), e1002890. https://doi.org/10.1371/journal.pmed.1002890

Jackson, M.I. (2015). Cumulative inequality in child health and academic achievement. *Journal of Health and Social Behavior, 56*(2), 262-280. https://doi.org/10.1177/0022146515581857

Johansson, S., Myrberg, E., & Toropova, A. (2022). School bullying: Prevalence and variation in and between school systems in TIMSS 2015. *Studies in Educational Evaluation, 74,* Article 101178. https://doi.org/10.1016/j.stueduc.2022.101178

Kilgore, J., Collins, A.C., Miller, J., & Winer, E.S. (2023). Does grit protect against the adverse effects of depression on academic achievement? *PLOS ONE, 18*(7), e0288270. https://doi.org/10.1371/journal.pone.0288270

Knopf, J.A., Finnie, R.K., Peng, Y., Hahn, R.A., Truman, B.I., Vernon-Smiley, M., Johnson, V.C., Johnson, R.L., Fielding, J.E., Muntaner, C., Hunt, P.C., Phyllis Jones, C., Fullilove, M.T., & Community Preventive Services Task Force. (2016). School-based health centers to advance health equity: A community guide systematic review. *American Journal of Preventive Medicine, 51*(1), 114-126. https://doi.org/10.1016/j.amepre.2016.01.009

Larson, S., Chapman, S., Spetz, J., & Brindis, C.D. (2017). Chronic childhood trauma, mental health, academic achievement, and school-based health center mental health services. *Journal of School Health, 87*(9), 675-686. https://doi.org/10.1111/josh.12541

Lawrence, E., Rogers, R., & Zajacova, A. (2016). Educational attainment and mortality in the United States: Effects of degrees, years of schooling, and certification. *Population Research and Policy Review, 35*(4), 501-525. https://doi.org/10.1007/s11113-016-9394-0

Lee, Y.L., Zhou, A.Q., Lee, R.M., & Dillon, A.L. (2020). Parents' functional health literacy is associated with children's health outcomes: Implications for health practice, policy, and research. *Children and Youth Services Review, 110,* Article 104801. https://doi.org/10.1016/j.childyouth.2020.104801

Li, J., Timpe, Z., Suarez, N.A., Phillips, E., Kaczkowski, W., Cooper, A.C., Dittus, P.J., Robin, L., Barrios, L.C., & Ethier, K.A. (2022). Dosage in implementation of an effective school-based health program impacts youth health risk behaviors and experiences. *Journal of Adolescent Health, 71*(3), 334-343. https://doi.org/10.1016/j.jadohealth.2022.04.009

Lintz, M.J., Sutton, B., & Thurstone, C. (2019). Associations between school-based substance use treatment and academic outcomes. *Journal of Child and Adolescent Psychopharmacology, 29*(7), 554-558. https://doi.org/10.1089/cap.2018.0178

Lipson, S.K., & Eisenberg, D. (2018). Mental health and academic attitudes and expectations in university populations: Results from the Healthy Minds Study. *Journal of Mental Health, 27*(3), 205-213. https://doi.org/10.1080/09638237.2017.1417567

Mahar, M.T. (2011). Impact of short bouts of physical activity on attention-to-task in elementary school children. *Preventive Medicine, 52*(1), S60-S64. https://doi.org/10.1016/j.ypmed.2011.01.026

Maughn, E.D., Cowell, J., Engelke, M.K., McCarthy, A.M., Bergren, M.D., Murphy, M.K., Barry, C., Krause-Parello, C.A., Luthy, K.B., Kintner, E.K., & Vessey, J.A. (2018). The vital role of school nurses in ensuring the health of our nation's youth. *Nursing Outlook, 66*(1), 94-96. https://doi.org/10.1016/j.outlook.2017.11.002

McClanahan, R., & Weismuller, P.C. (2015). School nurses and care coordination for children with complex needs: An integrative review. *Journal of School Nursing, 31,* 34-43. https://doi.org/10.1177/1059840514550484

McGill, N. (2016, August 1). Education attainment linked to health throughout lifespan: Exploring social determinants of health. *The Nation's Health, 46* (6), 1-19. https://www.thenationshealth.org/content/46/6/1.3

Meara, E.R., Richards, S., & Cutler, D.M. (2008). The gap gets bigger: Changes in mortality and life expectancy, by education, 1981-2000. *Health Affairs, 27*(2), 350-360. https://doi.org/10.1377/hlthaff.27.2.350

Merrick, M.T., Ford, D.C., Ports, K.A., Guinn, A.S., Chen, J., Klevens, J., Metzler, M., Jones, C.M., Simon, T.R., Daniel, V.M., Ottley, P., & Mercy, J.A. (2019). Vital signs: Estimated proportion of adult health problems attributable to adverse childhood experiences and implications for prevention—25 states, 2015-2017. *Morbidity and Mortality Weekly Report, 68*(44), 999-1005. https://doi.org/10.15585/mmwr.mm6844e1

Michael, S.L., Merlo, C.L., Basch, C.E., Wentzel, K.R., & Wechsler, H. (2015). Critical connections: Health and academics. *Journal of School Health, 85*(11), 740-758. https://doi.org/10.1111/josh.12309

Morrissey, T. (2019, April 25). *The effects of early care and education on children's health* (Health Affairs Healthy Policy Brief). https://doi.org/10.1377/hpb20190325.519221

Murphy, J.M. (2007). Breakfast and learning: An updated review. *Current Nutrition & Food Science, 3*, 3-36. https://doi.org/10.2174/1573401310703010003

National Academies of Sciences, Engineering, and Medicine. (2020). *School Success: An Opportunity for Population Health: Proceedings of a Workshop*. Washington, DC: The National Academies Press. https://doi.org/10.17226/25403

National Association of School Nurses. (2016). The role of the 21st century school nurse. *NASN School Nurse, 32*(1), 56-58.

National Association of School Nurses. (2017). *Definition of school nursing*. www.nasn.org/about-nasn/about

National Association of School Nurses & School-Based Health Alliance. (n.d.). *School nursing and school-based health centers in the United States: Working together for student success*. www.sbh4all.org/wp-content/uploads/2021/05/SBHA_JOINT_STATEMENT_FINAL_F.pdf

National Consensus for School Health Education. (2022). *National Health Education Standards: Model guidance for curriculum and instruction: 3rd edition*. www.schoolhealtheducation.org/

National Institute of Mental Health. (2022, January). *Major depression*. www.nimh.nih.gov/health/statistics/major-depression

Olshansky, S.J., Antonucci, T., Berkman, L., Binstock, R.H., Boersch-Supan, A., Cacioppo, J.T., Carnes, B.A., Carstensen, L.L., Fried, L.P., Goldman, D.P., Jackson, J., Kohli, M., Rother, J., Zheng, Y., & Rowe, J. (2012). Differences in life expectancy due to race and educational differences are widening, and many may not catch up. *Health Affairs, 31*(8), 1803-1813. https://doi.org/10.1377/hlthaff.2011.0746

Peña-Jorquera, H., Campos-Núñez, V., Sadarangani, K.P., Ferrari, G., Jorquera-Aguilera, C., & Cristi-Montero, C. (2021). Breakfast: A crucial meal for adolescents' cognitive performance according to their nutritional status. The Cogni-Action Project. *Nutrients, 13*(4), 1320. https://doi.org/10.3390/nu13041320

Pengpid, S., & Peltzer, K. (2020). Skipping breakfast and its association with health risk behaviour and mental health among university students in 28 countries. *Diabetes Metabolic Syndrome Obesity, 13*, 2889-2897. https://doi.org/10.2147/DMSO.S241670

Puma, M., Bell, S., Cook, R., Heid, C., Broene, P., Jenkins, F., Mashburn, A., & Downer, J. (2012). *Third grade follow-up to the Head Start Impact Study final report* (OPRE Report No. 2012-45). Office of Planning, Research and Evaluation, Administration for Children and Families, U.S. Department of Health and Human Services. www.acf.hhs.gov/sites/default/files/documents/opre/head_start_report_0.pdf

Raghupathi, V., & Raghupathi, W. (2020). The influence of education on health: An empirical assessment of OECD countries for the period 1995-2015. *Archives of Public Health, 78*(20), 1-18. https://doi.org/10.1186/s13690-020-00402-5

Raley, H.R., Naber, J.L., Cross, S., & Perlow, M.B. (2016). The impact of duration of sleep on academic performance in university students. *Madridge Journal of Nursing, 1*(1), 11-18. https://doi.org/10.18689/mjn-1000103

Raniti, M., Rakesh, D., Patton, G.C., & Sawyer, S.M. (2022). The role of school connectedness in the prevention of youth depression and anxiety: A systematic review with youth consultation. *BMC Public Health, 22*, Article 2152. https://doi.org/10.1186/s12889-022-14364-6

Rasberry, C.N., Tiu, G.F., Kann, L., McManus, T., Michael, S.L., Merlo, C.L., Lee, S.M., Bohm, M.K., Annor, F., & Ethier, K.A. (2017). Health-related behaviors and academic achievement among high school students—United States, 2015. *Morbidity and Mortality Weekly Report, 66*(35), 921-927. https://doi.org/10.15585/mmwr.mm6635a1

Reuter, P.R., & Forster, B.L. (2021). Student health behavior and academic performance. *PeerJ, 9*, e11107. https://doi.org/10.7717/peerj.11107

Robert Wood Johnson Foundation. (2016). *The relationship between school attendance and health*. Retrieved December 26, 2022, from www.rwjf.org/en/library/research/2016/09/the-relationship-between-school-attendance-and-health.html

Roy, B., Kiefe, C.I., Jacobs, D.R., Goff, D.C., Lloyd-Jones, D., Shikany, J.M., Reis, J.P., Gordon-Larsen, P., & Lewis, C.E. (2020). Education, race/ethnicity, and causes of premature mortality among middle-aged adults in 4 US urban communities: Results from CARDIA, 1985-2017. *American Journal of Public Health, 110*(4), 530-536. https://doi.org/10.2105/AJPH.2019.305506

Schmidt, R.E., & Van der Linden, M. (2015). The relations between sleep, personality, behavioral problems, and school performance in adolescents. *Sleep Medicine Clinics, 10*(2), 117-123. https://doi.org/10.1016/j.jsmc.2015.02.007

Shi, X., Tubb, L., Fingers, S.T., Chen, S., & Caffrey, J.L. (2013). Associations of physical activity and dietary behaviors with children's health and academic problems. *Journal of School Health*, *83*(1), 1-7. https://doi.org/10.1111/j.1746-1561.2012.00740.x

Sincovich, A., Moller, H., Smithers, L., Brushe, M., Lassi, Z.S., Brinkman, S.A., & Gregory, T. (2022). Prevalence of breakfast skipping among children and adolescents: A cross-sectional population level study. *BMC Pediatrics*, *22*, Article 220. https://doi.org/10.1186/s12887-022-03284-4

Solomon, B., Katz, E., Steed, H., & Temkin, D. (2018). Creating policies to support healthy schools: Policymaker, educator, and student perspectives. *Child Trends*. Retrieved December 26, 2022, from www.childtrends.org/wp-content/uploads/2018/10/healthyschool-stakeholderreport_ChildTrends_October2018.pdf.

Spernak, S.M., Schottenbauer, M.A., Ramey, S.L., & Ramey, C.T. (2006). Child health and academic achievement among former Head Start children. *Children and Youth Services Review*, *28*(10), 1251-1261. https://doi.org/10.1016/j.childyouth.2006.01.006

Stapp, A.C., & Karr, J.K. (2018). Effect of recess on fifth grade students' time on-task in an elementary classroom. *International Electronic Journal of Elementary Education*, *10*(4), 449-456. https://doi.org/10.26822/iejee.2018438135

Steiner, R.J., Sheremenko, G., Lesesne, C., Dittus, P.J., Sieving, R.E., & Ethier, K.A. (2019). Adolescent connectedness and adult health outcomes. *Pediatrics*, *144*(1), e20183766. https://doi.org/10.1542/peds.2018-3766

Stempel, H., Cox-Martin, M., Bronsert, M., Dickinson, L.M., & Allison, M.A. (2017). Chronic school absenteeism and the role of adverse childhood experiences. *Academic Pediatrics*, *17*(8), 837-843. https://doi.org/10.1016/j.acap.2017.09.013

Stempel, H., Cox-Martin, M.G., O'Leary, S., Stein, R., & Allison, M.A. (2019). Students seeking mental health services at school-based health centers: Characteristics and utilization patterns. *Journal of School Health*, *89*, 839-846. https://doi.org/10.1111/josh.12823

Temkin, D., Harper, K., Stratford, B., Sacks, V., Rodriguez, Y., & Bartlett, J.D. (2020). Moving policy toward a Whole School, Whole Community, Whole Child approach to support children who have experienced trauma. *Journal of School Health*, *90*, 940-947. https://doi.org/10.1111/josh.12957

United Health Foundation. (2022). *2021 health disparities report*. Retrieved December 26, 2022, from www.americashealthrankings.org/learn/reports/2021-disparities-report

Wade, T.J., & Guo, J.J. (2010). Linking improvements in health-related quality of life to reductions in Medicaid costs among students who use school-based health centers. *American Journal of Public Health*, *100*(9), 1611-1616. https://doi.org/10.2105/AJPH.2009.185355

Wald, A., Muennig, P.A., O'Connell, K.A., & Garber, C.E. (2014). Associations between healthy lifestyle behaviors and academic performance in U.S. undergraduates: A secondary analysis of the American College Health Association's National College Health Assessment II. *American Journal of Health Promotion*, *28*(5), 298-305. https://doi.org/10.4278/ajhp.120518-QUAN-265

Walker, S.C., Kerns, S.E., Lyon, A.R., Bruns, E.J., & Cosgrove, T.J. (2010). Impact of school-based health center use on academic outcomes. *Journal of Adolescent Health*, *46*(3), 251-257. https://doi.org/10.1016/j.jadohealth.2009.07.002

Westbrook, M., Martinez, L., Mechergui, S., & Yeatman, S. (2020). The influence of school-based health center access on high school graduation: Evidence from Colorado. *Journal of Adolescent Health*, *67*(3), 447-449. https://doi.org/10.1016/j.jadohealth.2020.04.012

Wilkins, N., Krause, K., Verlenden, J., Szucs, L.E., Ussery, E.N., Allen, C.T., Stinson, J., Michael, S.L., & Ethier, K.A. (2023). School connectedness and risk behaviors and experiences among high school students—Youth Risk Behavior Survey, United States, 2021. *MMWR Supplement*, *72*(1), 13-21. https://doi.org/10.15585/mmwr.su7201a2

Wingspread Declaration on School Connections. (2004). *Journal of School Health*, *74*(7), 233-234. https://doi.org/10.1111/j.1746-1561.2004.tb08279.x

Zimmerman, E., & Woolf, S.H. (2014). *Understanding the relationship between education and health* (NAM Perspectives Discussion Paper). National Academy of Medicine. https://doi.org/10.31478/201406a

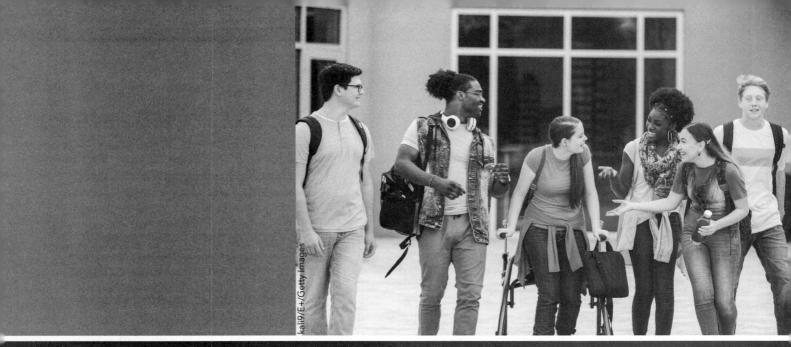

CHAPTER 5

Meeting the Needs of Diverse Students, Families, and Communities

Angelia M. Sanders

LEARNING OBJECTIVES

1. Analyze the diverse nature of students and communities.
2. Describe the rationale for addressing diversity, equity, and inclusion through the Whole School, Whole Community, Whole Child model.
3. Analyze considerations related to social justice–oriented schools.
4. Describe strategies that can be used to address diversity, equity, and inclusion in schools.

KEY TERMS

Anti-racist teaching
Critical race theory (CRT)
Cultural humility
Culturally responsive teaching
Diversity
Diversity, equity, and inclusion (DEI)

Equity
Inclusion
Intersectionality
Social justice
Social justice–oriented school

This chapter examines the interdependence of **diversity, equity, and inclusion (DEI)** and the Whole School, Whole Community, Whole Child (WSCC) model. Selected student groups who are disproportionately affected by poor education outcomes and poor health and well-being are examined. Among these groups are children living in poverty, experiencing homelessness or housing instability, and living with disabilities. The groups also include children who are dealing with adverse social conditions associated with their race, ethnicity, gender identity, or sexual orientation as well as students from families of immigrant status. Promoting DEI in schools is an important strategy for supporting these students. Position statements addressing DEI from organizations representing WSCC components are presented in the chapter. Specific strategies used to promote DEI are also presented, including programs, policies, and actions that lead to the development of **social justice–oriented schools**, **cultural humility**, family involvement, and community engagement. DEI commitment requires concerted efforts from schools to build genuine, effective partnerships with students, families, and communities to close academic achievement gaps and provide much-needed health services (Corsino & Fuller, 2021).

Students With Disproportionately Poor Education Outcomes

Being aware of diverse student groups, including their challenges and needs, is critical for meeting the needs of these students and implementing DEI strategies. Regardless of students' willingness and ability to learn, various interconnecting factors can affect their education outcomes (e.g., health and social determinants such as family, curriculum, school policies, communities, governance structure). Factors related to students' health, such as sensory perceptions, cognition, school connectedness, absenteeism, and dropping out or no longer enrolling in school, have been linked to educational achievement (Gardiner, 2020; Michael et al., 2015; National Academies of Sciences, Engineering, and Medicine, 2020). Education and health are associated with social determinants as well, which highlights the interrelated nature of children's health, their environment, and their education outcomes (Chang, 2019; Heard-Garris et al., 2021). The complex nature of this interconnection underscores the need to address academic, social, emotional, and physical health issues among students. The WSCC model can be used as a framework for this approach (Centers for Disease Control and Prevention [CDC], 2018; Michael et al., 2015). Although such comprehensive efforts benefit all students, special consideration is needed for students with disproportionately poor education outcomes (including higher dropout rates, lower graduation rates, poorer performance on standardized tests, and disproportionately more suspensions and expulsions). Students disproportionately affected by poor education and health outcomes include, among others, children living in poverty; students of color (e.g., Black or African American, Hispanic or Latino, Native American or Alaska Native children); children who are lesbian, gay, bisexual, transgender, queer, or questioning (LGBTQ+); students experiencing homelessness or housing instability; and children with disabilities (Chang, 2019; Heard-Garris et al., 2021; Parrott et al., 2022).

The overall public school population in the United States continues to change demographically. Approximately 16.5 percent of the U.S. population (about 55 million individuals) are children enrolled in prekindergarten through grade 12 (preK-12) in public and private schools (National Center for Education Statistics [NCES], 2022b). This population has experienced varying degrees of change since 2009. The greatest of these changes is that the percentage of Hispanic/Latino students enrolled in public school increased from 22 percent in 2009 to 28 percent in 2022 (NCES, 2022b). In contrast, the percentages of White (54 to 46 percent) and Black (17 to 15 percent) students decreased over those same years. The percentages of Asian students and of children of multiple races or ethnicities remained relatively stable, at approximately 5 percent each. In addition, the percentages of American Indian/Alaska Native and Native Hawaiian or other Pacific Islander enrollees remained steady at approximately 1 percent and less than 1 percent, respectively. Collectively, these figures indicate that although White students represent the largest group of public school enrollees, a little more than half of all students (about 54 percent) are from other racial or ethnic groups (NCES, 2022b).

Children Living in Poverty

Poverty is pervasive and affects all student population groups. The overall poverty rate in the United States for children younger than 18 years old was 16 percent in 2020 (NCES, 2022a). It was highest among American Indian/Alaska Native (28 percent), Black (28 percent), and Hispanic/Latino (23 percent) children. The poverty rate was about 16 percent, similar to the national rate, among Native Hawaiian or other Pacific Islander children and children of multiple races or ethnicities. The lowest poverty rates were among White (10 percent) and Asian (7 percent) children. The poverty rate for children was highest among those living in female parent–only households (35 percent), followed by those living in male parent–only households (17 percent). Children of immigrant families—especially children of color, specifically American Indian/Alaska Native, Black, and Hispanic/Latino children—have a high likelihood of living below the poverty line (NCES, 2022a). These student groups are also likely to experience economic and racial discrimination (Francis et al., 2018). Schools that promote DEI can influence the impact of these experiences.

Children living in poverty are disproportionately affected by physical and mental health issues (Francis et al., 2018). The impact of poverty on child health and well-being is extensive. Poverty has been associated with chronic disease, poor nutrition, environmental exposure (e.g., exposure to secondhand smoke or air pollutants), and other poor health conditions (Council on Community Pediatrics, 2016; Francis et al., 2018). Children living in poverty are more likely than children who are not impoverished to experience various hardships due to their poverty, including but not limited to racial and ethnic discrimination, homelessness or housing instability, substance use in the family, and violence (Francis et al., 2018). The chronic stress of living in impoverished conditions can be detrimental to children's health over the long term (Francis et al., 2018), which has implications for their learning and education outcomes (Council on Community Pediatrics, 2016).

Children of Color

Racial and ethnic minoritized students with disproportionately poor education outcomes (i.e., Black, Hispanic or Latino, Native American or Alaska Native students) experience various academic and health challenges. Despite decades of intervention, disparities continue to persist in health and health care among these student populations compared to their White and Asian counterparts (Gardiner, 2020; Office of Disease Prevention and Health Promotion, 2020). Such disparities may affect how they rate their quality of life. Wallander et al. (2019) found substantial disparities in health-related quality of life reported by racially and ethnically diverse youth in California, Alabama, and Texas; outcomes were particularly poor for Black and Hispanic youth. Many racial and ethnic minority children experience social and economic challenges such as language barriers, discrimination, and poverty (Ayalew et al., 2021; U.S. Department of Education, 2015). Collectively, these conditions have implications for students' academic achievement.

WSCC IN PRACTICE

Innovative Pilot Project Helps Reduce Chlamydia Rates Among Youth in Rural Florida County

The purpose of this project was to reduce sexual risk behaviors and lower rates of sexually transmitted disease (STD) among adolescents in Madison County, Florida. Using a WSCC approach, the University of South Florida, Florida Department of Education, and HIV/AIDS Prevention Education Program developed a project to address this problem with the support of the CDC's Division of Adolescent and School Health. Baseline data from the Youth Risk Behavior Surveillance System (YRBSS) survey showed that more than two-thirds of students in 12th grade in Madison County reported having had sexual intercourse at least once and that the county had the second highest rate of chlamydia in the state among youth ages 15 to 19 years old.

Several strategies that promote DEI were incorporated into the overall project. First, although the project would help address STD among all students, it was conducted in a medically disadvantaged setting (rural Madison County) among students who were mostly Black and disproportionately affected by higher rates of STD. Second, a strong community participatory approach was used that integrated the voice and leadership of the community into the development and implementation of the project. In addition to the Madison County School District and Madison County Health Department, several other groups representative of the community as members of the Healthy Start Coalition of Jefferson, Madison, and Taylor Counties were key partners. Third, cultural competence strategies were enacted through the use of age-appropriate sexual health education curricula and materials, which were also used in school and various community settings (e.g., a Boys and Girls Club, churches, a community center).

Overall project activities included using Positive Action curriculum kits in schools to promote a healthy school climate; providing funding and staff to implement Making Proud Choices, an evidence-based comprehensive sexual health education curriculum; training health department and coalition staff members on the Birds and the Bees curriculum so they could teach parents how to educate their children and become advocates for sexual and reproductive health education; and training a leadership task force to expand HIV and STD prevention education to parents and youth in community settings.

The findings of the STD pilot project were positive. Although Madison County started with the second highest rate of chlamydia among youth ages 15 to 19 years old, in four years it ranked 40th in the state. Collaboration among the partners was sustained, and numerous community members (youth, parents, community agency staff) were educated on sexual and reproductive health for youth. There are plans to use the project evaluation findings to develop an STD prevention guidance document that could be used across the state (Centers for Disease Control and Prevention, Division of Adolescent and School Health, 2013).

Children Experiencing Homelessness or Housing Instability

Children experiencing homelessness or housing instability are another student population with academic, health, and economic challenges (Parrott et al., 2022). Housing instability includes trouble paying rent, overcrowding, moving frequently, staying with relatives, or spending the bulk of the household income on housing (Frederick et al., 2014; Office of Disease Prevention and Health Promotion, 2020). Homelessness is housing deprivation in its most severe form (Office of Disease Prevention and Health Promotion, 2020). The McKinney-Vento Homeless Assistance Act of 1987 defines a person experiencing homelessness as one who lacks fixed, regular, and adequate nighttime residence. Research indicates that students experiencing homelessness or housing instability have disproportionately poor education outcomes (Parrott et al., 2022). Compared to their non-homeless counterparts, they are more likely to be retained in their grades, are more likely to have lower grades, and perform more poorly on tests (Masten et al., 2015). Furthermore, nearly three-fourths of all homeless students do not graduate from high school (Rahman et al., 2015). In addition, they experience more depression, anxiety, and withdrawal and physical illnesses (e.g., respiratory infections, ear infections, and stomach problems) compared to non-homeless children (Barnes et al., 2021; LoSchiavo et al., 2020; Parrott et al., 2022). Exposure to violence and other safety issues are also major concerns (Barnes et al., 2021). Many homeless youth have experienced abuse, including physical or emotional trauma (American School Counselor Association, 2022a). With approximately 1.5 million children experiencing homelessness or housing instability in the United States, it would be helpful if schools addressed not only their educational needs but also their unique health and social issues (Parrott et al., 2022).

LGBTQ+ Children

Children in the LGBTQ+ community are another group of students with special needs and unique challenges that include being at higher risk for poor academic outcomes and social-emotional well-being (American School Counselor Association, 2022b; Johns et al., 2020). LGBTQ+ students regularly feel unsafe in school because of their sexual orientation, gender identity, or gender expression and commonly experience prejudiced remarks, harassment, bullying, and sometimes attacks (Kosciw et al., 2020). Negative attitudes toward LGBTQ+ students place these children at increased risk for bullying and other forms of violence (Myers et al., 2020). Therefore, schools can be unsafe spaces for children, who may have to focus on safety and survival as priorities as opposed to education (Myers et al., 2020). Research indicates that LGBTQ+ students are at greater risk for depression and suicidal behavior compared to their non-LGBTQ+ counterparts (Johns et al., 2020). Thus, schools must effectively respond to these unique safety, health, and educational needs.

Children of Families With Immigrant Status

Children of families with immigrant status, specifically those who are poor and undocumented or who have family members who are, are another group with special needs. The 1982 U.S. Supreme Court ruling in *Plyler v. Doe* prohibits public schools from denying children with undocumented citizenship a kindergarten through grade 12 (K-12) education under the premise that if they are not supported, they are likely to experience a lifetime of hardship, which could potentially create a permanent underclass (American School Counselor Association, 2022e). Nonetheless, children of families with immigrant status who are poor or undocumented remain largely at risk for poor education and health outcomes (Chang, 2019; U.S. Department of Education, 2015). Many of these students and their families face multiple financial, social, and legal stressors (American School Counselor Association, 2022e; Ayalew et al., 2021; U.S. Department of Education, 2015). Schools implementing DEI strategies, such as cultural humility, community engagement, and a social justice–oriented education within the WSCC framework, provide an opportunity to meet students' needs by focusing on student health, safety, engagement, and support and appropriate levels of academic challenge (CDC, 2018; Michael et al., 2015).

Children With Disabilities

Students with disabilities are another group of students to whom special attention should be granted. These students already experience mental, emotional, or physical health issues that put them at risk for poor education outcomes, and their needs are sometimes insufficiently met in schools (Dembo & LaFleur, 2019; Fujita et al., 2022). Children with disabilities can receive special education services under the Individuals with Disabilities Education Act, which requires that public schools provide all

WSCC IN PRACTICE
Rhode Island Champions Safe Schools Through Anti-Bullying Mandate

The purpose of this project was to address bullying among high school students in Rhode Island by creating safer schools through school policy and legislative changes. Survey data from the YRBSS indicated that approximately one in five students (19.1 percent) reported being bullied at school, and 15 percent reported experiencing cyberbullying. Those who were bullied reported significantly higher health risks (e.g., issues with violence and injury, mental health, alcohol and drug use, sex, weight) than students who did not report being bullied.

Several strategies that promote DEI were incorporated into the overall project. First, although the project would help address bullying among all students, it was tailored specifically to students who were disproportionately affected by it: students from the LGBTQ+ community. The state's YRBSS survey data indicated that students who were bullied were more likely to be female; White; nonminority; or lesbian, gay, or bisexual. Second, a strong community participatory approach was used that integrated the voice and leadership of the priority population. LGBTQ+ students participated in a statewide LGBTQ+ anti-bullying forum during which their stories and bullying experiences were videotaped and shared statewide as part of the effort to increase awareness around bullying and support change. Third, in addition to the Rhode Island Department of Education (RIDE)/RIDE Board of Regents and the Rhode Island Senate Commission on Cyber-bullying, the LGBTQ+ community was directly involved as a key partner via Youth Pride, Inc., whose purpose is to meet the unique needs of youth and young adults affected by sexual orientation and gender identity or expression while also working to end homophobic and transphobic environments.

Overall project activities included conducting a statewide LGBTQ+ anti-bullying forum, providing extensive media coverage of the forum in partnership with a local NBC News affiliate, distributing video copies of voices from the field of LGBTQ+ youth and teachers describing their experiences, revising the Rhode Island school anti-bullying policy to include gender identity and expression and stronger language around antidiscrimination, and developing and passing the Safe Schools Act.

The project efforts generated positive results. Among the outcomes were prohibitions against bullying, cyberbullying, and retaliation; procedures for reporting bullying; procedures for responding to and investigating reports of bullying; and a range of disciplinary actions for bullying. In addition, the project led to the development of the Safe Schools Act that requires that all school districts, charter schools, career and technical schools, and others adopt the statewide anti-bullying policy. Finally, tools and resources have been provided to schools to help implement the state policy and promote anti-bullying within the school community (Centers for Disease Control and Prevention, Division of Adolescent and School Health, 2013).

---

students with a free and appropriate public education in the least restrictive environment (NCES, 2022c). Under this act, 7.2 million public school students are identified as having a disability and receive special education services (NCES, 2022c). The disabilities of these students are grouped into the following categories: specific learning disability (33 percent), speech or language impairment (19 percent), other health impairment (15 percent; e.g., chronic or acute health problems such as asthma, sickle cell anemia, epilepsy), autism (11 percent), developmental delay (7 percent), intellectual disability (6 percent), emotional disturbance (5 percent), multiple disabilities (2 percent), hearing impairment (1 percent), and orthopedic impairment (1 percent; NCES, 2022c). Other conditions, such as visual impairment, traumatic brain injury, and deaf-blindness, account for less than 0.5 percent of students served under the Individuals with Disabilities Education Act (NCES, 2022c). Qualifying students who have physical or mental impairments that substantially limit one or more major life activities are further protected under Section 504 of the Rehabilitation Act of 1973. Depending on the disability, many students experience stigma, discrimination, and bullying (Breau et al., 2018). A commitment to providing assistance and support while addressing both students' strengths and their challenges should be the focus of all schools (American School Counselor Association, 2022d).

PreK-12 public schools, as a whole, are very diverse and include various student groups with disproportionately poor education outcomes and needs. Students' identities can intersect with other factors and contexts (e.g., an LGBTQ+ student with a disability may reside in poverty), which might compound their problems. It is important to be cognizant of these intersections and the consequences they have. DEI efforts might help in addressing some of the educational disparities and social issues that affect students. As discussed previously, the WSCC model provides a framework for addressing these needs (CDC, 2018; Michael et al., 2015). Schools can play a key role in addressing children's health by implementing the WSCC model to positively affect all children, especially those with disproportionately poor health and education outcomes (CDC, 2018; Gardiner, 2020; Michael et al., 2015).

Diversity, Equity, and Inclusion

As indicated earlier, many students are faced with multiple and multilayered challenges that impede academic achievement, including poverty, racism, stigma, disabilities, poor health, and others. As U.S. schools become more racially and ethnically diverse (NCES, 2022b), it is important that school systems are able to adequately serve students without exacerbating existing disparities in education, health, and well-being or contributing to new ones. The incorporation of DEI considerations and actions within school systems and individual schools has the potential to have meaningful and positive impacts on the diverse students whom schools are designed to serve (Corsino & Fuller, 2021; Farmer et al., 2019; Padamsee et al., 2017).

DEI efforts in education involve the development, modification, and use of policies, standards, and practices that promote the representation and participation of members of all segments of the school community, with special focus on underrepresented groups (Thompson & Thompson, 2018). **Diversity** involves the representation of all ages, races, ethnicities, national origins, gender identities, sexual orientations, abilities, cultures, religions, citizenship types, and socioeconomic statuses as they are reflected in the broader community (Thompson & Thompson, 2018). It includes the presence of different types of people representing a range of identities and different perspectives and experiences (Padamsee et al., 2017). **Equity** involves providing voice and equal opportunity without discrimination or bias. It represents attempting to meet needs and challenges faced by all individuals and groups. However, it is important to note that equitable is not always equal. Taking an equitable approach may mean providing some students with more support and resources than others (Lehner, 2017). Equity is intended to ensure equally high outcomes (such as education outcomes), removing the predictability of success or failure that is associated with social and cultural factors (Padamsee et al., 2017). **Inclusion** involves a commitment to serving underrepresented communities and individuals with unique backgrounds, circumstances, needs, and perspectives (Thompson & Thompson, 2018). It involves seeking ways to cultivate a sense of belonging among staff, students, partners, and the communities served by creating an environment of involvement, respect, and connection (Padamsee et al., 2017).

DEI efforts often go beyond providing standard quality education and normal school services. Yet there are many benefits of doing so. DEI efforts focus on creating a positive culture that embraces all, building better support for students, strengthening community, developing opportunities for students to feel free to express themselves without fear of judgment, and providing equitable services and treatment to all (Padamsee et al., 2017). When organizations are diverse, equitable, and inclusive, they tend to have higher levels of satisfaction and engagement, stronger staff retention, higher productivity, and a heightened sense of belonging (U.S. Department of Education, 2022). Learning in multicultural environments provides meaningful opportunities for developing cultural awareness, understanding, empathy, and cross-cultural skills (Byrd, 2016; Chen et al., 2022; Tanase, 2022; Vassallo, 2022; Woodley et al., 2017). Implementing strategies that increase DEI can be beneficial to all.

DEI efforts that value human differences, promote fairness that results in access for all, and create open environments are critical to students' success. Given that racial and ethnic minority students are the numeric majority (approximately 54 percent) in U.S. public schools (NCES, 2022b), it is especially important to consider DEI strategies. Using DEI approaches within a WSCC framework can be effective and lead to improved educational and health outcomes among students (CDC, 2018; Michael et al., 2015).

WSCC IN PRACTICE
Ohio's Our Child, Our Future

The Ohio Department of Education has customized the WSCC model to reflect Ohio's strategic plan for education in an effort called "Our Child, Our Future." Ohio's version of the WSCC model, identified as Ohio's Whole Child Framework, addresses the needs of the whole child that are fundamental to children's intellectual and social development so they can engage fully in learning and in school.

Ohio's version of the infographics in the white band that surrounds the whole child and the Whole Child tenets in the WSCC model includes "coordinate policy, processes and practices" and "practice cultural responsiveness, equity and continuous improvement." The Ohio Department of Education (2020) describes the white band and its contents as follows:

> *Students thrive in schools and districts committed to aligning their work with the needs of the populations they serve through a thoughtful, systemic approach. To best coordinate resources, districts should* coordinate policy, processes and practices, practice cultural responsiveness, *deliberately focus on* equity *and dedicate time and resources to structured* continuous improvement *[emphasis added] (p. 7).*

These practices represent systemic approaches that districts and schools throughout Ohio use to strengthen the Whole Child tenets and support students and families.

To support and address the needs of the whole child, an Ohio Improvement Process is presented to school districts and schools for consideration. The process emphasizes that one size does not fit all and that special consideration should be given to rural and Appalachian communities, students with disabilities, and vulnerable populations (including students involved in the court system, children experiencing homelessness, students in foster care, English learners, and students in military families). It is recommended that to serve vulnerable student populations using a Whole Child approach, districts and schools provide the following (Ohio Department of Education, 2020):

- An established system for regularly identifying vulnerable students
- Ongoing professional development for school personnel around meeting the unique needs and circumstances of individual populations
- Established partnerships with community-based organizations and local service providers to provide wraparound supports
- Opportunities for two-way communication between the school and vulnerable students and families

Position Statements on Diversity, Equity, and Inclusion

Many national organizations support DEI, which are sometimes reflected in their position statements. Because such statements set the tone for action, they can help cultivate inclusive academic environments as well as influence curricula (Walton-Fisette & Sutherland, 2020). Though not an exhaustive list, table 5.1 lists some organizations that provide DEI-related position statements that affect K-12 students. The relationship of each agency or organization is linked to one or more of the

TABLE 5.1 DEI Position Statements

Professional organization or national agency	WSCC component	Year	Statement title or DEI focus
American Academy of Pediatrics (AAP)	Health services	2018	AAP Diversity and Inclusion Statement
American Board of Pediatrics (ABP)	Health services	2020	Diversity, Equity, and Inclusion (DEI)
American Counseling Association (ACA)	Counseling, psychological, and social services	2017	Social Justice and Human Rights Statements • A Basic Human Right: Access to Public Restrooms That Match an Individual's Gender Identity • Liberty and Justice for All • Preventing Discrimination and Harassment
American Psychological Association (APA) APA Task Force on Psychological Practice With Sexual Minority Persons	Counseling, psychological, and social services Social and emotional climate	2021	Guidelines for Psychological Practice With Sexual Minority Persons
American Public Health Association (APHA)	All WSCC components	2016-2022	APHA Policy Statements • Promoting Transgender and Gender Minority Health Through Inclusive Policies and Practices, Policy #20169, 2016 • Public Health and Early Childhood Education: Support for Universal Preschool in the United States, Policy #20173, 2017 • Achieving Health Equity in the United States, Policy #20189, 2018 • Addressing Environmental Justice to Achieve Health Equity, Policy #20197, 2019 • Structural Racism Is a Public Health Crisis: Impact on the Black Community, Policy #LB20-04, 2020 • Sexual and Gender Minority Demographic Data: Inclusion in Medical Records, National Surveys, and Public Health Research, Policy #202111, 2021 • Racism as a Public Health Crisis: A Declaration to Action, 2022

> *continued*

TABLE 5.1 > *continued*

Professional organization or national agency	WSCC component	Year	Statement title or DEI focus
American School Counselor Association (ASCA)	Counseling, psychological, and social services Social and emotional climate	2018-2022	ASCA Position Statements • Children Experiencing Homelessness, 2018 • Equity for All Students, 2018 • Supporting Students in Foster Care, 2018 • Students Experiencing Issues Surrounding Undocumented Status, 2019 • Gender Equity, 2020 • Anti-Racist Practices, 2021 • Cultural Diversity, 2021 • LGBTQ+ Youth, 2022 • School–Family–Community Partnerships, 2022 • Students With Disabilities, 2022 • Transgender and Nonbinary Youth, 2022
American School Health Association (ASHA)	All WSCC components	2016, 2018, 2019	ASHA Position Statements • School Administrators Enhance Student Achievement by Supporting the Whole Child, 2016 • Building Effective School–Family Partnerships, 2018 • An Update on ASHA's Diversity Efforts (for ASHA Membership), 2019
Association for Counselor Education and Supervision (ACES)	Counseling, psychological, and social services	2021	ACES Statement: Drafted by the ACES Human Rights and Social Justice Committee Under the Leadership of Dr. Harvey Peters
National Association of Secondary School Principals (NASSP)	Physical environment Social and emotional climate	2019	Position Statement: Culturally Responsive Schools
National PTA	Community involvement Family engagement	2002, 2017, 2022	• Citizenship and Equality, 2002 • Rights and Services for Undocumented Children, 1996, 2017 • Inclusive Curriculum in K-12 Schools, 2022 • Say Their Names: Addressing Systemic or Institutional Racism, 2022
Society for Public Health Education (SOPHE)	Health education	2020, 2022	Strategies 1 and 3, SOPHE Strategic Plan 2021-2025, 2020 • Strengthen health education and promotion capacity to achieve health equity • Promote and advocate for health-equity enhancing systems and policies SOPHE Value Statement • Embracing Diversity, 2022

Professional organization or national agency	WSCC component	Year	Statement title or DEI focus
Society of Health and Physical Educators (SHAPE America)	Health education Physical education and physical activity	2013, 2018, 2020	• Promoting Equity and Reducing Health Disparities Among Racially/Ethnically Diverse Adolescents, 2013 • The Healthcare Needs and Rights of Youth Experiencing Homelessness, 2018 • Racism and Its Harmful Effects on Nondominant Racial-Ethnic Youth and Youth-Serving Providers: A Call to Action for Organizational Change, 2018 • Promoting Health Equity and Nondiscrimination for Transgender and Gender-Diverse Youth, 2020
U.S. Department of Education Office of Inspector General	All WSCC components	2019	Diversity and Inclusion Strategic Plan FY [fiscal years] 2019-2022
U.S. Secretary of Education Miguel A. Cardona, EdD	All WSCC components	2021	Policy Statement on Diversity, Equity, Inclusion, and Accessibility

WSCC components: health education; nutrition environment and services; employee wellness; social and emotional climate; health services; counseling, psychological, and social services; community involvement; family engagement; physical environment; and physical education and physical activity (CDC, 2018). Collectively, these components ensure students are healthy, safe, engaged, supported, and challenged, which are the five tenets of the WSCC model (CDC, 2018).

Considerations Related to Social Justice–Oriented Schools

A social justice–oriented focus is linked to the WSCC model in that the model advocates for equitable, respectful, and culturally appropriate instruction and services and promotes social, educational, and systemic change (Chitiyo & Pietrantoni, 2023; Shriberg & Clinton, 2016). The overall goal of **social justice** is to promote

full and equal participation of all groups in a society that is mutually shaped to meet their needs. Social justice includes a vision of society in which the distribution of resources is equitable and all members are physically and psychologically safe and secure. (Bell, 2013, p. 21)

Thus, in the context of education, social justice focuses on equal access to educational resources and equitable opportunities for participation in educational activities and programs (Chitiyo & Pietrantoni, 2023). It also centers on dismantling hierarchies of power and systemic barriers that negatively affect educational achievement and student well-being, especially among marginalized students. Action might be taken through policy, legislation, and other efforts to address these barriers

(Chitiyo & Pietrantoni, 2023). Moreover, social justice emphasizes the importance of diversity as well as the inclusion of and respect for all students regardless of their race, ethnicity, gender, sexual orientation, or economic background (Chitiyo & Pietrantoni, 2023). Several strategies can be used to achieve social justice in education.

Instruction can be viewed as an instrument of social justice (Dixson & Anderson, 2018). Among strategies that can promote social justice through instruction are **culturally responsive teaching**, **anti-racist teaching**, and **critical race theory (CRT)**.

Culturally Responsive Teaching

Culturally responsive teaching incorporates principles of diversity and inclusion and requires that teachers understand the relationship between students' culture and learning (Gay, 2018; Tanase, 2022). It involves incorporating diverse students' knowledge, prior experiences, frames of reference, and performance styles into educational experiences to make these experiences more relevant and effective (Gay, 2018). A primary tenet of culturally responsive teaching is the linkage of instruction to students' personal experiences, their culture, and their community context (Gay, 2018). This can be achieved in a number of ways. At the individual level, it involves teachers being aware of and knowledgeable about various learning and communication styles among their students and cultural influences on their lives (Abacioglu et al., 2020). This involves in-depth learning about their students' culture as it pertains to families and familial experiences, communities, language, religion, customs, traditions, events, artifacts, and so on. Methods of achieving this level of knowledge can include making home visits, asking students to write stories about their experiences, having classroom discussions, and so on (Abacioglu et al., 2020; Byrd, 2016; Gay, 2018).

In addition, culturally responsive teaching involves directly affecting the curriculum and instruction to make it more diverse and inclusive. It is expected that teachers reflect on their curriculum to ensure that it does not present exclusively mainstream cultural conceptions of students' culture and be intentional about incorporating multiculturalism into their teaching (Abacioglu et al., 2020; Tanase, 2022). For example, instructional activities could be based on or include a song that is relevant to students' culture. Culturally responsive teaching builds a sense of community among students (Byrd, 2016; Chen et al., 2022; Gay, 2018; Woodley et al., 2017) that can be facilitated by team-building activities among students and teachers that promote social cohesion or a sense of solidarity (Abacioglu et al., 2020). Essentially, this strategy focuses on the assets students bring to education and helps make learning relevant to them. Culturally responsive teaching has been associated with increased engagement and educational achievement among minoritized students and can positively affect all students (Aronson & Laughter, 2016; Byrd, 2016; Gay, 2018).

Anti-Racist Teaching

Anti-racist teaching, a type of instruction that counters racist patterns and expressions, is another strategy that can help promote a social justice–oriented school (Arneback, 2022). In this strategy, educators participate in anti-racist pedagogy by identifying and fighting biases, addressing power dynamics, promoting equity, and bringing awareness to prejudice and racism while also promoting respect for and the value of differences (Cheesman, 2022; Kishimoto, 2018). Teaching through an anti-racist lens aids students in understanding the origins, manifestations, and impact of racism (past and present) so they can be countered or addressed. The WSCC model is particularly relevant in this regard, given that an anti-racist curriculum promotes the well-being and academic engagement of all students, especially those of color and other minoritized students (CDC, 2018).

Key elements of anti-racist teaching and an anti-racist curriculum are visibility, recognition, and empathy (Helmsing, 2022), which are also DEI principles. In anti-racist teaching, student voices and experiences are amplified and respected (Cheesman, 2022). Educators incorporate students' knowledge and culture into their pedagogy and collaborate with students in their learning. They also create space for minoritized children to feel safe, included, and welcomed (Helmsing, 2022). For instance, it can be effective to use group agreements in class discussions, in particular those that address power dynamics, create safe spaces, and promote open dialogue for students to express themselves (Massicotte, 2023). Examples include emphasizing to students that identity and background are reflected in individuals' opinions; that all opinions matter; and that students have the right to pass or not engage in classroom discussions.

Additional examples of anti-racist teaching include the following:

- Obtaining feedback from minoritized students to inform curricular and programmatic decisions (Massicotte, 2023)
- Including literature and other instructional materials by authors of diverse racial and ethnic backgrounds (Samuels et al., 2020)
- Using culturally relevant scenarios in curriculum content, which involves viewing subject matter through a culturally relevant lens to avoid homogenizing and generalizing about student groups and communities (Massicotte, 2023)
- Taking advantage of opportunities to embed racial history into curriculum content, even if only briefly (Massicotte, 2023)

Overall, anti-racist teaching can be helpful for promoting a social justice–oriented school. Professional development among teachers that promotes knowledge and implementation of anti-racist practices is important to implementing this approach (Cheesman, 2022).

Critical Race Theory

CRT, which addresses the role of race and racism in U.S. education, provides another framework for examining policies, practices, and services in education as they pertain to social justice (Gillborn, 2015; Milner & Laughter, 2015; Murray et al., 2015). Although it is not a curriculum itself, CRT draws attention to long-standing patterns of exclusion and other forms of structural racism—especially those unnoticed or taken for granted—and provides avenues for action (Gillborn, 2015; Milner & Laughter, 2015; Murray et al., 2015). With regard to educational disparities, CRT shifts the focus from a deficiency-focused model to "an approach that uncovers how inequities in access, power, and resources in the educational system perpetuate the achievement gap" (Hernández, 2016, p. 170). Some basic tenets of CRT include the following:

- Race and racism should be continually centered in education discourse (Milner & Laughter, 2015).
- Dominant ideologies (e.g., neutrality, objectivity, color blindness, meritocracy) should be challenged or problematized (Dixson & Anderson, 2018; Laughter & Han, 2019).
- The experiential knowledge of underrepresented students and minoritized communities is appropriate, valid, and essential (Delgado & Stefancic, 2017).
- Consideration should be given to **intersectionality**, which occurs when inequality and identity are influenced or affected by overlapping or interconnecting drivers, such as race, socioeconomic class, gender, and disability (Crenshaw, 2015; Gillborn, 2015).
- An interdisciplinary perspective is needed whereby race and racism are placed in both contemporary and historical contexts (Dixson & Anderson, 2018).
- A commitment to social justice is expected (Dixson & Anderson, 2018).

CRT promotes a social justice–oriented school by acknowledging the pervasiveness of racism, enhancing the understanding of individual experiences, challenging dominant ideologies, acknowledging and valuing experiential knowledge and voice, using interdisciplinary perspectives, advancing an understanding of intersectionality, and committing to social justice (Delgado & Stefancic, 2017; Hernández, 2016; Murray et al., 2015).

A social justice–oriented school can be facilitated through the use of culturally responsive teaching, anti-racist teaching, and CRT, among other educational frameworks and strategies. The concept of a social justice–oriented school directly links to the WSCC model in that it advocates for equitable, respectful, and culturally appropriate educational instruction, practices, services, and policies that affect the 10 WSCC components. In addition, the strategies discussed here also pertain to the WSCC tenets: healthy, safe, engaged, supported, and challenged. Professional development and training can help school staff members have a sense of what a social justice–oriented WSCC program looks like and aid them in understanding the impact on students and schools of institutional racism and other forms of structural discrimination. The WSCC model provides a useful framework for promoting a social justice–oriented school that ensures appropriate educational services for all (CDC, 2018).

Promoting Diversity, Equity, and Inclusion Through Cultural Humility

Cultural humility is a process in which teachers gain an awareness and understanding of their own beliefs, values, and biases as well as the influence of these on their ability to effectively engage and teach diverse students (Fisher, 2020; Habashy & Cruz, 2021). This introspection creates a humble curiosity about other cultures along with a goal of improving one's relationship with individuals from those cultures. Cultural humility "involves a lifelong process of self-awareness, critical reflection, and development of personal attitudes and beliefs" that allows teachers to engage and build relationships with students from various backgrounds (Fisher, 2020, p. 54). It involves approaching others and situations with openness and humility, including a disposition to understand across cultural differences (Fisher-Borne et al., 2015; Habashy & Cruz, 2021; Mosher et al., 2017).

Culturally humble teachers value all aspects of students' identities, respect students and their community's expertise on themselves, and strive to build effective interactions and partnerships in which students feel empowered (Foronda et al., 2016). Cultural humility is important for effective intercultural interactions (Haynes-Mendez & Engelsmeier, 2020). It also provides a filter or lens through which teachers gain an awareness and understanding of the impact of past and current biases and discrimination and other social determinants (e.g., income, health, family resources) on their students (Fisher, 2020). When interacting with students and families from different cultural backgrounds, culturally humble teachers are open and respectful of them and do not interpret their own cultural beliefs and practices as being superior or more meaningful (Haynes-Mendez & Engelsmeier, 2020). Cultural humility also involves being aware of one's own values, beliefs, and practices and engaging in a lifelong process of self-reflection and critique (Haynes-Mendez & Engelsmeier, 2020). Such an approach has implications for student–teacher relationships as well as for developing or using relevant curricula and activities.

According to Habashy and Cruz (2021), humility can be learned and, by extension, taught. For instance, professional development and trainings can provide opportunities for teachers to learn how to transform their knowledge, skills, and abilities for working with diverse children through guided critical reflection, real-life situations, and field experiences (Brown et al., 2016). Similarly, cultural humility can be instilled in students through carefully planned service-learning experiences, self-reflection activities, creative projects, and extracurricular activities that promote meaningful student involvement. Implementing a pedagogy of cultural humility can promote global learning through a variety of educational interventions (Habashy & Cruz, 2021). Given the fact that global society is increasingly diverse and interconnected, there is a growing need for culturally humble educators and students.

Incorporating Diversity, Equity, and Inclusion Into Family Engagement

Family engagement in schools promotes inclusion among students and families and is a component of WSCC (CDC, 2018). The benefits of family engagement (or family involvement) for academic success and school readiness are well documented (Castillo, 2022; Epstein et al., 2019; Hill et al., 2018; Marti et al., 2018; Zolkoski et al., 2018). Family engagement is associated with increased school readiness, student achievement, attendance, and student resilience as well as an enhanced school climate (American School Counselor Association, 2022c; Castillo, 2022; Hill et al., 2018; Marti et al., 2018).

Many parents of racial and ethnic minority students report feeling isolated, stereotyped, and discriminated against in their interactions with schools (Yull et al., 2014). Without intervention, this can lead to low parent involvement or family engagement. With regard to DEI, intentional efforts to be inclusive are needed to engage families of racial and ethnic minority students as well as families of children living in poverty and children within the LGBTQ+ community. Research indicates that the following strategies were helpful in schools that successfully demonstrated diverse family involvement:

- A focus on trust and collaborative relationships
- Concerted attempts to recognize, respect, and address the needs of diverse families, including their socioeconomic and cultural differences
- A philosophy that embraces shared power and responsibility with families (Epstein et al., 2019; Hill et al., 2018; Zolkoski et al., 2018)

Low income, poor parental literacy, inflexible work schedules, and language limitations are frequently cited barriers to family involvement in schools (Francis et al., 2018; Hornby & Blackwell, 2018; Keller et al., 2021; Sim et al., 2021). These conditions have implications for families in terms of attending school events, being able to pay for their children's extracurricular activities, volunteering at school, and being involved in other school-related activities and meetings. Examples of DEI strategies that can help low-income families be more engaged with schools include providing creative volunteer opportunities, varying times for school events, low-cost school activities, financial assistance for students, and alternative methods of providing academic support to students without overburdening parents. To address inadequate parental literacy, schools can develop and use materials written at appropriate literacy levels and include pictures or other illustrations, audiovisuals, and varying formats when appropriate. Schools can also partner with local organizations (e.g., adult basic education programs) to offer literacy programs, health literacy seminars, GRE courses, and so on to families. With regard to language barriers, it would be helpful for parents to know there is someone at school events who can aid them in their communication (Sim et al., 2021). Providing forms and materials in other languages is also an important strategy.

Promoting Diversity, Equity, and Inclusion Through Community Involvement

Communities can be valuable assets to the schools, children, and families they serve. Research has shown the benefits of community involvement (or community engagement; Cummings & Olson, 2020; Stanley & Gilzene, 2023). Community involvement is associated with increased buy-in, trust, partnership, capacity building, and program sustainability (Cummings & Olson, 2020; Stanley & Gilzene, 2023). These approaches have been especially helpful in working with racial and ethnic diverse communities (Kervick et al., 2022; Stanley & Gilzene, 2023). Communities offer a wealth of resources that can contribute to the curriculum and other educational needs of diverse students and families.

Community involvement in school efforts can be formal or informal and can include a number of strategies, such as partnering with community members or organizations to sponsor school or community events, establishing a community advisory board, focusing curricula on topics deemed important to the community, and inviting community members to provide presentations to students and families. Examples of community organizations that can be engaged are parent organizing groups, faith communities, universities and colleges, businesses, social service agencies, and nonprofit organizations (Cummings & Olson, 2020; Kervick et al., 2022; Stanley & Gilzene, 2023).

DEI strategies can be incorporated into community involvement efforts. One example is building a diverse school staff and volunteer pool that reflect the diversity in the community (Goldhaber et al., 2019; Nevarez et al., 2019; Yull et al., 2014). For instance, in one study Black and Latinx students who were taught by teachers of similar racial or ethnic backgrounds had fewer discipline referrals and improved academic outcomes than students taught by teachers of non-similar races and ethnicities (Goldhaber et al., 2015). As another DEI-focused effort, schools can engage representatives from sectors associated with the social and structural drivers of education and health inequities. Examples might include, among others, local housing entities; social justice, civil, and human rights organizations; advocacy groups; and employment or job training agencies.

Another DEI consideration is the use of a community participatory approach, which is characterized by genuine collaboration between the academic and community partners. In this approach, not only is significant input expected from the community, but its contribution is valued (Jung et al., 2021; Kervick et al., 2022). The project is mutually beneficial to the partners. In one approach, community-based participatory research (CBPR), there is a long-term commitment to this partnership (Minkler & Wallerstein, 2008). In CBPR, decision-making is shared between the partners, and the community is involved in each step of the process. In addition, in CBPR, co-learning occurs, and capacity building among community members is encouraged (Minkler & Wallerstein, 2008). Community participatory approaches, in general, result in increased participation, meaningful and relevant projects, and successful project outcomes (Baquerizo et al., 2023; Jung et al., 2021; Kervick et al., 2022; Núñez et al., 2015; Waters et al., 2018). An example of CBPR in education might be the formulation of an LGBTQ+ community advisory board that includes members from the high school LGBTQ+ community and others (e.g., a college student representing a university LGBTQ+ organization, a school counselor, a therapist in the community, a representative from a community-based LGBTQ+ organization). The community advisory board would be an equal partner with the school in developing its LGBTQ+ advocacy, implementing programs, being informed of project results and other pertinent information, and deciding what information is shared with the broader school and community.

Summary

As the United States becomes more culturally diverse, it is important that school systems and their communities be responsive to the needs of students by promoting DEI. Presently, many student populations experiencing disproportionately poor education outcomes are faced with complex, multilevel, interrelated challenges that hinder the effectiveness of traditional educational methods. Given persistent disparities in health among students, other approaches and models of involvement are needed. Although such efforts require significant commitment and time, the WSCC approach can serve as a meaningful framework for DEI implementation.

The focus of the WSCC model is on keeping youth healthy, safe, engaged, supported, and challenged (its five tenets), which is consistent with DEI principles and strategies (CDC, 2018). For instance, strategies that promote a social justice–oriented school (e.g., culturally responsive teaching) can be helpful in promoting an emotionally safe space for children and providing opportunities for personalized learning experiences from qualified, trained teachers (two WSCC tenets). Some DEI strategies (e.g., family engagement and community involvement) are components of the WSCC model, whereas others (e.g., cultural humility) are embedded within its components.

Several professional organizations and national agencies address components of the WSCC model and have called for DEI-related efforts as indicated in their policy statements. Specific and effective DEI strategies recommended in the literature involve genuine collaboration and culturally appropriate strategies. DEI efforts require mutual respect, trust, and shared power and decision-making among students, families, communities, and partners. Sufficient strategies that support DEI and that are incorporated into WSCC components and tenets are recommended to help achieve equitable educational and health outcomes for children.

LEARNING AIDS

GLOSSARY

anti-racist teaching—A style of teaching that focuses on helping students gain an understanding of the origins of racism and past and present racism to move them toward actions that oppose and disrupt systemic racism and other forms of discrimination.

critical race theory (CRT)—A theory that holds that racism results not only from individual bias and prejudice but also from systemic racism present in laws, policies, processes, practices, and institutions. CRT is not a course but an interdisciplinary approach to teaching that is intended to examine the history and impact of systemic racism in the United States and its effect on individuals and communities.

cultural humility—A commitment to learning about another's culture, including examining one's own beliefs related to other cultures. Cultural humility involves a willingness to learn about others' culture, a recognition of the effects of power and systemic discrimination on various cultures, and a desire to support and address social justice–oriented change.

culturally responsive teaching—A style of teaching that incorporates students' culture, life experiences, frames of reference, and performance styles to enhance the authenticity and relevance of teaching and learning. Culturally responsive teaching involves teaching to and through the strengths of students and is relevant to the life experiences of students, their families, and their community.

diversity—All types of difference among individuals and groups, including differences in race, ethnicity, ability, sex, gender, gender identity, sexual orientation, socioeconomic status, place of residence, and religion or spirituality.

diversity, equity, and inclusion (DEI)—When used in reference to schools, the policies, processes, practices, and climate that support and promote DEI to foster health, education, and overall well-being among students and school staff.

equity—Fairness and an attempt to meet the needs and unique challenges faced by all individuals and groups. Equity is sometimes confused with equality, in which all individuals or organizations receive the same thing. In the case of schools, however, equity means that schools, students, and families receive the resources and support needed to promote academic success. In equitable situations, resources and support are provided according to need rather than all receiving the same amount.

inclusion—In the school setting, referring to a school community in which all members are and feel respected, connected, and able to achieve to their potential.

intersectionality—Additive forms of discrimination experienced by individuals with multiple social identities that influence their perceptions of their lived experiences. The social identities might emanate from the intersection of some combination of race, ability or disability status, gender, sexual orientation, socioeconomic status, place of residence, or so on.

social justice—The presence of full and equal participation of all groups in a society that is mutually shaped to meet their needs. This requires an equitable distribution of resources which leads to the opportunity for the physical and psychological health and safety of all members.

social justice–oriented school—A school that demonstrates a commitment to meeting the needs of all to ensure equitable access to economic, educational, political, and social rights and opportunities.

APPLICATION ACTIVITIES

1. Develop a five- to eight-minute presentation for your class on the current state of diversity in schools in the United States. Present the most recent data on the percentages of students of different races or ethnicities, experiencing homelessness or housing instability, of immigrant status, living in poverty, identifying as LGBTQ+, and with a disability. Following your presentation, lead a discussion among your peers that focuses on their thoughts on benefits, challenges, needed actions by schools, and other perspectives related to meeting the educational and health needs of diverse student populations.

2. Use the information presented in the chapter and your own personal perspective to develop a list of 5 to 10 characteristics of a social justice–oriented school. For each characteristic on your list, provide an example of how it is demonstrated or applied in one of the 10 WSCC components. Present the examples in table or chart format.

3. Select three WSCC components from those presented in table 5.1. Review the position statements and websites for each organization listed for the three selected components. In addition to the position statement, review other information related to DEI and social justice that is on the organization's website. Prepare a report based on your review. The report should include a summary of the information you found for each component, the additional information on each website, and your personal reaction to the organization's approach to DEI and social justice. In your reaction include your thoughts on the quality and thoroughness of the information and any questions you may have based on your review.

REFERENCES

Abacioglu, C.S., Volman, M., & Fischer, A.H. (2020). Teachers' multicultural attitudes and perspective taking abilities as factors in culturally responsive teaching. *British Journal of Educational Psychology, 90,* 736-752.

American School Counselor Association. (2022a). *ASCA position statements: The school counselor and children experiencing homelessness* (pp. 19-20). www.schoolcounselor.org/getmedia/d597c40b-7684-445f-b5ed-713388478486/Position-Statements.pdf

American School Counselor Association. (2022b). *ASCA position statements: The school counselor and LGBTQ youth* (pp. 51-53). www.schoolcounselor.org/getmedia/d597c40b-7684-445f-b5ed-713388478486/Position-Statements.pdf

American School Counselor Association. (2022c). *ASCA position statements: The school counselor and school-family-community partnerships* (pp. 78-79). www.schoolcounselor.org/getmedia/d597c40b-7684-445f-b5ed-713388478486/Position-Statements.pdf

American School Counselor Association. (2022d). *ASCA position statements: The school counselor and students with disabilities* (pp. 88-89). www.schoolcounselor.org/getmedia/d597c40b-7684-445f-b5ed-713388478486/Position-Statements.pdf

American School Counselor Association. (2022e). *ASCA position statements: The school counselor and working with students experiencing issues surrounding undocumented status* (pp. 108-110). www.schoolcounselor.org/getmedia/d597c40b-7684-445f-b5ed-713388478486/Position-Statements.pdf

Arneback, E. (2022). Becoming an anti-racist teacher: Countering racism in education. *Teachers and Teaching, 28*(3), 357-368.

Aronson, B., & Laughter, J. (2016). The theory and practice of culturally relevant education: A synthesis of research across content areas. *Review of Educational Research, 86*(1), 163-206.

Ayalew, B., Dawson-Hahn, E., Cholera, R., Falusi, O., Haro, T.M., Montoya-Williams, D., & Linton, J.M. (2021). The health of children in immigrant families: Key drivers and research gaps through an equity lens. *Academic Pediatrics, 21*(5), 777-792.

Baquerizo, H., Munoz, S., Sahu, N., & Chen, P.H. (2023). Novel community participatory approach to violence intervention program for Latino youth. *The Columbia University Journal of Global Health, 13*(1). 1-5. https://journals.library.columbia.edu/index.php/jgh/article/view/10698/5519

Barnes, A.J., Gower, A.L., Sajady, M., & Lingras, K.A. (2021). Health and adverse childhood experiences among homeless youth. *BMC Pediatrics, 21*, 164, 1-10.

Bell, L.A. (2013). Theoretical foundations. In M. Adams, W.J. Blumenfeld, C. Castañeda, H.W. Hackman, M.L. Peters, & X. Zúñiga (Eds.), *Readings for diversity and social justice* (3rd ed., pp. 21-26). Routledge.

Breau, L.M., Aston, M., & MacLeod, E. (2018). Education creates comfort and challenges stigma towards children with intellectual disabilities. *Journal of Intellectual Disabilities, 22*(1), 18-32.

Brown, E.L., Vesely, C.K., & Dallman, L. (2016). Unpacking biases: Developing cultural humility in early childhood and elementary teacher candidates. *Teacher Educators' Journal, 9*, 75-96.

Byrd, C.M. (2016). Does culturally relevant teaching work? An examination from student perspectives. *SAGE Open, 6*(3). https://doi.org/10.1177/2158244016660744

Castillo, B.M. (2022). "Equity work is messy": Exploring a family and community partnership in one school district. *Education and Urban Society, 55*(2), 201-221.

Centers for Disease Control and Prevention, Division of Adolescent and School Health. (2013). *2012 Division of Adolescent and School Health success stories: State and local organization examples.* www.cdc.gov/healthyschools/stories/pdf/ss_booklet_0713.pdf

Centers for Disease Control and Prevention, Division of Adolescent and School Health. (2018). *The Whole School, Whole Community, Whole Child (WSCC) model.* www.cdc.gov/healthyyouth/wscc/model.htm

Chang, C.D. (2019). Social determinants of health and health disparities among immigrants and their children. *Current Problems in Pediatric and Adolescent Health Care, 49*(1), 23-30.

Cheesman, E. (2022). *Exploring BIPOC student experiences and the teacher's role in anti-racist pedagogy.* https://vc.bridgew.edu/honors_proj/503

Chen, X., Fletcher, L., Castagno-Dysart, D., Popp, J.S., Rose, C., & Holyoke, E.S. (2022). Teacher educators' culturally sustaining pedagogy and activism in practice: A multi-institutional collaborative self-study. *New Waves, 25*(2), 32-52.

Chitiyo, J., & Pietrantoni, Z. (2023). Preface. In J. Chitiyo & Z. Pietrantoni (Eds.), *Social justice and culturally-affirming education in K-12 settings* (pp. xvi-xviii). IGI Global.

Corsino, L., & Fuller, A.T. (2021). Educating for diversity, equity, and inclusion: A review of commonly used educational approaches. *Journal of Clinical and Translational Science, 5*(1), e169.

Council on Community Pediatrics. (2016). Poverty and child health in the United States. *Pediatrics, 137*(4), e20160339.

Crenshaw, K. (2015, September 24). Why intersectionality can't wait. *The Washington Post.* www.washingtonpost.com/news/in-theory/wp/2015/09/24/why-intersectionality-cant-wait/

Cummings, M.I., & Olson, J.D. (2020). The importance and potential of community partnerships in urban schools in an era of high-stakes accountability. *Improving Schools, 23*(2), 109-124.

Delgado, R., & Stefancic, J. (2017). *Critical race theory: An introduction.* New York University Press.

Dembo, R.S., & LaFleur, J. (2019). Community health contexts and school suspensions of students with disabilities. *Children and Youth Services Review, 102*, 120-127.

Dixson, A.D., & Anderson, C.R. (2018). Where are we? Critical race theory in education 20 years later. *Peabody Journal of Education, 93*(1), 121-131.

Epstein, J.L., Sanders, M.G., Sheldon, S.B., Simon, B.S., Salinas, K.C., Jansorn, N.R., Van Voorhis, F.L., Martin, C.S., Thomas, B.G., Greenfeld, M.D., Hutchins, D.J., & Williams, K.J. (2019). *School, family, and community partnerships: Your handbook for action* (4th ed.). Corwin Press.

Farmer, T.W., Hamm, J.V., Dawes, M., Barko-Alva, K., & Cross, J.R. (2019). Promoting inclusive communities in diverse classrooms: Teacher attunement and social dynamics management. *Educational Psychologist, 54*(4), 286-305.

Fisher, E.S. (2020). Cultural humility as a form of social justice: Promising practices for global school psychology training. *School Psychology International, 41*(1), 53-66.

Fisher-Borne, M., Montana Cain, J., & Martin, S.L. (2015). From mastery to accountability: Cultural humility as an alternative to cultural competence. *Social Work Education, 34*(2), 165-181.

Foronda, C., Baptiste, D., Reinholdt, M.M., & Ousman, K. (2016). Cultural humility: A concept analysis. *Journal of Transcultural Nursing, 27*(3), 210-217.

Francis, L., DePriest, K., Wilson, M., & Gross, D. (2018). Child poverty, toxic stress, and social determinants of health: Screening and care coordination. *Online Journal of Issues in Nursing*, 23(3), 1-14.

Frederick, T.J., Chwalek, M., Hughes, J., Karabanow, J., & Kidd, S. (2014). How stable is stable? Defining and measuring housing stability. *Journal of Community Psychology*, 42(8), 964-979.

Fujita, M., Francis, G.L., & Duke, J. (2022). I'm not prepared: Experiences of professionals working with students with disabilities and co-occurring mental health disorders. *Journal of the American Academy of Special Education Professionals*, 17(2), 26-44.

Gardiner, T. (2020). Supporting health and educational outcomes through school-based health centers. *Pediatric Nursing*, 46(6), 292-299.

Gay, G. (2018). *Culturally responsive teaching: Theory, research, and practice* (3rd ed.). Teachers College Press.

Gillborn, D. (2015). Intersectionality, critical race theory, and the primacy of racism: Race, class, gender, and disability in education. *Qualitative Inquiry*, 21(3), 277-287.

Goldhaber, D., Roddy, T., & Tien, C. (2015). *The theoretical and empirical arguments for diversifying the teacher workforce: A review of the evidence* (CEDR Working Paper No. 2015-9). Center for Education & Data Research.

Goldhaber, D., Theobald, R., & Tien, C. (2019). Why we need a diverse teacher workforce. *Phi Delta Kappan*, 100(5), 25-30.

Habashy, N., & Cruz, L. (2021). Bowing down and standing up: Towards a pedagogy of cultural humility. *International Journal of Development Education and Global Learning*, 13(1), 16-31.

Haynes-Mendez, K., & Engelsmeier, J. (2020). Cultivating cultural humility in education. *Childhood Education*, 96(3), 22-29.

Heard-Garris, N., Boyd, R., Kan, K., Perez-Cardona, L., Heard, N.J., & Johnson, T.J. (2021). Structuring poverty: How racism shapes child poverty and child and adolescent health. *Academic Pediatrics*, 21(8), S108-S116.

Helmsing, M.E. (2022). Teaching beyond racialized national fantasies for anti-racist curriculum: A portrait of a high school civics course. *Curriculum and Teaching Dialogue*, 24(1-2), 67-81.

Hernández, E. (2016). Utilizing critical race theory to examine race/ethnicity, racism, and power in student development theory and research. *Journal of College Student Development*, 57(2), 168-180.

Hill, N.E., Witherspoon, D.P., & Bartz, D. (2018). Parental involvement in education during middle school: Perspectives of ethnically diverse parents, teachers, and students. *Journal of Educational Research*, 111(1), 12-27.

Hornby, G., & Blackwell, I. (2018). Barriers to parental involvement in education: An update. *Educational Review*, 70(1), 109-119.

Johns, M.M., Lowry, R., Haderxhanaj, L.T., Rasberry, C.N., Robin, L., Scales, L., Stone, D., & Suarez, N.A. (2020). Trends in violence victimization and suicide risk by sexual identity among high school students—Youth Risk Behavior Survey, United States, 2015-2019. *Morbidity and Mortality Weekly Report*, 69(Suppl. 1), 19-27.

Jung, Y., Burson, S.L., Julien, C., Bray, D.F., & Castelli, D.M. (2021). Development of a school-based physical activity intervention using an integrated approach: Project SMART. *Frontiers in Psychology*, 12, Article 648625.

Keller, J.G., Miller, C., LasDulce, C., & Wohrle, R.G. (2021). Using a community-based participatory research model to encourage parental involvement in their children's schools. *Children & Schools*, 43(3), 149-158.

Kervick, C.T., Haines, S.J., Green, A.E., Reyes, C.C., Shepherd, K.G., Moore, M., Healy, E.A., & Gordon, M.E. (2022). Engaging interdisciplinary service providers to enhance collaboration to support refugee families whose children have special health care needs. *Educational Action Research*, 30(5), 768-790.

Kishimoto, K. (2018). Anti-racist pedagogy: From faculty self-reflection to organizing within and beyond the classroom. *Race Ethnicity and Education*, 21(4), 540-554.

Kosciw, J.G., Clark, C.M., Truong, N.L., & Zongrone, A.D. (2020). *The 2019 National School Climate Survey: The experiences of lesbian, gay, bisexual, transgender, and queer youth in our nation's schools*. GSLEN.

Laughter, J., & Han, K.T. (2019). Introduction and overview. In K.T. Han & J. Laughter (Eds.), *Critical race theory in teacher education: Informing classroom culture and practice* (pp. 1-12). Teachers College Press.

Lehner, P. (2017). Money doesn't ensure equity. *Education Week*, 36(33), 20.

LoSchiavo, C., Krause, K.D., Singer, S.N., & Halkitis, P.N. (2020). The confluence of housing instability and psychosocial, mental, and physical health in sexual minority young adults: The P18 Cohort Study. *Journal of Health Care for the Poor and Underserved*, 31(4), 1693-1711.

Marti, M., Merz, E.C., Repka, K.R., Landers, C., Noble, K.G., & Duch, H. (2018). Parent involvement in the Getting Ready for School Intervention is associated with changes in school readiness skills. *Frontiers in Psychology*, 9, Article 759.

Massicotte, L.M. (2023). Implementing anti-racist strategies in the evidence-based sexuality education classroom. *American Journal of Sexuality Education*, 18(1), 149-169.

Masten, A.S., Fiat, A.E., Labella, M.H., & Strack, R.A. (2015). Educating homeless and highly mobile students: Implications of research on risk and resilience. *School Psychology Review*, 44(3), 315-330.

Michael, S.L., Merlo, C.L., Basch, C.E., Wentzel, K.R., & Wechsler, H. (2015). Critical connections: Health and academics. *Journal of School Health*, 85(11), 740-758.

Milner, H.R., & Laughter, J.C. (2015). But good intentions are not enough: Preparing teachers to center race and poverty. *Urban Review*, 47(2), 341-363.

Minkler, M., & Wallerstein, N. (2008). *Community-based participatory research for health: From process to outcomes.* Wiley.

Mosher, D.K., Hook, J.N., Captari, L.E., Davis, D.E., DeBlaere, C., & Owen, J. (2017). Cultural humility: A therapeutic framework for engaging diverse clients. *Practice Innovations, 2*(4), 221-233.

Murray, M.M., Mereoiu, M., Cassidy, D., Vardell, R., Niemeyer, J.A., & Hestenes, L. (2015). Not Black like me: The cultural journey of an early childhood program. *Early Childhood Education Journal, 44*(5), 429-436.

Myers, W., Turanovic, J.J., Lloyd, K.M., & Pratt, T.C. (2020). The victimization of LGBTQ students at school: A meta-analysis. *Journal of School Violence, 19*(4), 421-432.

National Academies of Sciences, Engineering, and Medicine. (2020). *Promoting positive adolescent health behaviors and outcomes: Thriving in the 21st century.* National Academies Press.

National Center for Education Statistics. (2022a). *Characteristics of children's families.* www.nces.ed.gov/programs/coe/indicator/cce/family-characteristics

National Center for Education Statistics. (2022b). *Racial/ethnic enrollment in public schools.* https://nces.ed.gov/programs/coe/indicator/cge

National Center for Education Statistics. (2022c). *Students with disabilities.* https://nces.ed.gov/programs/coe/indicator/cgg

Nevarez, C., Jouganatos, S., & Wood, J.L. (2019). Benefits of teacher diversity: Leading for transformative change. *Journal of School Administration Research and Development, 4*(1), 24-34.

Núñez, A., Robertson-James, C., Reels, S., Jeter, J., Rivera, H., & Yusuf, Z. (2015). Exploring the role of gender norms in nutrition and sexual health promotion in a piloted school-based intervention: The Philadelphia Ujima™ experience. *Evaluation and Program Planning, 51,* 70-77.

Office of Disease Prevention and Health Promotion. (2020). *Housing instability.* Healthy People 2030. https://health.gov/healthypeople/priority-areas/social-determinants-health/literature-summaries/housing-instability#:~:text=Healthy%20People%202030%20organizes%20the%20social%20determinants%20of,a%20key%20issue%20in%20the%20Economic%20Stability%20domain

Ohio Department of Education. (2020). *Ohio's Whole Child framework.* https://education.ohio.gov/getattachment/Topics/Student-Supports/Ohios-Whole-Child-Framework/Whole-Child-Framework.pdf.aspx?lang=en-US

Padamsee, X., Crowe, B., Hurst, L., Johnson, E.T., Louie, L., Messano, F., & Paperny, T. (2017). *Unrealized impact: The case for diversity, equity and inclusion.* www.promise54.org/wp-content/uploads/2020/10/Unrealized_Impact-Final-072017.pdf

Parrott, K.A., Huslage, M., & Cronley, C. (2022). Educational equity: A scoping review of the state of literature exploring educational outcomes and correlates for children experiencing homelessness. *Children and Youth Services Review, 143,* Article 106673.

Rahman, M.A., Turner, J.F., & Elbedour, S. (2015). The U.S. homeless student population: Homeless youth education, review of research classifications and typologies, and the U.S. federal legislative response. *Child & Youth Care Forum, 44*(5), 687-709.

Samuels, S., Wilkerson, A., Chapman, D., & Watkins, W. (2020). Toward a conceptualization: Considering microaffirmations as a form of culturally relevant pedagogy and academic growth for K-12 underserved populations. *Journal of Negro Education, 89*(3), 298-311.

Shriberg, D., & Clinton, A. (2016). The application of social justice principles to global school psychology practice. *School Psychology International, 37*(4), 323-339.

Sim, W.H., Toumbourou, J.W., Clancy, E.M., Westrupp, E.M., Benstead, M.L., & Yap, M.B.H. (2021). Strategies to increase uptake of parent education programs in preschool and school settings: A Delphi study. *International Journal of Environmental Research and Public Health, 18,* Article 3524.

Stanley, D.A., & Gilzene, A. (2023). Listening, engaging, advocating and partnering (L.E.A.P): A model for responsible community engagement for educational leaders. *Journal of Research on Leadership Education, 18*(2), 253-276.

Tanase, M.F. (2022). Culturally responsive teaching in urban secondary schools. *Education and Urban Society, 54*(4), 363-388.

Thompson, D.L., & Thompson, T. (2018). Educational equity and quality in K-12 schools: Meeting the needs of all students. *Journal for the Advancement of Educational Research International, 12*(1), 34-46.

U.S. Department of Education. (2015). *Resource guide: Supporting undocumented youth.* www2.ed.gov/about/overview/focus/supporting-undocumented-youth.pdf

U.S. Department of Education. (2022). *U.S. Department of Education strategic plan fiscal years 2022-2026.* www2.ed.gov/about/reports/strat/plan2022-26/strategic-plan.pdf

Vassallo, B. (2022). Leading the flock: Examining the characteristics of multicultural school leaders in their quest for equitable schooling. *Improving Schools, 25*(1), 22-36.

Wallander, J.L., Fradkin, C., Elliott, M.N., Cuccaro, P.M., Tortolero, E.S., & Schuster, M.A. (2019). Racial/ethnic disparities in health-related quality of life and health status across pre-, early-, and mid-adolescence: A prospective cohort study. *Quality of Life Research, 28*(7), 1761-1771.

Walton-Fisette, J.L., & Sutherland, S. (2020). Time to SHAPE up: Developing policies, standards and practices that are socially just. *Physical Education and Sport Pedagogy, 25*(3), 274-287.

Waters, E., Gibbs, L., Tadic, M., Ukoumunne, O.C., Magarey, A., Okely, A.D., de Silva, A., Armit, C., Green, J., O'Connor, T., Johnson, B., Swinburn, B., Carpenter, L., Moore, G., Littlecott, H., & Gold, L. (2018). Cluster randomised trial of a school-community child health promotion and obesity prevention intervention: Findings from the evaluation of Fun 'n Healthy in Moreland! *BMC Public Health, 18*(1), 1-16.

Woodley, X., Hernandez, C., Parra, J., & Negash, B. (2017). Celebrating difference: Best practices in culturally responsive teaching online. *TechTrends, 61*(5), 470-478.

Yull, D.G., Blitz, L.V., Thompson, T., & Murray, C.T. (2014). Can we talk? Using community-based participatory action research to build family and school partnerships with families of color. *School Community Journal, 24,* 9-32.

Zolkoski, S.M., Sayman, D.M., & Lewis-Chiu, C.G. (2018). Considerations in promoting parent and family involvement. *Diversity, Social Justice, and the Educational Leader, 2*(1), 1-17.

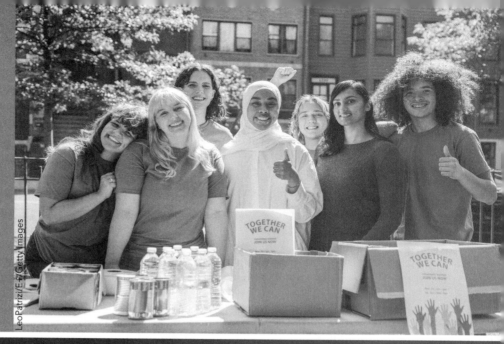

CHAPTER 6

Developing and Maintaining Collaborations

Bonni C. Hodges • Donna M. Videto

LEARNING OBJECTIVES

1. Describe the benefits of using collaborations for Whole School, Whole Community, Whole Child (WSCC) programming.
2. Recognize major barriers and challenges to successful collaborations.
3. Analyze important characteristics of WSCC-based collaborations.
4. Describe actions that can be used to sustain successful collaborations.

KEY TERMS

ASCD's nine levers of school change
Bicultural individual
Collaboration
Credibility
Education support professional (ESP)
Interrelatedness
Siloing

Social determinants
Socioecological approach
Socioeconomic
Solution-focused approach
Sustainability
Systems approach

The authors sincerely thank Lisa Angermeier for contributing certain content in this chapter to the first edition of this book.

> Schools are an ideal setting to transform kids' health and wellness, as the locations where children spend more than 1,200 hours each year—more than anywhere else besides their homes. Schools are a reflection of the local community and are places to support, cultivate, and maximize student potential. For kids to develop the lifelong habits necessary to become healthy and successful adults, schools, families, and communities must commit to working together to build a culture that supports the whole child. (Action for Healthy Kids, 2020, p. 1)

Developing and maintaining **collaborations** involves connecting groups and individuals from the school district, families, and the community. These connections are essential for supporting and advancing the Whole School, Whole Community, Whole Child (WSCC) model. Often collaborating within the district consists of reaching out to committed parents and staff who are often active in a number of committees and activities. Traditionally partners outside the school or district consist of a few local businesses, local colleges and universities, and service-learning or internship opportunities (Rooney et al., 2015). Putting the WSCC model into action requires broader outreach than to just the "usual suspects," involving school staff, families, and community members in providing input, resources, and collaboration to support the child at the center (Centers for Disease Control and Prevention [CDC], 2022b).

Integral to a broad **socioecological approach** to youth health and academic development is this supportive role of the greater community (Bronfenbrenner, 1979; CDC, 2022b). Engaging community members, agencies, and families as partners in collaborations allows schools and communities to more effectively address the health and academic challenges that face our young people (CDC, 2022b; Rooney et al., 2015). Moreover, collaboration among and across the 10 components of the WSCC model is integral to the full realization of the benefits of WSCC (CDC, 2022b; Kolbe, 2019).

Strong collaborations among school, family, and community members can serve to support the foundation of the WSCC model, ASCD's Whole Child approach, and the Healthy School Communities initiative (ASCD, 2015; Kolbe, 2019; Ng'andu & Elstein, 2020). ASCD's Whole Child approach, to ensure that each and every child is healthy, safe, engaged, supported, and challenged (ASCD, 2015), includes collaborations as one of its primary indicators. Adelman and Taylor (2011) pointed to the need for a paradigm shift from a "marginalized and fragmented set of student services" (p. 437) to a multifaceted system of coordinated and interconnected supports to provide students ways to get around the myriad and complex barriers that interfere with learning. The Southwest Educational Development Laboratory identified a need for a "shift from a patchwork of random acts of involvement to a systemic approach" (Ferguson et al., 2010, p. 18) enabling family and community members to serve multiple roles supportive of WSCC while sharing responsibility for student learning. Yet a scan of the professional literature in school health and education suggests that most work is being done within WSCC components rather than from a true collaborative model across multiple components (Howley & Hunt, 2020).

This chapter addresses many aspects related to building school–family–community collaborations and the benefits to WSCC of engaging in collaborations. In addition, it provides recommendations for developing successful collaborations, presents a theoretical approach to supporting quality collaborations, describes barriers and challenges to collaborations, discusses recruiting partners for collaborations, and makes suggestions for implementing and sustaining collaborations, all with the intent of developing and advancing the WSCC model.

School–Family–Community Collaborations

Put simply, collaboration is working together for a common purpose. In this chapter, the focus is collaboration among partners, who are those individuals, groups, agencies, institutions, or organizations that decide to work with another toward this common purpose. Collaboration that weaves together responsibilities and resources is the focus of this discussion. In true collaboratives, partners trust each other and share risk, reward, resources, and responsibility while working toward a common purpose (Kolbe, 2019; Mashek & Nanfito, 2015). An example of a common purpose for both the school and the community is promoting the **interrelatedness** of learning and health, which is a foundational understanding of the WSCC model (Hunt et al., 2015). The CDC (2022b) describes this common purpose among education leaders and the health sector as the desire to improve each child's cognitive, physical, social, and emotional development.

Collaborations can take different forms. Partners can work within their own spheres or sectors toward their own defined part of a common goal or work together across areas. For example, one area may take on the role of another, such as when a school contracts with a health agency to provide health services on school grounds (New York City Department of Education, 2022). In this example, the school benefits from the services provided by the health agency because students are able to receive services they might not otherwise have received. The health agency is able to provide the services it was funded to support with access to potential clients. In a true collaboration, as in this example, the form of the collaboration is agreed on by all partners, and all partners share in planning the agreed-on actions to be taken.

Seeking out partnerships for developing collaborations brings many benefits for advancing WSCC. Partners can certainly share resources, including funding, staffing, space, expertise, and credibility, as well as bring fresh ideas to the arrangement. When the school, families, and the community are included, there are opportunities to increase awareness and coordination across the school and community while building connections and sharing responsibility for the success of young people (Pittman et al., 2020). Collaborations help families and the community support and reinforce healthy behaviors while creating additional health champions and advocates. Collaborations may help to move initiatives forward, strengthen capacity, and improve the chances of efforts becoming sustainable (CDC, 2022b).

Developing Successful Collaborations

Developing successful collaborations is important to ensuring effective efforts and making sure the results of the relationships are a win for all. Sufficient time and a real commitment are required to develop and maintain a productive and trusting partnership (Rooney et al., 2015). In successful collaborations, members take the time to set goals and objectives and work together to meet them. Although a number of partners may agree to work together, this does not mean the collaboration will be successful. What should partners do to ensure a successful collaboration? A number of hallmarks common to successful school–family–community collaborations have been identified in the professional literature. Partners involved in successful collaborations do the following:

- Have mutual trust and respect while recognizing each other's priorities (Action for Healthy Kids [AFHK], 2020)
- Identify common values, find a shared vision, and establish common goals (Abt Associates, 2016; AFHK, 2020), with all partners able to clearly describe and communicate the vision and goals of the collaboration (Mashek & Nanfito, 2015)
- Learn about their partners' disciplines, scope, structures and policies, perspectives and experiences, and connections to healthy youth (Abt Associates, 2016; AFHK, 2020)
- Identify communication pathways and structures (Mashek & Nanfito, 2015)
- Identify and use a variety of communication technologies and strategies (AFHK, 2020; Dewane, 2015; Hunt et al., 2015)
- Communicate on a regular basis (Hunt et al., 2015)
- Use a shared governance model for planning and decision-making (California

School Boards Association, 2009; Center for Mental Health in Schools at UCLA [CMHS], 2015)
- Provide relevant professional skills development for coalition participants (Abt Associates, 2016; Dewane, 2015)
- Engage in needs and asset assessment followed by evaluation activities (CMHS, 2015) to inform collaboration activities (Abt Associates, 2016)
- Establish an accountability and evaluation system that includes tracking tasks and progress toward goals along with achievements of outcomes (Abt Associates, 2016; CMHS, 2015; Mashek & Nanfito, 2015)

The Southwest Educational Development Laboratory has outlined characteristics of effective school–family–community collaborations (Ferguson et al., 2010, pp. 15-18). When these characteristics are adapted to WSCC, the potential exists to create effective WSCC collaborations that result in the following:

- *Shared responsibility for the health and education of youth among school staff, families, and the larger community.* Institutions, organizations, and individuals acknowledge and support that they all, individually and collectively, have a responsibility and a role in fostering healthy youth. These stakeholders demonstrate this responsibility by engaging in shared planning and decision-making (National School Climate Center, 2017). The vision of the school is expanded to include the family and the community (Health Equity Works, 2022), and schools, families, and community entities reach out to one another. The Center for Communities That Care (2022) provides resources for communities that realize that preventing underage drinking, tobacco use, violence, delinquency, school dropout, and substance abuse is a community-wide responsibility. Center for Communities That Care community groups and schools work together through a coalition structure to determine each community's priority prevention needs in these areas and the best way to use their collective resources.

- *Seamless and continuous support for developing good health and health-enhancing behaviors from birth to career in schools, at home, and in the community.* Opportunities to practice health and academic skills intended to develop self-efficacy and reinforce knowledge are created and embedded throughout the community. The ability to practice health-related skills in a variety of real-world situations is an important factor in becoming confident and comfortable in using the skills (Bandura, 1986). School–family–community collaborations are an important tool for creating formal and informal opportunities to practice these skills across socioecological levels (Bronfenbrenner, 1979).

- *Pathways that honor and attend to the dynamic and multiple factors that contribute to health.* Education and health are affected by many common **social determinants**, such as housing and poverty levels (Health Equity Works, 2022). Identifying the systems and pathways that affect these social determinants shows how school and non-school systems are connected to the common determinants and illuminates how changes in one system can affect and change others. Complex interrelated challenges require comprehensive solutions, and these solutions need to be integrated into school improvement plans (Adelman & Taylor, 2011). School–community collaborations provide individuals working in schools the opportunity to work with noneducators to create new pathways to support health and healthy behaviors. For example, a school health team can work with local grocery stores to establish learning centers within the stores for youth and their parents to apply skills and knowledge, or the team can work with the local restaurant association to improve children's menus and create placemats with health-related learning activities for children to play with while waiting for food. By engaging a wide variety of community partners in the determination and creation of these pathways, the entire community may see improved health, which reinforces the goals of WSCC (CDC, 2022b).

- *A supportive culture for health both in the classroom and throughout the community.* Collaborations do a better job of creating family- and community-wide social norms for health behavior than single entities do because families with their children—and community collaborators with their nonstudent employees, clients, customers, and so on—can reinforce a universal positive health message.

• *Opportunities and processes to foster advocacy for student health and healthy communities.* Collaborations foster opportunities for all stakeholders to advocate for health and can be powerful tools for creating healthy communities. Family members, community members, youth, and educators can all be advocates for health and the WSCC approach with schools and the community through such actions as participating in school board meetings, working with parent–teacher organizations, and speaking in favor of funding that supports youth health and WSCC at local government meetings.

• *Quality health status and health behaviors for every child.* The WSCC approach can help create structural supports and systems within and outside school buildings through collaborations. For example, partners can align curricula across grades, identify and align additional services to support students and their families, and strengthen communication among school and parent systems that support quality health status and health behaviors. Collaborators both within and outside the school should understand that school health should happen not just in the health education classroom but across the school, the district, families, and the community (Videto & Dake, 2019).

Supporting Quality Collaborations

Quality collaborations can increase and improve the efficiency and effectiveness of programs and services for all collaborators and create structure supporting the Whole Child tenets, which are foundational to advancing the WSCC model (ASCD, 2015). Collaborations can be improved by using a **systems approach**, such as in the socioecological framework or in ASCD's nine levers of school change.

Socioecological Framework

Bronfenbrenner (1979) provided a landmark framework that illustrates how important quality school, family, and community collaborations can be for advancing WSCC (see figure 6.1). This socioecological framework nests the

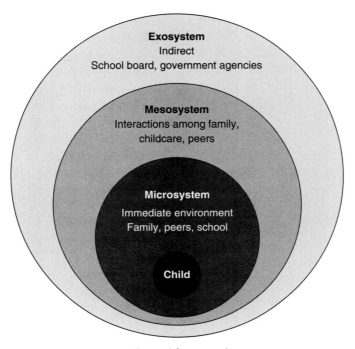

FIGURE 6.1 Socioecological framework.
Adapted by permission from U. Bronfenbrenner (1979).

child in the center of layers of broadening environments that have direct and indirect effects on the child's development. The layer that immediately surrounds the child, the microsystem, directly affects the child's development. This layer consists of such elements as the child's family, peers, and school. The interactions among elements within this layer create the next outward layer, the mesosystem. The mesosystem also has a direct effect on the child. Surrounding these two layers is the exosystem. One can think of the exosystem as containing the many systems that shape how the child's life is experienced but with which the child has no direct interaction. Representation across areas of the socioecological framework creates connectedness and increases the **credibility** of, buy-in for, follow-through on, and institutionalization of the resulting collaborative programs and services (Hodges & Videto, 2012).

Consider the area of nutrition and diet. The socioecological framework suggests that what an elementary school-age child eats is directly affected by what the parents and school serve the child at meal and snack times (microsystem), that what is appropriate for school snack time can be affected by parents and schools working together to determine a healthy snack policy (mesosystem), and that what is served for school lunches can be affected by community cultural norms (exosystem).

At the very center of the WSCC model is the whole child surrounded by 10 components that are supported by the community. Quality WSCC efforts can clearly demonstrate the influence of Bronfenbrenner's ideas. The positive effects of the impact of these systems on the health and academic development of children are greater when the systems are in alignment and working together (Pittman et al., 2020). Beyond these outcomes, increased efficiency arises through sharing services, staff, expertise, funding, space and facilities, and programming among community members and with community organizations. This sharing assists schools, community organizations, families, and caregivers in being able to fully use resources available to them to support the health, academic growth, and overall development of youth (Ferguson et al., 2010).

ASCD's Nine Levers of School Change

ASCD's nine levers of school change were identified to provide guidance for schools in moving toward a Whole Child approach by changing the culture of the school community through a systems approach to school improvements (ASCD, 2010; see figure 6.2). The levers are considered approaches within a project or program that contribute to positive change in the school community culture. The goal of the study associated with the identification of the nine levers of school change was to determine what factors (programs, policies, and processes) enabled a school to most easily facilitate and successfully implement programming supportive of the whole child and ultimately the WSCC model (ASCD, 2010).

FIGURE 6.2 ASCD'S NINE LEVERS OF SCHOOL CHANGE

Principal as leader
Active and engaged leadership
Distributive leadership

Integration with the school improvement plan
Effective use of data for continuous school improvement
Ongoing and embedded professional development

Authentic and mutually beneficial community collaborations
Stakeholder support of the local efforts
The creation or modification of school policy related to the process

Adapted from ASCD (2010).

Running through the nine levers is the thread of community stakeholder engagement and collaboration, the essential element necessary for making school improvements for advancing health and academic success. As is evident in the nine levers, for quality collaborations to be successful, family and community stakeholders need to be engaged in meaningful problem-solving through all phases of the planning, implementation, and evaluation of these collaborations.

Barriers and Challenges to Collaboration

It is useful to identify and important to understand common barriers and challenges to effective school, family, and community collaborations. A number of barriers within and outside the school have been identified by people working to improve school–community collaborations (see figure 6.3).

FIGURE 6.3 BARRIERS AND CHALLENGES TO SCHOOL–COMMUNITY COLLABORATIONS

Siloing in the school district

Unclear or undefined leadership for school health (where school health efforts are driven by individuals, not the district)

Lack of recognition of shared vision, values, and goals

Lack of effective communication

Perceived or real budgetary constraints

A perceived need to protect one's turf

Past negative experiences

Failure to recognize health systems and links to academic success

Infrastructure and implementation issues

Adapted from Hodges and Videto (2015); Lohman et al. (2018).

Broad barriers and challenges exist around the **siloing** that often occurs within schools and school districts as well as between schools and community agencies and institutions. Siloing tends to take place in environments where people focus narrowly on their own piece or what they think is their piece, missing opportunities to enhance their abilities to realize common goals and objectives that have a positive effect on outcomes for which they are directly responsible (Hodges & Videto, 2015; Willgerodt et al., 2021). Siloing within school districts creates several disincentives for school–family–community collaborations (Rooney et al., 2015; Willgerodt et al., 2021). Community agencies have reported that negotiating the multiple levels of approval that are often required to do work in schools (e.g., from building-level individuals or committees, the district, the board of education) is a lengthy process that can have a deleterious effect on timely program and policy development and implementation and serves as a disincentive to working in collaboration with schools. For some, there is a perception that schools and school districts choose to remain in their silos and only connect with community organizations when these organizations can do something for them.

The first step in moving out of the silo should be for schools to have a stronger, more active presence in existing coalitions or other groups in which they are currently represented. Community groups have reported that schools have a seat on most community coalitions that involve youth development and health but often are not active with these groups (Hodges & Videto, 2012; Hodges et al., 2011). Schools can seek out collaborations with relevant and appropriate groups and stakeholders to engage in two-way relationship building. Schools seeking collaborations need to be inclusive and involve a wide range of stakeholders in planning potential collaborations (Health Equity Works, 2022). Once established, these collaborations should work toward moving beyond the joint projects stage.

Barriers specific to school–family collaborations may include some of the barriers identified to school–community collaborations (see figure 6.3) as well as others that are unique to them. A literature review conducted by Lohman et al. (2018) concerning barriers to family–school collaborations included family issues such as lack of transportation, work schedule and other time constraints, and turmoil (including homelessness, unemployment, substance abuse, and spousal abuse). Additional barriers specific to the relationship between families and schools included teachers' lack of collaboration skills, a lack of communication from schools, and an excessive amount of negative communication from schools as well as past negative experiences with schools (Lohman et al., 2018).

Lack of clear administrative leadership for school health is a barrier to both developing school–family–community collaborations as well as establishing a fully functioning WSCC approach within a district (Green, 2018; Hodges & Videto, 2015). This lack of administrative leadership may take the form of a clear separation between WSCC components, such as with health-related services and classroom health education, or the absence of a full and functioning school health team. Without clear administrative leadership it is not apparent to potential collaborators with whom they need to connect. Moreover, without school health leadership, promising collaborative initiatives are not seen as a priority for implementation and can get lost in a maze of approvals and requests for resources. Lack of clear administrative leadership creates school health initiatives that are driven by individuals rather than the district. Individual-driven initiatives result in school health that is neither collaborative nor systematic, decreasing the impact and greatly hampering the sustainability of successful initiatives.

As part of their role and responsibilities in active leadership of WSCC, school administrators, along with school boards, are vital to fostering welcoming structures for school–family–community collaborations. School boards and school administrators can provide leadership for collaboration in school health by creating policies and structures that enable WSCC to be fully implemented (Adelman & Taylor, 2011; Green, 2018). Identifying those involved with the WSCC approach, both within and outside the school structure, and communicating their roles and responsibilities provide entry points for those seeking to collaborate. School administrators are key players in identifying and connecting with potential collaboration partners (Green, 2018).

Lack of recognition of shared vision, values, and goals among schools and community agencies and organizations is another barrier to collaboration. This lack of recognition may be the result of the use of different terminology that creates the appearance of differences in vision, values, and goals. Without a common vision, a climate can be created that prevents schools from recognizing how numerous institutions are charged with improving the health of youth and working to do so. Schools that expand the concept of *school* to include the entire community are more likely to look for and see where community groups share similar vision, values, and goals. Active participation in community coalitions by school representatives can help schools see commonalities. Schools and community agencies and groups should help each other understand the meanings of discipline and group-specific jargon and move toward the development of common terminology for their efforts so all stakeholders understand what they are working toward.

A lack of effective communication among school staff, families, community members, and community organization staff makes it difficult to establish and sustain collaborations and initiatives. This barrier may take the form of, for example, lacking communication within and outside the organization or school about vision, values, and goals, making it difficult to see where they may be shared; not involving a wide enough representation of stakeholders early in the visioning or planning process; or communicating messages ineffectively to their intended targets. Ensuring transparent and broad communication among all stakeholders within and outside schools, including community organizations, requires delivering communication through multiple channels to those for whom it is intended. Schools and organizations should work to determine and establish the best channels of communication with intended audiences and with each other. Follow-up systems should be created to confirm that messages have been received and understood by the intended audience.

Budgetary constraints, both real and perceived, may prevent the establishment, functioning, or sustainability of school–community collaborations (Grier & Bradley-King, 2011; Sepanik & Brown, 2021; Weist et al., 2012). Rather than seeing collaboration as a means of using resources efficiently and as an avenue for obtaining funding for school and community health goals, stakeholders may think that schools and community agencies do not have funds for nonacademic initiatives in the schools. Funding may not, in fact, be available, but school–community collaborations can make a powerful argument for allocating funding through planned school health advocacy. Real budgetary constraints may exist but should not act as barriers to relationship building; collaborative joint projects may create efficiencies that can relieve some budgetary constraints for all involved. An examination of shared vision, values, and goals as a part of relationship building will help to clarify perceptions and assist in identifying where joint projects may bring about budgetary efficiencies.

Schools and community agencies are sometimes reluctant to engage with others because they feel they must protect their turf (CMHS, 2015; Weist et al., 2012). In times of economic challenge and budgetary constraints, many in schools and community agencies feel that collaboration may indicate that their job or program is not necessary or can be taken over by or outsourced to someone or something else. Staff working in schools may also think of schools as safe spaces for children and feel that collaborating with others outside the school compromises this safe space (Hodges et al., 2011; Hodges & Videto, 2012). When there is a focus on the broader common goal of healthy youth and communities, collaboration and shared resources can make programs stronger and broader in scope while providing support for institutionalization.

For some, one or more past negative experiences trying to collaborate creates reluctance to do so again (Lohman et al., 2018). Potential collaborators should review historical records for evidence of past collaborative efforts and their outcomes and engage in open communication around past experiences in collaboration, both good and bad. Acknowledge the past but focus on the present and future with open communication, systematic planning, and shared decision-making. Family members who have had negative experiences will benefit from positive outreach from schools and communication strategies that focus on shared goals and the avenues for achieving them (Lohman et al., 2018).

Community members may feel as if they do not see a place for themselves in working with schools because they are not parents or family members of school-age youth. Even though they may not have children in the schools, helping community members see the value of their role in developing or supporting the whole child is important in establishing collaborative relationships.

The failure of people working in schools and community agencies to recognize health systems and their links to academic success makes it difficult for them to see the need to collaborate (Hodges & Videto, 2015). Many within and outside schools think that a knowledge-focused health education class constitutes school health (Videto & Dake, 2019) and therefore that school health has nothing to do with their own roles or with broader academic success. The development of school–community collaborations can be assisted by advocating for and implementing strong health promotion policies, practices, and processes. Raising awareness of the links between the health status of children and families and academic success within both school district systems and the community can also assist in the creation of school–family–community collaborations by helping academic and health stakeholders see shared outcomes. For example, for a number of years school districts in one county in central New York had been documenting a rise in mental health issues among students. At the same time, local mental health service providers were tracking growth in the prevalence of mental health issues in the county. Accessing mental health services was a challenge for students, and service providers faced difficulty gaining greater access to clients. Concerned individuals within the schools and the community worked to connect the prevalence of mental health issues with challenges to academic performance. A partnership was formed between a local nonprofit counseling services agency and county school districts and resulted in the provision of school-based counseling.

Real and perceived implementation issues can prevent new collaborations from forming and prevent existing ones from moving beyond the information-sharing stage (Hodges & Videto, 2012). Lack of adequate or compatible infrastructure to support collaboration, such as technology and space, can pose challenges to implementing collaborations and partnerships. Differences in conditions and incentives for participation can also be a challenge to implementation (Bates et al., 2019; CMHS, 2015). For example, work schedules and expectations for attending work-related meetings outside core work hours may differ across existing and potential partners, posing barriers to the recruitment and retention of participants. Learning about the work expectations and work cultures of potential partners, exploring and communicating incentives for participation, and using technology may help.

Putting policy and initiatives into action is hard work that requires good planning, teamwork, and coordination with others outside the collaboration partners. Many stakeholders have been involved in collaborations that have not realized goals and objectives and initiatives that may have been developed but never enacted. These potential collaborators may see new collaborative initiatives as a waste of time. In these cases, new leadership and new collaborations may entice partners. Once operational, members of the collaboration need to work together to prioritize goals and objectives, focus on small achievable steps, and celebrate and publicize achievements.

Recruiting Partners for Collaborations

Recruiting partners from the district or school is an important consideration for creating effective collaborations. All school staff members, including faculty across disciplines, view themselves as serving students. Representatives of WSCC components, such as school food service directors, health education teachers, guidance counselors, and parent–teacher association representatives, are traditionally engaged in school activities and need to be considered for collaborative efforts. In addition, recruiting and including **education support professionals (ESPs)**, such as bus drivers, school food workers, custodians, or classroom paraprofessionals, and faculty such as special education teachers can provide different perspectives on factors affecting student health and academic performance critical to goal setting, program planning, and evaluation. ESPs are very visible and may observe different patterns of behaviors than what teachers see in a classroom, providing insights into student well-being

WSCC IN PRACTICE
Collaboration and Partnership in Massachusetts

The Brockton Healthy Schools Team, formed in February 2021, saw the extreme need for mental health resources and wellness support for students, parents, and other community members. As the Brockton Public Schools district navigated the challenges of remote learning, the wellness team began to research and vet resources, specifically mental health and food assistance resources, to share in the resource guide it was developing. This team partnered with Pinnacle Partnerships, a technical assistance provider for Massachusetts grantees, to produce a website resource with direct links to organizations and other communication products for the resource guide, and a print version of the guide to be shared with schools, community partners, and families. The Brockton Resource Area Guide project demonstrates the value of having a district-wide focus and highlights the importance of collaboration and partnership building. (CDC, 2022a, paras. 1-2)

(Long, 2022). Moreover, they often live in the community and also may be parents, and so have multiple perspectives to share (Pittman et al., 2020; Rosales, 2017a). ESPs can play an important role as partners and collaborators when intentionally included and respected (Capp et al., 2021; Long, 2022; Pittman et al., 2020; Rosales, 2017a, 2017b).

Partnerships and collaborations should strive to represent the demographics of the school district (Lewis, 2023). When individual partners and their organizations reflect the values and cultural and **socioeconomic** characteristics of the district and community, the resulting programs and policies are more likely to be successful (McMullen & Walton-Fisette, 2022; Pittman et al., 2020). In considering whom to involve in a partnership or coalition, one should reflect on and identify any preconceived notions one might have about who might want to be involved and to what extent and how potential partners might think about specific issues (Dewane, 2015). Taking a **solution-focused approach** to building a representative collaboration might mean, for example, minimizing language and cultural barriers by recruiting bilingual and **bicultural individuals** as partners, providing for interpretation during meetings, or providing translations of online and hard-copy school documents. Representatives of local health departments or agencies bring a community-wide perspective and access to skills and data that may not be easily available to school personnel, yet often schools believe these representatives do not have the time or interest to partner (Hodges & Videto, 2015).

Partnering and collaborating with only the usual suspects risks missing pieces of the picture important to successful efforts to support and improve student health and academics. The Healthy Schools Toolkit (Health Equity Works, 2022) suggests using social network analysis to aid in identifying key individuals for building partnerships. The toolkit provides a template and directions for conducting this type of analysis. A social network analysis can be particularly helpful for identifying ESPs and respected community members outside of official positions who could bring different perspectives valuable to WSCC assessment and program planning. When moving beyond the usual suspects it is important to plan for the full engagement of all members of the group. This may involve agreeing to such actions as meeting outside school hours, meeting in various locations in the community, and providing for virtual participation and transportation as necessary.

Implementing and Sustaining Collaborations

An initial set of partners have been identified and recruited for collaboration. Now what? Whether partners were identified and recruited for something as broad as "supporting the health and academic achievement of youth in this community" or as narrow as "addressing mental health issues in our youth," developing a statement of shared purpose needs to be an initial step (Mashek & Nanfito, 2015). Inviting, documenting, and considering the thoughts

---

Seeking Potential Partners for a WSCC Collaboration

1. Identify community agencies and organizations with a similar or shared vision, mission, or history.
2. Build a roster of individuals with an interest in health and youth within and outside these agencies and organizations. Ask others for suggestions. Ensure that the individuals and community agencies identified reflect the diverse demographics of the student population.
3. Invite participation in the collaboration. Review potential shared goals and benefits.
4. Conduct follow-up communication, confirm participation, and plan for an organizational meeting.

and perspectives of all partners in developing a shared purpose clarifies the issue or opportunity and the level of urgency needed for action. Establishing and documenting clear roles and responsibilities for partners invited to sit on councils, committees, or teams sets the stage for a more effective implementation process. It is recommended that an operating agreement be developed (Society for Public Health Education, 2020). Operating agreements define relationships among and outline the roles and responsibilities of group members. Whether a group is newly formed, or new members have been added to an existing group, previous efforts related to the purpose of the collaboration and their effectiveness, acceptance, and stakeholder support should be reviewed (Mashek & Nanfito, 2015). This may involve the review of existing documents such as meeting minutes, annual reports, evaluation reports, and recent community health improvement plans. These documents along with any recent health-related needs assessments can help the group further define its purpose.

An assessment of the levels of group and individual professional skills (e.g., in leadership, communication, technology) needed for the collaboration to be successful should be part of implementation. A plan for professional development and boosters can then be developed. Professional development activities not only help the collaboration function well but also can provide incentives for participation.

Developing a plan and a timeline for periodic check-ins of the elements of a successful collaboration should be part of implementation and will contribute to the success and sustainability of the initiative (RMC Health, 2020). This should include making time in meetings to check in on group dynamics and functioning.

Having coleaders will improve the **sustainability** of the collaboration (RMC Health, 2020). Staggering the terms of the coleaders will ensure the group always has an experienced leader. Periodically reassessing whether the right people are at the table is important in sustaining collaborations. As the goals and objectives of the collaboration's projects are met or as needs change, other groups and individuals may need to be added; moreover, some existing members may not have an interest in new directions. Sustainability can be supported by establishing protocols for how members are replaced.

Planning and taking actions to sustain a collaboration will contribute to improving and maintaining the health and academic performance of youth in the community. However, sometimes it is appropriate to disband a collaboration. How does one know when to wind down a collaboration? A clear indication it may be time to disband a specific collaboration is when the goals and objectives of the effort have been met. Celebrate the successes, thank the partners, and move on (RMC Health, 2020). A loss of stakeholder support for the collaboration and its activities, diminishing resources, lack of active participation by partner representatives, a lack of progress toward goals and objectives, and unresolved conflict among partners signal a need to seriously consider disbanding the group. Therefore, celebrate any successes, thank the partners, and move on.

Sample Collaboration Operating Agreement

- We, the group leaders, will create an agenda for every meeting and circulate it at least five days prior to the meeting. We will rotate responsibility for taking meeting minutes. Meeting minutes will be circulated no later than one week after the meeting.
- We will create a task list at every meeting.
- We will address conflict by talking directly and privately with the other person involved.
- We will make every effort to attend all team meetings. If we are absent, we will take responsibility to get caught up with team decisions within 48 hours.

Adapted from SOPHE (2020).

WSCC IN PRACTICE
Partners for Breakfast in the Classroom: Suggestions for Success

Some of the most successful breakfast after the bell programs are built on strong stakeholder engagement from the very start. They are also built on ensuring that all members of the school community know what to do, how to do it, and have the training and resources they need. Successful programs don't stop there—school stakeholders work hard to sustain the program, including making changes and adjustments as needed. Successful programs commit to communicating with families and the community on an ongoing basis. This includes providing them with information and soliciting their feedback on the program [involving the state or local affiliates of the organizations representing school staff]. (Partners for Breakfast in the Classroom, 2019, p. 1)

"Stakeholders include anyone who will be involved in the program, who can help support it, and who has an interest in feeding children" (p. 2). Such individuals include administrators, food service staff, teachers, para-educators, custodians, nurses, parents or guardians, and community anti-hunger advocates.

Summary

Strong collaborations among schools, families, and community members allow schools and communities to effectively support the health and academic development of youth. Building and sustaining successful collaborations and partnerships require a well-thought-out plan. The plan should consider how to overcome common barriers to the establishment and sustainability of coalitions and partnerships, involve wide representation from the community, include processes for identifying and developing skills needed by coalition members, and consider what assessment and evaluation data are needed and how they will be obtained and used.

LEARNING AIDS

GLOSSARY

ASCD's nine levers of school change—A series of nine levers identified by a team of ASCD evaluators that can change the culture of school communities to focus more on promoting health:

1. The principal as leader
2. Active and engaged leadership
3. Distributive leadership
4. Integration with the school improvement plan
5. Effective use of data for continuous school improvement
6. Ongoing and embedded professional development
7. Authentic and mutually beneficial community collaborations
8. Stakeholder support of the local efforts
9. The creation or modification of school policy related to the process

These levers work in concert to support the implementation and sustainability of efforts to advance the WSCC model.

bicultural individual—A person with the cultural attitudes, customs, history, and language of two peoples, groups, or nations.

collaboration—The act of working together for a common purpose or common goal in a relationship with shared power and trust.

credibility—The quality of being trustworthy.

education support professional (ESP)—The subgroup of employees in kindergarten through grade 12 or higher education who are not classroom teachers; this group may include persons in skilled trades, counselors, office support staff, nurses, and any others employed in the educational setting necessary to ensure quality education.

interrelatedness—A state of being mutually related or connected.

siloing—The case in which a group or department isolates itself from others in a way that restricts or hinders communication and cooperation. From the term *silo*.

social determinants—Conditions in which people are born or live that typically affect their health outcomes. These conditions and their outcomes are shaped by money, power, and resources.

socioecological approach—Involves individuals' interaction with and response to the environment around them and how these interactions affect society and the environment as a whole.

socioeconomic—Describes the interaction between the social and economic habits of a group of people.

solution-focused approach—A future-focused, goal-directed approach that highlights the importance of searching for solutions rather than focusing on problems.

sustainability—The ability to continue at a certain rate or level so as to maintain or support a process continuously over time.

systems approach—The use of different methods to achieve a goal through connections and interactions between subsystems of a whole.

APPLICATION ACTIVITIES

1. Select a community near you and, while reviewing the chamber of commerce website, state or national health and demographic data for the community, and school district websites, conduct a community audit. Identify agencies, institutions, and organizations in the community to which one could reach out for a potential collaboration. Determine the demographic breakdown so potential partners can be identified that reflect the makeup of the community. For each selection, write a three- to four-sentence rationale for why that organization would be a good source of partners. Then select faculty, staff, or administrators in the school district who would be potential partners for sitting on school teams or committees to support WSCC efforts.

2. Take the following communication for establishing a collaboration and customize the health and academic issues to represent a local school or district. Identify one local agency or organization that has a mission or agenda reflective of WSCC to which the script could be directed. Describe why you feel the agency you have selected would be a potential partner for working with the school or district on advancing the WSCC model.

Our recent school health assessment found the following health issue _____ and the following academic issue _____ . We know that this is also an area of concern for you and your agency. We would like to work together with you to improve this situation. We are meeting next week to discuss what steps we can take to move forward. Can we count on your help?

3. Interview two local school or district administrators and ask about collaboration success stories or successful strategies they have used in the past. Develop a presentation for the class and share those successes.

REFERENCES

Abt Associates. (2016, October). *Successful school-based partnerships: What does it take?* https://williampennfoundation.org/sites/default/files/reports/Successful%20School-Based%20Partnerships_What%20Does%20it%20Take_%20Oct%202016%20high%20res.pdf

Action for Healthy Kids. (2020). *Collaborating for healthy schools: Building an effective school-family partnership.* www.actionforhealthykids.org/wp-content/uploads/2020/11/AFHK-Collaboration-Guide-FINAL.pdf

Adelman, H., & Taylor, L. (2011). Expanding school improvement policy to better address barriers to learning. *Policy Futures in Education, 9*(3), 431-446. https://doi.org/10.2304/pfie.2011.9.3.4

ASCD. (2010). *Healthy school communities.* www.ascd.org/ASCD/pdf/siteASCD/products/healthyschools/ltl_may2010.pdf

ASCD. (2015). *About the Whole Child approach.* www.wholechildeducation.org/about

Bandura, A.C. (1986). *Social foundations of thought and action: A social cognitive theory.* Prentice Hall.

Bates, S.M., Mellin, E., Paluta, L.M., Anderson-Butcher, D., Vogeler, M., & Sterling, K. (2019). Examining the influence of interprofessional team collaboration on student-level outcomes through school-community partnerships. *Children and Schools, 41*(2), 111-122. https://doi.org/10.1093/cs/cdz001

Bronfenbrenner, U. (1979). *The ecology of human development: Experiments by nature and design.* Harvard University Press.

California School Boards Association. (2009). *Building healthy communities: A school leaders guide to collaboration and community engagement.* www.saferoutespartnership.org/resources/toolkit-report-case-study/building-healthy-communities

Capp, G.P., Astor, R.A., & Moore, H. (2021). Positive school climate for school staff? The roles of administrators, staff beliefs, and school organization in high and low resource school districts. *Journal of Community Psychology, 50,* 1060-1082. https://doi.org/10.1002/jcop.22701

Center for Communities That Care. (2022). *The science behind the programs.* www.communitiesthatcare.net/prevention-science/

Center for Mental Health in Schools at UCLA. (2015). *Working collaboratively: From school-based teams to school-community connections. Introductory packet.* http://smhp.psych.ucla.edu/pdfdocs/worktogether/worktogether.pdf

Centers for Disease Control and Prevention. (2022a). *Massachusetts.* www.cdc.gov/healthyschools/achievement_stories/massachusetts.htm

Centers for Disease Control and Prevention. (2022b). *Whole School, Whole Community, Whole Child (WSCC).* www.cdc.gov/healthyschools/wscc/index.htm

Dewane, C.J. (2015). Solution-focused supervision: A go-to approach. *Social Work Today, 15*(5), 24.

Ferguson, C., Jordan, C., & Baldwin, M. (2010). *Working systematically in action: Engaging family and community.* Southwest Educational Development Laboratory. https://sedl.org/ws/ws-fam-comm.pdf

Green, T.L. (2018). School as community, community as school: Examining principal leadership for urban school reform and community development. *Education and Urban Society, 50*(2), 111-135.

Grier, B.C., & Bradley-King, K.L. (2011). Collaborative consultation to support children with pediatric health issues: A review of the biopsychoeducational model. *Journal of Educational and Psychological Consultation, 21*(2), 88-105. https://doi.org/10.1080/10474412.2011.571522

Health Equity Works. (2022). *Healthy schools toolkit.* Washington University in St. Louis. https://healthyschoolstoolkit.wustl.edu/

Hodges, B., & Videto, D. (2012, November 1). *Connecting silos: Uniting institutions for healthy schools and communities* [Webinar]. American Association for Health Education.

Hodges, B., & Videto, D. (2015, November 2). *School-community collaborations improve school health systems: Results from the School Health Systems Change Project* [Conference session]. American Public Health Association Annual Meeting, Chicago, IL, United States.

Hodges, B., Videto, D.M., & Greeley, A. (2011, October 13). *Working to create limitless possibilities in limited environments* [Conference session]. American School Health Association Conference, Louisville, KY, United States.

Howley, N.L., & Hunt, H. (2020). Every school healthy: Policy, research, and action. *Journal of School Health, 90*(12), 903-906.

Hunt, P., Barrios, L., Telljohan, S.K., & Mazyck, D. (2015). A whole school approach: Collaborative development of school health policies, processes, and practices. *Journal of School Health, 85*(11), 802-809. https://doi.org/10.1111/josh.12305

Kolbe, L.J. (2019). School health as a strategy to improve both public health and education. *Annual Review of Public Health, 40*, 443-463.

Lewis, A. (2023). Getting to institutional level change. *ASCD Educational Leadership, 80*(6). www.ascd.org/el/articles/getting-to-institutional-level-change

Lohman, M.J., Hathcote, A.R., & Boothe, K.A. (2018). Addressing the barriers to family-school collaboration: A brief review of the literature and recommendations. *International Journal of Early Childhood Special Education, 10*(1), 25-31. https://doi.org/10.20489/intjecse.454424

Long, C. (2022, May 10). Education support professionals often first to see student mental health struggles. *NEA Today*. www.nea.org/advocating-for-change/new-from-nea/education-support-professionals-often-first-see-student-mental-health-struggles

Mashek, D., & Nanfito, M. (2015). *People tools and processes that build collaborative capacity*. www.researchgate.net/profile/Debra-Mashek/publication/284672867_People_Tools_and_Processes_that_Build_Collaborative_Capacity/links/5655efcd08aefe619b1cf505/People-Tools-and-Processes-that-Build-Collaborative-Capacity.pdf

McMullen, J., & Walton-Fisette, J. (2022). Equity-minded community involvement and family engagement strategies for health and physical educators. *Journal of Physical Education, Recreation and Dance, 93*(2), 46-50. https://doi.org/10.1080/07303084.2022.2020055

National School Climate Center. (2017). *Connecting communities of courage: Building inclusive, safe, and engaging schools—A summit recap report*. https://schoolclimate.org/wp-content/uploads/2021/05/NSCC_SummitRecap.pdf

New York City Department of Education. (2022). *School-based health centers*. www.schools.nyc.gov/school-life/health-and-wellness/school-based-health-centers

Ng'andu, J., & Elstein, J. (2020). A vision for healthy schools: Children and families at the center. *Journal of School Health, 90*(12), 901-902.

Partners for Breakfast in the Classroom. (2019, November). *Best practices: Tips for teachers and education support professionals*. https://live-breakfastintheclassroom.pantheonsite.io/wp-content/uploads/2019/11/BP_Tips_for_Teachers_and_ESPs_Final.pdf

Pittman, K., Moroney, D.A., Irby, M., & Young, J. (2020). Unusual suspects: The people inside and outside of school who matter in Whole School, Whole Community, Whole Child efforts. *Journal of School Health, 90*(12), 1038-1044. https://doi.org/10.1111/josh.12966

RMC Health. (2020). *The guidebook: Creating a culture of learning and health*. www.rmc.org/wp-content/uploads/2020/01/District-Level-Destination.pdf

Rooney, L.E., Videto, D.M., & Birch, D.A. (2015). Using the Whole School, Whole Community, Whole Child model: Implications for practice. *Journal of School Health, 85*(11), 817-823. https://doi.org/10.1111/josh.12304

Rosales, J. (2017a). Positive school cultures thrive when support staff included. *NEA Today*. www.nea.org/advocating-for-change/new-from-nea/positive-school-cultures-thrive-when-support-staff-included

Rosales, J. (2017b). School custodians help students through mentoring—one at a time. *NEA Today*. www.nea.org/advocating-for-change/new-from-nea/school-custodians-help-students-through-mentoring-one-time

Sepanik, S., & Brown, K.T. (2021, November). *School-community partnerships: Solutions for educational equity through social and emotional well-being*. MDRC. https://eric.ed.gov/?id=ED616007

Society for Public Health Education. (2020). *WSCC team: Teams training script: Organizing for success: Establishing your Whole School, Whole Community, Whole Child (WSCC) team*. www.sophe.org/wp-content/uploads/2020/03/SOPHE-WSCC-Script-Teams.pdf

Videto, D.M., & Dake, J.A. (2019). Promoting health literacy by defining and measuring quality school health education. *Health Promotion Practice, 20*(6), 824-833.

Weist, M.P., Mellin, E.A., Chambers, K.L., Lever, N.A., Haber, D., & Blaber, C. (2012). Challenges to collaboration in school mental health and strategies for overcoming them. *Journal of School Health, 82*(2), 97-105. https://doi.org/10.1111/j.1746-1561.2011.00672.x

Willgerodt, M.A., Walsh, E., & Maloy, C. (2021). A scoping review of the Whole School, Whole Community, Whole Child model. *Journal of School Nursing, 37*(1), 61-68.

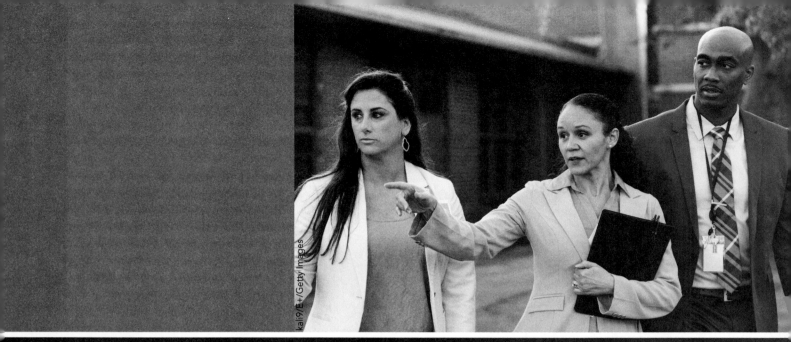

CHAPTER 7

Planning and Evaluating WSCC

Donna M. Videto • Bonni C. Hodges

LEARNING OBJECTIVES

1. Examine the role of a needs assessment and asset analysis approach to prepare for program planning for Whole School, Whole Community, Whole Child actions.
2. Describe the three actions recommended for program planning along with examples of data collected in each action.
3. Analyze the four methods of data collection and match them to the types of data being collected (primary, secondary, qualitative, and quantitative).
4. Explain the steps in the Centers for Disease Control and Prevention's framework for program evaluation.
5. Analyze considerations for developing process and outcome evaluation questions.

The authors sincerely thank Robert F. Valois for contributing certain content in this chapter to the first edition of this book.

KEY TERMS

Academic performance data
CDC framework for program evaluation
External evaluator
Focus group
Formative evaluation
Impact evaluation
Institutionalizing
Internal evaluator
Key informant interview
Logic model
Needs assessment and asset analysis
Outcome evaluation
PRECEDE–PROCEED model
Primary data
Process evaluation
Program evaluation
Qualitative data
Quantitative data
School district health and wellness profile
Secondary data
Snowball sampling
Summative evaluation
Windshield tour
Youth Risk Behavior Surveillance System (YRBSS)

This chapter begins by describing how to conduct a **needs assessment and asset analysis** and then moves to the analysis of the assessment data for the creation of a comprehensive school district health and wellness profile. The resulting profile serves as a foundation for planning programs to advance the Whole School, Whole Community, Whole Child (WSCC) model. The actions described in this chapter should be the work of a planning committee under the direction of a school health coordinator, if one has been identified at this point. For the process to be effective, it is important to appoint a coordinator to oversee the 10 WSCC components and to facilitate the planning process and beyond (Centers for Disease Control and Prevention [CDC], 2019b). The chapter also addresses planning for how to monitor programs once put into place and then how to evaluate the outcome of the efforts being used to build or enhance WSCC efforts. Note that the word *programs* is used in this chapter as an inclusive word covering practices, policies, and processes as well as programs.

A recommended set of actions is presented to help planners identify data sources, obtain and collect data, and analyze and interpret the assessment data. The steps presented in this chapter serve as a framework for planning WSCC-related activities with the use of the **PRECEDE–PROCEED model**, which is designed to facilitate the development of programming to address a health problem or problems through a step-by-step process (Center for Community Health and Development [Center for Community], 2023a; Green & Kreuter, 2005). The evaluation of WSCC programs through the use of steps adopted from the **CDC framework for program evaluation** (CDC, 2017) is presented as well.

Systematic Planning

The WSCC approach requires the identification and coordination of numerous assets and health and wellness systems within schools, districts, and communities. Program planning models are important tools for ensuring a systematic planning approach and helping districts or schools plan for and assess initial or expanded WSCC efforts while determining the best path forward. The needs assessment and asset analysis, which are the first step in high-quality program planning, should be comprehensive enough to identify the multiple avenues linking school health and academic performance by including information about the community in which the district and its schools are located, in addition to systems that work within the school and district (Hodges & Videto, 2011). Using a planning model can help guarantee that the scope of the needs assessment and asset analysis is broad enough to capture the full picture of WSCC-linked gaps or needs to possibly fill as well as assets that could support programming efforts (Green & Kreuter, 2005; National Healthy Schools Collaborative, 2022).

A comprehensive **school district health and wellness profile** includes community, health, and academic data compiled from a variety of sources during the needs assessment and asset analysis. The profile identifies school health and community assets and needs that are suggested by the data. It can assist in illustrating connections between health and academic performance, reveal district and community assets that can be built on to improve health and academic performance, and provide a platform for the establishment of more efficient and effective school health systems and collaborations (CDC, 2023b; Hunt et al., 2015). A list of potential needs and assets to consider is presented later in this chapter in the section titled A Word About Data and Their Use.

Conducting a needs assessment and asset analysis that results in the creation of an extensive profile of the school district's health and wellness systems is a critical initial step in WSCC planning. It is essential for schools and districts to identify needs or gaps and what they already have in place across the WSCC components, using multiple information collection strategies where feasible, before making program and policy recommendations and implementing further action (Hunt et al., 2015; Rooney et al., 2015). A variety of existing instruments or tools that provide relatively user-friendly frameworks for looking at the components of WSCC are described in this chapter. It has been our experience as practitioners, consultants, researchers, and professors in school health that schools and districts often select and use only one, if any, of the popular tools used to assess the components of WSCC (see table 7.1). Using multiple tools and infor-

TABLE 7.1 WSCC-Related Assessment Tools

Assessment	Assessment focus	Source
School Health Index (SHI; 2017 edition)	Online self-assessment and planning tool to improve health and safety programs and policies	CDC
School Improvement Tool (SIT)	Online assessment of Whole Child tenets and indicators along with WSCC model components	ASCD
WellSAT 3.0	Online tool to assess and improve school district wellness policies	Partnership between the University of Connecticut (UConn) Rudd Center for Food Policy and Health and UConn's Collaboratory on School and Child Health
WellSAT-I (2021)	Interview that measures how fully a district or school is implementing wellness practices; the WellSAT-I is designed to be used with the WellSAT 3.0	
WellSAT WSCC 2.0	Comprehensive online tool to assess policies related to each of the 10 WSCC components	
CDC Health Education Curriculum Analysis Tool (HECAT)	Assessment tool to help school districts assess school health curriculum and related policies	CDC
Physical Education Curriculum Analysis Tool (PE-CAT)	Assessment tool to help school districts assess physical education curriculum and related policies	CDC
Youth Risk Behavior Surveillance System (YRBSS)	System of surveys at the national and local levels that monitors six categories of health-related behaviors that contribute to the leading causes of death and disability among youth and adults	CDC
SCHOOL CLIMATE ASSESSMENTS		
Education School Climate Survey (EDSCLS)	School climate surveys for middle and high school students, instructional staff, non-instructional staff, and parents or guardians that measure three domains of school climate: engagement, safety, and environment	U.S. Department of Education
Comprehensive School Climate Inventory (CSCI)	Nationally recognized school climate survey that provides an in-depth profile of a school's community strengths as well as areas in need of improvement	National School Climate Center at Ramapo for Children

Adapted from Videto and Dake (2019); ASCD (2023); CDC (2023a); National School Climate Center (2021); U.S. Department of Education (2023).

mation-gathering strategies together to assist in school health planning will enable a more holistic look at gaps and strengths related to WSCC efforts, setting the stage for programs and policies best suited to the school or district (Center for Community, 2023f; Rooney et al., 2015).

The job of constructing an extensive health system and wellness profile of a school district and the communities it serves may seem overwhelming to school district personnel. This initial task should not be the responsibility of one person. Schools or districts should use their school health coordinator, school health advisory council, school health team, or other similar groups to plan and direct the construction of the profile. The roles of the school health coordinator, school health advisory councils, and school health teams are discussed in more detail in chapter 8. Representatives of local health departments and health-related agencies are important collaborators for consideration on the council and teams because they can identify and provide access to useful information and data and often have experience in conducting needs assessments (Rooney et al., 2015).

In addition, collaborations between school districts and higher education institutions can provide the guidance and assistance needed to undertake the comprehensive assessment necessary to develop the profile as well as to develop and then implement the evaluation plan (Center for Community, 2023f; Rooney et al., 2015). The district or school needs to decide early on whether to work with an **internal** or **external evaluator**; evaluator selection may depend on available resources as the hiring of an external evaluator may come at a high cost. Seeking a volunteer evaluator from a local college or university may help to keep such costs down and provide a more objective option than an internal evaluator. The evaluation plan will need to be put into motion as implementation begins and therefore needs to be developed once the evaluator has been selected and the initial assessment data have been collected and analyzed (Center for Community, 2023e).

Creating a Comprehensive Profile for Program Planning

Comprehensive school district health and wellness profiles need to identify and include the multitude of factors that contribute to the health and academic success of students. The PRECEDE portion of the PRECEDE–PROCEED framework provides useful guidance for identifying districtwide and school building–based health-related assets and needs required for quality WSCC-related program planning (Center for Community, 2023a; Green & Kreuter, 2005).

WSCC IN PRACTICE

Kentucky Healthy Schools Needs Assessment and Professional Development

With CDC support, the Kentucky Healthy Schools team began a multiyear systemic process of planning, implementing, and evaluating professional development to expand WSCC efforts across the state. During the first year, a professional development needs assessment was administered to school nurses, food service directors, district and school administrators, teachers, and so on in selected school districts. The following are some of the key findings from that needs assessment:

- June and July were the preferred months for professional development.
- Tuesday, Wednesday, and Thursday were the preferred days of the week for professional development.
- The three most preferred methods of professional development were a three-hour face-to-face training, a one-hour virtual session, and a six-hour face-to-face training (Kentucky Department of Education, 2020).

PRECEDE helps to identify specific data points needed for inclusion in the profiles. This half of the model includes four phases of data gathering useful in developing a comprehensive school health and wellness profile. Figure 7.1 shows examples of such data points.

FIGURE 7.1 PRECEDE FRAMEWORK SAMPLE DATA POINTS

Social Assessment Data Points (Phase 1)

Community

Demographic data and trend data
Socioeconomic data and trend data
Employment rates and trend data
Crime rates and trend data
Housing characteristics
Land area and geographic characteristics
Local government structure
Community resources: health, educational, other
Community engagement: rates, civic organization membership, community events attendance

School District

District student demographic information and trend data
District and school building needs designation
Free or reduced lunch enrollment and trend data
Academic performance and trend data
Students with disabilities classification rates and trend data
Students with special needs rates and trend data
Graduation and college enrollment rates and trend data

Epidemiological, Behavioral, and Environmental Assessment Data Points (Phase 2)

Morbidity and mortality data (incidence, prevalence, death rates, and trends)
Adult and youth health-related behavior information, including Behavioral Risk Factor Surveillance System and Youth Risk Behavior Surveillance System data
Environmental contributors to morbidity and mortality priorities

Educational and Ecological Assessment Data Points (Phase 3)

Predisposing

Knowledge of health condition and its contributing factors
Attitudes toward health condition and its contributing factors
Beliefs and perceptions of health condition and its contributing factors
Confidence in one's ability to engage in health-enhancing behaviors

Reinforcing

Health-enhancing and health-risk behaviors modeled by peers, important others (e.g., teachers, parents, caregivers, coaches), and media
Levels of social support for health-enhancing behaviors
Cultural expectations
Reinforcement of health-enhancing and health-risk behaviors

> *continued*

FIGURE 7.1 > continued

Enabling

Levels of health-related skills

Opportunities for students to practice healthy behaviors and skills during the school day

Enforcement of existing WSCC, wellness, and health-related policies and procedures

Availability and accessibility of health services and health education

Administrative and Policy Diagnosis Data Points (Phase 4)

School district structure

WSCC organization and leadership

WSCC implementation and function

Level of integration of WSCC with academic mission and planning

WSCC resources: faculty and staff, funding, collaborations, educational resources

Knowledge of, attitudes toward, and perceptions of WSCC and its tenets among faculty, staff, administrators, and parents

Perceptions of the role of schools in the health of youth

Perceptions of the role of schools in the health of the community

Attitudes of school administrators, staff, and parents regarding the role of being healthy in students' academic success

Strength of belief in the tie between health and academic performance

Support of WSCC initiatives among school administrators, staff, parents, and community members

Resources designated for WSCC

Intraschool and extraschool communication systems and efficacy

Level of WSCC coordination skill

Adapted from Center for Community Health and Development (2023a); Green and Kreuter (2005); Rooney et al. (2015).

Because school districts can be considered both as part of communities and communities unto themselves, it is useful to gather information on social indicators for the communities a district serves as well as school-specific district indicators. This action will assist planners in identifying social assets and needs that represent or are affected by health-related situations in the school and the community. Under *social assessment* (phase 1 in figure 7.1), a list of community and school-specific data sources is presented that can reveal broad assets and needs within a community and a school district. It is important to consider both current data and trend data from the past several years. Trend data allow a look at whether a situation is getting better, getting worse, or staying the same and are important in determining priorities for programming efforts (Center for Community, 2023a; CDC, 2023b).

Epidemiological, behavioral, and environmental assessment (phase 2 in figure 7.1) indicates the need to gather specific health-related data on youth and adults. Information about the types and spread of illness and other health problems in school district communities, as well as causes of death and death rates for specific health problems, is needed to set health priorities to be addressed through WSCC programming. Adult morbidity and mortality data can guide decisions regarding prevention (Center for Community, 2023a; CDC, 2023b). Data on morbidity and mortality may be found in reports such as community health assessments or community health improvement plans developed by county or local health departments, often in conjunction with local hospitals (National Association of County and City Health Officials, 2022).

Data collected by school nurses on student conditions, screening results, and health indicators provide a more specific picture of the health status of youth in schools. Data that provide information on the incidence and prevalence of mental and emotional health diagnoses among students are included in the *epidemiological, behavioral, and environmental phase*. School and community environmental factors along with behavioral contributors to these health conditions should also be determined (Rooney et al., 2015).

Most WSCC programs and policies are directed at changing those factors that contribute to behaviors and environments responsible for elevated levels of morbidity and mortality—addressing those factors is key to improving academic performance. A district or school must determine which factors contribute most to behavioral and environmental challenges to health in the district or school to identify specific and realistic targets for change. These contributors in the *educational and ecological assessment* (phase 3 in figure 7.1) include access to and affordability of services, social support and modeling, skill levels, and policy enforcement, along with knowledge, attitudes, and beliefs associated with behaviors and environments that compromise health (CDC, 2018; Rooney et al., 2015).

The administrative and policy diagnosis (phase 4 in figure 7.1) provides direction for looking at current structures within the district, policies, leadership, existing collaborations, and resources. It is important in this phase to review information from the initial identification of assets already in place across the WSCC components. In addition, it is useful to examine the knowledge of, attitudes toward, and perceptions of school health among school faculty, staff, administrators, students, parents, family members, guardians, and community members to help explain the existing level of WSCC and the five Whole Child tenets (Center for Community, 2023a; CDC, 2023b). Among the questions to be pursued are the following:

- Is there accurate understanding of what school health is and can be?
- What is the existing level of support for school health?
- What resources are currently available for school health?
- What skills do people directly and indirectly associated with school health have or need that can be built on or developed?
- Which WSCC components are implemented fully? Partially? Not at all?
- Which components are included in collaborations?

Actions for Collecting Needs Assessment Profile Data

The needs assessment and asset analysis data points described in the PRECEDE framework can be collected through a series of three actions for locating existing data and collecting additional data:

- *Action 1.* Collect information and data to develop an understanding of school and community health and academic needs and assets. (PRECEDE phases 1-3)
- *Action 2.* Conduct a district and school wellness policy review. (PRECEDE phase 4)
- *Action 3.* Review current WSCC implementation levels. (PRECEDE phase 4)

The three actions described here to identify and collect the data on needs and assets are suggested as ways to organize and conduct the assessment and complete the data collection for the school district health and wellness profile, thus setting the stage for informed policy, process, and program planning. Data-gathering strategies need to provide breadth and depth yet also need to be acceptable to and achievable by school personnel. A review of the professional literature, consultation with state education department staff members and local or county health department staff, and discussions with public school administrators and staff are useful avenues for informing the data-gathering procedure (Center for Community, 2023g; CDC, 2023b). Table 7.2 provides an overview of a general process we have used in several public school districts to collect the necessary information for developing the school district health and wellness profile.

TABLE 7.2 Actions for Developing a School District Health and Wellness Profile

Action	Data-gathering activities
1. Develop an understanding of the school and community	Review of documents in the public domain, review of existing data reports • Demographic information • Vital statistics • Crime rates • Local government structure • Community issues and initiatives • Epidemiological data • Health and human services resources • School structure and function • Academic performance data • Windshield tour • Physical environment data
2. Conduct a wellness policy review	WellSAT assessment
3. Review WSCC implementation	CDC School Health Index assessment Review of existing report(s) Interviews with key informants • School district personnel • Parents and families • Youth • Community members Focus group discussions • School district personnel • Parents and families • Youth • Community members

Action 1: Develop an Understanding of the School and Community

It is necessary to develop an understanding of the school district, the youth within the district, and the surrounding community to understand the context in which the school district functions. Community assets can be leveraged by school health programs through collaborations to assist in addressing the needs of the school and the nearby communities. This action begins with the generation of a list of necessary information about the youth, the school district, and the communities it serves. Figure 7.1 and table 7.2 serve as general guidelines, but data specific to the communities and district need to be identified within the broad categories listed. After the data list is finalized, potential sources for the information on the list are brainstormed. The state education department, school district, and local government and health-related agency stakeholders should be consulted to refine, validate, and finalize potential sources of information. Community understanding can be built largely through existing documents and information in the public domain, yet the most recent or current information needs to be accessed. Connecting with stakeholders may reveal sources of information and documents not generally known but that will be useful, such as internal reports from community agencies that may not be posted online. After the data list and sources have been finalized, the data can be obtained. Community demographic and public health data are easily obtained through federal, state, and local government websites, such as those for departments of labor; city or county legislatures; and state, county, and local health departments. Websites or hard copy documents of the local chamber of commerce, local and regional newspapers, local health and human service agencies, local health care providers, and local telephone directories are also good data sources (Center for Community, 2023a; CDC, 2023b; Rooney et al., 2015).

Given the nature of school district structure and functioning, some district-related data—but not all—are publicly available and easy to find and obtain. For example, **academic performance data** (such as student assessment results) can often be obtained through either the district website or state education department school report cards. School district websites should be accessed and reviewed for other pertinent information. When available, district or school newsletters and board of education minutes for the past three to five years should be reviewed for trends, issues, and initiatives. Providing key administrators and staff with a list of information needed from the school district will often produce the required data (Center for Community, 2023a; CDC, 2023b; Rooney et al., 2015). See chapter 4 for more on academic data and links to WSCC.

School districts should be asked to provide information and documents related to district and school health structure and functioning. Specifically, requests should be made to districts for the most current district wellness policy; any policies related to alcohol, tobacco, and other drugs; policies on parent involvement; nutrition and food service policies, school health services policies, and any additional local health-related policies; a diagram of the reporting hierarchy and governance structure of the district; available district data on student health, including mental, social, and emotional health as well as social-emotional learning; student behavioral health data (Youth Risk Behavior Survey [YRBS] data or other reports); school climate data; and the most recent School Health Index (SHI) or School Improvement Tool data and report if one has been done within the past two to three years (CDC, 2019a, 2023c; Hunt et al., 2015).

Systematic **windshield tours** of school districts and the communities associated with them provide a way to get a sense of the physical environment and to confirm some of the existing data. Windshield tours are conducted by driving throughout the community and recording notable observations about the environment, such as the quantity and quality of walkways, playgrounds, parks, restaurants, and food stores (Center for Community, 2023d).

WSCC IN PRACTICE
Using Assessment Tools to Improve a District Wellness Policy

This case study involving assessment tools took place in Buffalo, the second largest urban school district in New York State. Tools such as the YRBS, the WellSAT, and the SHI were used to ensure a "strong equitable wellness policy" (p. 1045) and to improve health and education outcomes for students. The school district's Whole Child Health Committee created a wellness policy shaped by the WSCC model and used the WellSAT 3.0 to assess the policy. The wellness policy is assessed every three years with the most recent edition of the WellSAT and feedback from stakeholders and school well-being teams prior to final revisions and adoption by the board of education (Baldwin & Ventresca, 2020).

Action 2: Conduct a Wellness Policy Review

The Child Nutrition and WIC Reauthorization Act, mandated by Congress in 2004 (Food Research and Action Center, 2022), required school districts that participate in federal school meal programs to create and implement school wellness policies by 2006. The policies needed to address nutrition education, nutrition standards for foods sold, and physical activity. All policies needed to include measures for evaluating the effectiveness of the policy (Rudd

Center, 2021). Although new legislation is due, the program continues to operate (Food Research and Action Center, 2022). One tool for conducting this evaluation is the WellSAT 3.0, an assessment tool that can provide districts with guidance and resources for making improvements to strengthen existing wellness policies based on best practices (Rudd Center, 2021).

Wellness policies are available through either school district websites or district office administrators. Although one person can conduct the review using the WellSAT or another assessment tool, ideally the review should be conducted by more than one individual, such as by members of the school health advisory council, the school health or wellness team, or a team of researchers and administrators. We recommend that, if possible, two different individuals conduct the assessment, then compare the WellSAT scores and reach a consensus on ratings for each of the sections, which include the following:

- Nutrition education
- Standards for U.S. Department of Agriculture child nutrition programs and school meals
- Nutrition standards for competitive and other foods and beverages
- Physical education and activity
- Wellness promotion and marketing
- Implementation, evaluation, and communication (Rudd Center, 2021)

Other tools or processes may be useful for conducting a wellness policy review; we have used the WellSAT 3.0, and our experience is described in this chapter. A WellSAT WSCC tool (which differs from the WellSAT 3.0) that assesses districtwide policies in each of the 10 components of WSCC is available for conducting a broader policy review and is offered through the University of Connecticut's Institute for Collaboration on Health, Intervention, and Policy in conjunction with the Rudd Center (2021). The school or district conducting the review will need to select what works best for meeting its needs and provides the necessary data for this action.

Action 3: Review WSCC Implementation

A specific systematic assessment of the current or potential level of implementation and functioning is a critical component of planning for WSCC. The SHI is an assessment and planning tool that districts or schools can use to improve health and safety policies and programs by using the self-assessment modules that reflect the 10 components of WSCC. The SHI also takes the district and school through a process that involves planning for making improvements to any existing WSCC approach (CDC, 2019b).

Districts and school buildings that either have never undertaken an assessment using the SHI or a similar tool or have not completed one in the past three years should conduct such an assessment. See table 7.1 for assessment tools available at the national level; state or local options may also be available. The WellSAT-I, which is an interview that helps measure how fully a school or district is implementing wellness practices and is designed to be used in combination with the WellSAT 3.0, is also a tool to consider using for this action (University of Connecticut, n.d.). When selecting a tool for conducting the assessment, the team should consider the following:

- Available resources, such as the time, cost, and equipment needed to complete and process the survey and the availability of personnel required to complete the survey
- Linkage, or the idea that the items covered on the survey match the assessment needs
- The match or link between characteristics of the survey population, the wording and formatting of items, and data collection goals
- The age of existing data (if data are recent, then a new survey may not be needed)

In addition to using assessment tools during the WSCC implementation process, taking the time to talk with people about school health can unearth previously unidentified assets and needs, reveal potential barriers to expanding or **institutionalizing** school health within the school structure and community, and provide context for priority setting. **Key informant interviews** and **focus groups** involving people from the school district and the communities it serves are suggested (Center for Community, 2023c).

Key Informant Interviews

Carrying out key informant interviews is a common practice when collecting baseline data or conducting a needs assessment (CDC, 2023b). A key informant is a person in the community or school district who has direct knowledge of a group or has access to information about a group (Center for Community, 2023c). A school district can be asked to provide a list of names of key school, parent, family, youth, and community contacts for interviews. Some recommended participants for interviews include the school district superintendent, the school nurse, school principals, faculty leaders, parent–teacher organization officers, local government officials, the head of the chamber of commerce, student group leaders, and others.

Key informant interviews may be conducted in person, via videoconferencing software, or by telephone. It is recommended that interviews be recorded, once permission is obtained, so exact responses will be available during data analysis. See figure 7.2 for a list of sample key informant interview questions to ask during the interviews.

FIGURE 7.2   KEY INFORMANT INTERVIEW QUESTIONS

Questions for All Informants (except students; see Student-Specific Questions)

Q1: When I say the term *school health*, what do you think I am referring to?

Q2: On a scale from 1 (extremely poor) to 5 (outstanding), where would you place the general health of students in your district? Faculty and staff? The greater community? Why?

Q3: What policies does the district have that support a broad range of health and wellness programs and services?

Q4: Does the district or your school building use a shared decision-making process? If yes, is shared decision-making done with school health issues? Describe how that might be done.

Q5: Does the district actively plan and build partnerships with the community (groups)? If so, would you consider this systematic planning? Why or why not? If so, are any partnerships associated with school health? What are they?

Q6: Can you point to and share examples of how the current school health system contributes to positive health outcomes for students? Faculty and staff? Parents? The greater community?

Q7: Can you point to and share examples of something that occurs within the current school district or building that you believe might have a negative effect on student learning?

Q8: With regard to school health in this district or building, what works particularly well? What is in particular need of improvement?

Q9: How important do you think having good health is to being a successful student?

Q10: Does the district or specific buildings have health or wellness councils? If so, who sits on them? List their titles or the type of people. Who facilitates them?

Q11: Does the district or specific buildings have leadership teams that meet on a regular basis to address health, mental health, and safety issues? How do these leadership groups differ from any health or wellness council? What types of issues do they address?

Q12: Do health or wellness school teams write annual or five-year program plans that contain goals and objectives? If so, describe how goals and objectives are selected.

> continued

FIGURE 7.2 > continued

Parent-Specific Questions

PQ13: Describe how your child's school contributes to his or her health.

PQ14: How important do you think having good health is to being a successful student?

PQ15: How are parents involved in creating a healthy school building or district?

PQ16: What makes it easy to get involved in creating a healthy school building or district?

PQ17: What makes it difficult to get involved in creating a healthy school building or district?

PQ18: What do you see as the role of school districts or buildings in creating healthy youth and adolescents?

PQ19: What do you see as the role of school districts or buildings in creating healthy communities?

Community Leader–Specific Questions

CLQ13: How are community members who are not parents of students involved in creating a healthy school building or district?

CLQ14: What stands in the way of community members who are not parents of students from getting involved in creating a healthy school building or district?

CLQ15: What do you see as the role of school districts or buildings in creating healthy youth and adolescents?

CLQ16: What do you see as the role of school districts or buildings in creating healthy communities?

Student-Specific Questions

SQ1: When I say the term *school health*, what do you think I am referring to?

SQ2: On a scale from 1 (horrible) to 5 (outstanding), where would you place the general health of other students in your district? Faculty and staff? The greater community? Why?

SQ3: Can you point to and share examples of how the current school health system contributes to positive health outcomes for students? Faculty and staff? Parents? The greater community?

SQ4: Can you point to and share examples of something that occurs within the current school district or building that you believe might have a negative effect on student learning?

SQ5: With regard to school health in this district or building, what works particularly well? What is in particular need of improvement?

SQ6: What do you see as the role of school districts or buildings in creating healthy youth and adolescents?

SQ7: What do you see as the role of school districts or buildings in creating healthy communities?

SQ8: How important do you think having good health is to being a successful student?

SQ9: Does the district or specific buildings have health or wellness councils? If so, who sits on them? List their titles or the type of people. Who facilitates them?

SQ10: How are students involved in creating a healthy school building or district?

SQ11: What makes it easy to get involved in creating a healthy school building or district?

SQ12: What makes it difficult to get involved in creating a healthy school building or district?

Focus Groups

Focus groups are frequently used in health education. Hosting a focus group is a qualitative approach to learning about an intended audience (Center for Community, 2023b). Hodges and Videto (2011) recommended running several focus groups representing subgroups of the population as part of the needs assessment process. School district and community agency personnel can be requested to use **snowball sampling** to provide contacts for setting up focus group discussions with groups representing members of the community; parents, families, youth, and guardians; and school faculty, staff, and administrators (Kennedy-Shaffer et al., 2021). Focus group questions are developed to elicit participants' understanding and perceptions of the strengths and challenges of school health.

Focus groups of parents and school faculty, staff, and administrators should be conducted at both the elementary and secondary levels. Focus groups of students at the elementary and secondary levels can also be helpful. Focus group facilitators should have training in the use of follow-up questions, the need to ask primary questions in a uniform way, and the importance of confidentiality. See figure 7.3 for a list of sample focus group questions.

FIGURE 7.3   FOCUS GROUP QUESTIONS

1. When I say the term *school health*, what do you think I am referring to?
2. Keeping in mind that health has physical and psychological aspects, on a scale from 1 (extremely poor) to 5 (outstanding), where would you place the general health of youth and adolescents in your city or town? Why?
3. We want to get a sense of how you think the schools in this district contribute to the health of youth in this community.
   - What are some examples of how the schools contribute positively to the health of youth in this community?
   - What are some examples of how the schools may interfere with or hinder the health of youth in this community?
4. Do you have any suggestions for how the schools might better address the health needs of children in this community?
5. Do you think that healthy children or youth are more likely to be successful students? Why do you think the way you do?
6. [Show and briefly explain the Whole School, Whole Community, Whole Child model.]
   - When you think about the whole child and school health as including all these pieces, which pieces do you see as working particularly well in this school or this district? Why? Can you provide one or two specific examples?
   - What is in particular need of improvement? Why? Can you provide one or two specific examples?
7. How are community members who are not parents involved in creating a healthy school building or district?
8. What might community members who are not parents do to be more involved in creating a healthy school building or district?
9. On a scale from 1 (no responsibility) to 10 (complete responsibility), how much responsibility should the public schools have in creating healthy youth and adolescents? Why did you pick that number? Can you identify one or two specific examples of how public schools should be creating healthy youth and adolescents?
10. On a scale from 1 (no responsibility) to 10 (complete responsibility), how much responsibility should the public schools have in creating healthy communities? Why did you pick that number? Can you identify one or two specific examples of how public schools should be creating healthy communities?

> **WSCC IN PRACTICE**
> ### Using Comprehensive School Health and Wellness Profiles
>
> Looking at a variety of health status, school health, and academic data together allows school district decision-makers and stakeholders to understand the connections between health and academic performance not as something abstract but as something with real implications for their school districts. Comprehensive school health and wellness profiles can bring into view a number of existing situations for support or alteration that are often hidden when health and academic data are segregated (within school districts and between school districts and community health agencies). In our research, focus group and key informant interview data with school personnel in two school districts in New York suggested that mental health issues in student and student family populations had a negative impact on students' ability to make academic progress. Parent interview data suggested a negative impact of student mental health issues on the classroom and school environment and their children's ability to learn.
>
> We found that data on community health status supported mental health as an issue of concern in youth and adult populations, identified inadequate access to the diagnosis and treatment of mental health issues (in particular in youth), and suggested likely sociocultural contributors to mental health issues. The school districts had processes to consider the influence of mental health on the academic performance of individual students, yet there appeared to be no mechanism for addressing possible mental health issues. For example, there were neither districtwide goals related to improving the mental health of the student population nor any mention of mental health in school improvement plans. The current silo structure in these communities and within the school districts appeared to have created the following situation:
>
> - Community health agencies and organizations and schools worked largely in isolation on what was a communal problem at a time when resources were scarce.
> - Classroom teachers felt unprepared and unsure of their role in managing students who exhibited socioemotional mental health issues and assisting those students with their struggles, even though the effect of their struggles on academic performance was apparent.
> - Community mental health agencies, for the most part, were reluctant to approach school districts to explore collaborative interventions because of past negative experiences working with school districts and a feeling of being unwelcome.
>
> Following the school health assets and needs presentations, school and community members in attendance discussed how it was clear that the mental health status of the student population was having a deleterious effect on academic performance and that to do something about it, the district would have to seek help from outside agencies and organizations.

A Word About Data and Their Use

As described previously, a number of different types of data should be collected during the three actions for conducting the health and wellness profile. Identifying and collecting different types of data from different sources helps to provide the holistic picture of the district needed to plan quality WSCC-based programs. Understanding a bit about the why, where, and how of data can help guide the data collection for the needs assessment, their use, and the analysis, which can be easily used to set goals and objectives.

As described, both **primary** and **secondary data** should be collected. Primary data are collected directly from the school district, family, or community members through, for example, windshield tours, key informant interviews, or focus groups. Secondary data are collected by another source, such as the state health department, the CDC (in the case of state-level YRBS data), the local health department, or state departments of education (CDC, 2023b, 2023c).

A variety of data are needed to provide a complete understanding of the existing programs, processes, and policies as well as to evaluate the implementation and outcomes of the resulting efforts. Both **qualitative** and **quantitative data** are needed. Qualitative data, which are primarily words and pictures, are descriptive in nature and are obtained by conducting interviews, running focus groups, or observing and describing behaviors, such as food selection in the school cafeteria. Quantitative data, such as high school grade point averages, the percentage of students who use marijuana on a weekly basis, or the yearly school dropout rate, are numerical and can undergo statistical operations. Some examples of CDC national databases that offer quantitative data are the results from the Adolescent Behaviors and Experiences Survey, YRBSS, and the National Health and Nutrition Examination Survey (CDC, 2023a, 2023c).

The community profile, SHI or School Improvement Tool data along with the resulting recommendations, academic performance data, WellSAT results, and results of the key informant interviews and focus groups are reviewed collectively by the assessment group. Once the data are reviewed, then a list of school health assets and needs for the district can be generated.

Assets and Needs: Identified From the Data

Assets are items such as the following:

- A community physical environment conducive to physical activity and recreation
- Low rates of particular health conditions or engagement in health-risk behaviors
- Abundant health resources in the community
- Varied cultural opportunities
- Diverse, active parent groups
- A willingness among community agencies to partner with schools
- Present or past success with school–community partnerships
- Physical education that meets or exceeds recommended minutes
- Existing resources and processes within the school structure for supporting students experiencing health issues

Needs are items such as the following:

- Low socioeconomic status
- Limited access to health care in the community
- Low graduation rates
- High rates of particular health conditions or engagement in health-risk behaviors
- Lack of effective communication across schools and between central administrators and schools
- Lack of institutional belief in a connection between health and well-being and academic performance
- Lack of evidence of using health data in decision-making (policy, programs, strategic planning)
- Lack of community programs for youth

Additional needs might be the lack of a WSCC structure or only partial implementation of WSCC, such as weak or nonexistent health education or neighborhood safety issues.

School health assets and needs identified through the process should be disseminated to the district through presentations and a report intended for selected administrative and instructional personnel. Each district presentation should prompt a discussion of the realities of what the data suggest compared to the perceptions of school personnel, any disconnect between school health and academic initiatives, and the effect that WSCC programming could have on academic performance. These discussions should be followed up with priority setting and action planning initiatives. The data are used to drive the development of goals and objectives for school health councils and teams, to develop programming and policy, to make decisions related to the selection of curricula, to support internal and external funding requests, and to shape the missions and school improvement plans of schools and districts (CDC, 2023b; Rudd Center, 2021).

The Logic Model: After the Data, Now What?

After the data examination, efforts then go into making programming decisions. At this stage a **logic model** can be used to both plan and evaluate a program and to help the planners, evaluation team, and stakeholders visualize the program to determine potential barriers and needed resources (CDC, 2023b). Figure 7.4 shows a sample logic model for programming efforts to increase the graduation rate in a district by 10 percent.

Evaluating WSCC

As the needs assessment data are collected and reviewed and plans are being made to enhance or develop new efforts based on the assessment, plans for the evaluation of those efforts need to be made. **Program evaluation** is an ongoing process that indicates whether the program, policy, or process is being implemented as planned; whether efforts are creating change; and whether the outcome is what the district had hoped to achieve (CDC, 2023b).

Evaluation is not just a process of collecting baseline data in the planning phase and again at the end of the activity. As stated by the CDC, evaluation is "a systematic method for collecting, analyzing, and using data to examine the effectiveness and efficiency of programs and, as importantly, to contribute to continuous program improvement" (CDC, 2023b, "What Is Program Evaluation?"). Questions that an effective evaluation can address include the following:

- Was the program, policy, or process implemented as planned?
- Did the effort that was implemented have the value, effect, or impact expected or desired?
- Did the program, policy, or process work?

Without the information that is obtained in an evaluation, the planning, resources, and efforts are but a waste of time. It is critical that stakeholders and planners have a sense of when to make adjustments and when actions are working or not (CDC, 2023b).

The information collected must address the evaluation question, which is the reason for the evaluation in the first place. For example, if the

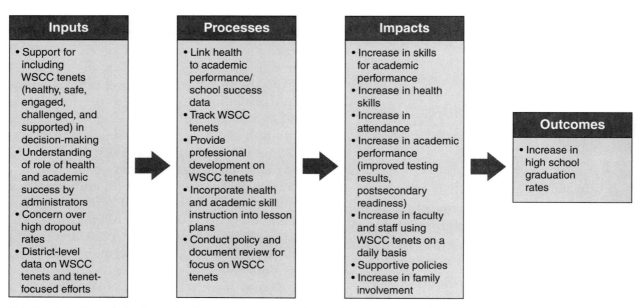

FIGURE 7.4 Sample logic model for WSCC programming to increase graduation rates.

evaluation question is "Did the programming efforts increase the high school graduation rate by 10 percent?" then the information being collected needs to answer that question. The quality, validity, and accuracy of the information are important, and the information must be informative for stakeholders. Information on programming efforts (e.g., those that are being offered to address dropout rates) needs to provide credible evidence for accepting the evaluation's conclusion (CDC, 2023b).

Types of Evaluation

As seen in the CDC framework for program evaluation, evaluation actions take place throughout the planning and implementation process. When evaluation occurs and what the evaluation team is looking for at that time are determined by the type of evaluation being conducted (CDC, 2023b).

Formative Evaluation

At the beginning of the process, **formative evaluation** produces information gathered during the planning and implementation phase. As described earlier in this chapter, the data collected prior to implementation (baseline data) are identified as the needs assessment. Once the programming begins, then ongoing **process evaluation** begins (CDC, 2023b).

Process evaluation documents whether a program has been implemented as intended and whether revisions or changes to programming are necessary. Process evaluation is an examination of whether the activities are taking place, who is conducting the activities, who is reached through the activities, and whether the resources and actions have been allocated as necessary. Process evaluation measures whether the programming efforts were implemented as planned and helps to identify barriers and supporting factors to program success (CDC, 2023b; Rooney et al., 2015).

Summative Evaluation

Summative evaluation is a broad term that refers to evaluation conducted to determine whether a program was effective and met its goals and objectives (CDC, 2023b; Rooney et al., 2015). Summative evaluation looks at how successful the outcome of the program was and thus may be referred to as **outcome evaluation**. The CDC describes outcome evaluation by using terms such as *short-term*, *intermediate*, and *long-term outcomes* (2023b).

Within the PRECEDE–PROCEED model, summative evaluation is divided into impact and outcome evaluation, with **impact evaluation** referring to the desired impact (short term and intermediate) and outcome evaluation being the long-term desired outcome or project goal (Center for Community, 2023a). Depending on the stage of development of the program and the purpose of the evaluation, outcome evaluations may include any or all outcomes, including the following:

- Changes in people's attitudes and beliefs
- Changes in health risk factors or protective behaviors
- Changes in the environment, including policies, enforcement of rules and regulations, and the influence of social norms
- Changes in trends in morbidity and mortality
- Changes in academic status, including grades and retention rates

In sum, process evaluation and outcome evaluation are the two main types of evaluation. Figure 7.5 from the CDC demonstrates what the evaluation team looks at during each type of evaluation.

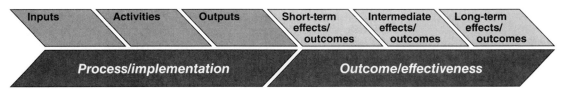

FIGURE 7.5 The focus of two types of evaluation.
From CDC (2012).

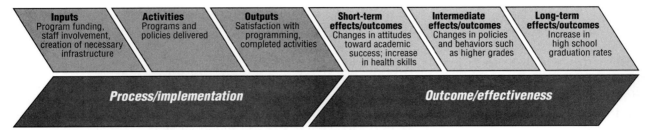

FIGURE 7.6 Types of evaluation with examples for increasing high school graduation rates.
Adapted from CDC (2012).

With figure 7.5 in mind, consider a programming goal of increasing the high school graduation rate by 10 percent. The evaluation sequence might look like what is presented in figure 7.6.

Planning for Program Evaluation

In planning for the evaluation of programming efforts, decisions regarding what information or data needs to be collected and when it will be collected are key to the evaluation process. An evaluation plan and timeline will help to ensure the necessary data are collected and used for improving the WSCC process and the outcome of all efforts. When planning an evaluation of WSCC efforts it is important to select a model or tool to guide the evaluation steps. A program evaluation process or tool such as the CDC framework (see figure 7.7) is useful for helping to identify and summarize the essential elements needed in an effective program evaluation (CDC, 2017). Use of the framework will assist the people involved in planning and modifying programs, policies, and processes and will help to show the effects of WSCC-related efforts and resources (CDC, 2017). The six recommended steps in the CDC framework for program evaluation (CDC, 2017), depicted in figure 7.7, are as follows:

1. Engage stakeholders
2. Describe the program
3. Focus evaluation design
4. Gather credible evidence
5. Justify conclusions
6. Ensure use and share lessons

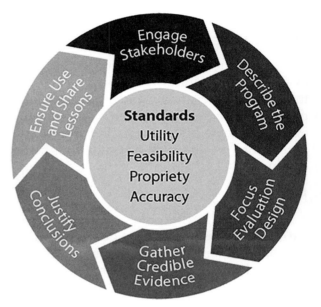

FIGURE 7.7 The CDC's framework for program evaluation.
From CDC (2017).

Step 1: Engage Stakeholders

From as early on as possible in the process it is important to involve stakeholders (Center for Community, 2023e; CDC, 2017). Stakeholders are those people or organizations that feel that the WSCC model and the health and well-being of children and youth are important and that are concerned about the academic success of youth. The success of WSCC and of the evaluation process requires representation from all segments of the community. Representatives from each of the WSCC components—the school, the district, families, youth, and the local community—need to be members of the evaluation team (Center for Community, 2023e; CDC, 2017, 2023b).

It is important that the voices of a wide range of stakeholders are heard and that their perspective is taken into consideration from the beginning of this process. Early involvement helps to build ownership and helps to ensure the evaluation findings are taken seriously and are not ignored (Center for Community, 2023e; CDC, 2017, 2023b).

Step 2: Describe the Program

It is important that the planners work together to describe the program and what they hope the program will achieve. If a program is developed to reduce the high school dropout rate, make sure all involved in the planning process agree that the program being implemented was designed to achieve the stated outcome (CDC, 2017, 2023b).

Step 3: Focus Evaluation Design

The evaluation plan is designed to answer a series of questions being asked within the scope of the resources available. For example, in the logic model presented in figure 7.4, the outcome evaluation question is "Did the programming efforts decrease the high school dropout rate by 10 percent?" The evaluation question needs to be important to the stakeholders and needs to reflect the point of the evaluation (CDC, 2017, 2023b).

Evaluation needs to follow proper protocol regarding when and how data are collected while protecting human subjects. Consider the following four issues when developing the evaluation:

1. *Purpose:* Why is the evaluation being conducted? Are you trying to gain insight into the program or assess the effects of the program?
2. *Users:* Who will be receiving the findings of the evaluation, and who will gain from being a part of the evaluation process?
3. *Questions:* What questions are the evaluation strategies trying to answer?
4. *Methods:* What evaluation procedures will be used that will give the evaluation team and the stakeholders the information they need to answer the question or questions?

An evaluation plan can provide guidance for the process and will help to identify what data are needed to best answer evaluation questions. In addition, an evaluation plan will help the team to come up with a realistic timeline for collecting the necessary information (CDC, 2017, 2023b). See table 7.3 for a sample evaluation plan.

TABLE 7.3 Sample Evaluation Plan

Evaluation question	Indicators or performance measure	Methods of data collection	Data sources	Frequency	Whose responsibility?
Process evaluation—Is the district wellness policy being implemented as planned?	Description and update of activities described in the policy	Key informant interviews, document reviews, observations	Interview scripts, reports, observation checklists	Every three months	School principal and school teams (with help from health and wellness peer mentors)
Outcome evaluation—Are students eating healthier food?	Results from the Youth Risk Behavior Survey nutrition section, sales data from the school cafeteria and store	Surveys and sales	Survey responses, sales receipts	Yearly	School health coordinator and school teams

Adapted from CDC (2011).

Step 4: Gather Credible Evidence

It is important to collect information that provides a comprehensive picture of the program being evaluated and that is seen as credible by the stakeholders (CDC, 2023b). In the sample logic model (figure 7.4), the actions under *processes* would be those efforts or actions that the district has implemented to increase the high school graduation rates, and the evaluation will try to determine their impact on those rates. Sources such as district and school-level documents on chronic absenteeism, retention rates, grade point average, and yearly graduation rates would provide multiple sources of evidence to help answer the evaluation question and evaluate the results of the programming efforts (Rooney et al., 2015).

Step 5: Justify Conclusions

Once the evaluation information is gathered, it is then reviewed and analyzed. The stakeholders will need to agree with confidence on the results and what the evidence means. Do the data show that the programming was worth it and justified? Did the program achieve the desired results? After the stakeholders have agreed on the interpretation of the data and have made a judgment regarding the value or significance of the program, recommendations for further action will need to be considered (CDC, 2017, 2023b). In other words, where does the program go from here?

Step 6: Ensure, Use, and Share Lessons

The evaluation findings and the lessons learned during the evaluation process need to be shared with the district community. How the findings will be shared with the public and in what form or format will need to be considered (CDC, 2017, 2023b). Will there be opportunities to collect feedback from the greater community? Will the findings be tailored to the various stakeholders? How will the evaluation team ensure that the findings will be used to make future programming decisions? These are some of the questions that will need to be addressed as the findings are prepared to be communicated to all potential stakeholders.

Summary

Data-informed school health planning provides a strong foundation for updating or implementing WSCC, and using the four phases of the PRECEDE model to determine needs and assets is valuable in that process. Moreover, a broad ecological scan of school and community data can illuminate the importance of school health to the health of the community and to academic performance.

Three actions—developing community understanding, conducting a wellness policy review, and reviewing WSCC implementation—can be performed to collect the data needed for the needs assessment for making initial programming planning decisions and the evaluation plan. Evaluation can follow the CDC framework for program evaluation for a systematic and effective approach. Once implementation takes place, process evaluation can then help to determine whether all is going as planned. Process evaluation can be used to make necessary adjustments as the program evolves and, along with the needs assessment, makes up the formative evaluation. Summative evaluation includes looking at short-term, intermediate, and long-term effects or outcomes. The results help the evaluation team determine whether the programming being examined was successful.

LEARNING AIDS

GLOSSARY

academic performance data—Data related to the performance of schools or youth (e.g., student assessment results or state-issued report cards) that indicate how well they are doing in regard to a set of academic standards.

CDC framework for program evaluation—A tool that guides health professionals in the use of program evaluation. The framework is designed to summarize and to organize essential elements of program evaluation.

external evaluator—A person carrying out an evaluation who is outside the focus of the evaluation or outside the agency or institution in which the evaluation is occurring.

focus group—A qualitative approach to learning about a group of people that is often used in health education and health promotion to collect information for program planning. Participants in the group are usually alike on one or more characteristics, although the composition of the group depends on the purpose of the discussion.

formative evaluation—A type of evaluation used to modify or improve programs, activities, or interventions based on feedback obtained during the planning, development, and implementation of a health promotion program.

impact evaluation—A measurement of the extent to which a program or intervention has caused intended short-term changes in the group or community being addressed.

institutionalizing—The process of embedding a program or policy in an organization so that it continues after the initial effort ends.

internal evaluator—A person carrying out an evaluation who is inside the focus of the evaluation or inside the agency or institution in which the evaluation is occurring.

key informant interview—A key informant is a person in a community or school district who has direct knowledge of a group or has access to information about a group. In a key informant interview, the identified person is interviewed to provide information to the person collecting the data for the purposes of developing or assessing a program or policy.

logic model—A graphic description of the relationship of the resources, activities, strategies, impacts, and outcomes for a program. Seen as an effective tool for planning, implementation and evaluation of a proposed program.

needs assessment and asset analysis—A process of identifying needs and inventorying assets to move toward workable solutions that result in improvement in a group or community. A goal of a community assessment is to develop an informed understanding of the gaps or needs that exist within a community and their effect on the community members.

outcome evaluation—A measurement of the extent to which a program causes intended long-term changes in a population. Outcome or effectiveness evaluations measure program effects in a target population by assessing progress on the sequence of outcomes the program is meant to address. Program planners may describe this sequence using terms such as *short-term*, *intermediate*, and *long-term outcomes*.

PRECEDE–PROCEED model—A planning model developed by Green and Kreuter that offers a framework for identifying intervention strategies for achieving objectives. The model provides a comprehensive structure for assessing health and quality-of-life needs and for designing, implementing, and evaluating health promotion and other public health programs to meet those needs. PRECEDE (predisposing, reinforcing, and enabling constructs in educational diagnosis and evaluation) outlines a diagnostic planning process to assist in the development of targeted public health programs. PROCEED (policy, regulatory, and organizational constructs in educational and environmental development) guides the implementation and evaluation of programs designed using the PRECEDE part of the model.

primary data—Data generated by the researcher themselves through methods such as a survey, interview, focus group, or observation.

process evaluation—A type of evaluation conducted to explain why a program or intervention may or may not have been effective. The evaluation often includes monitoring of the implementation, measurement of progress toward goals and objectives, assessment of satisfaction levels, staff performance reviews, and resource reviews. In general, process evaluation looks at how program activities were delivered.

program evaluation—A systematic method for collecting, analyzing, and using information to answer questions about projects, policies, and programs. The CDC describes effective program evaluation as a systematic means of improving and accounting for public health actions.

qualitative data—Data that are descriptive and nonnumeric. Qualitative data are often in the form of narratives and descriptions that result from observations, key informant interviews, and focus groups.

quantitative data—Data that are empirical and numerical (such as data collected with the CDC's Youth Risk Behavior Surveillance System). Quantitative data can undergo mathematical and statistical operations.

school district health and wellness profile—A comprehensive school audit that provides an overview of a school district's health and wellness. The profile may include community, health, and academic data compiled from a variety of tools and sources. It identifies school health and community assets and needs that are suggested by these kinds of data.

secondary data—Data that have been collected by someone other than the primary user. Data collected by agencies at the local, state, and federal levels are examples of sources of secondary data.

snowball sampling—A method of sampling in which existing study subjects recruit future subjects from among their friends and acquaintances. The sample grows in snowball fashion, hence the name of the technique.

summative evaluation—A type of evaluation used to determine whether a program or policy was effective. It includes the use of measures to draw conclusions about the policy or program that was implemented. It is often used to answer the question "Did it work?"

windshield tour—A process of collecting data through direct observation of (e.g., driving a car through) a community or area where a program or intervention is being developed or assessed.

Youth Risk Behavior Surveillance System (YRBSS)—The YRBSS monitors priority health-risk behaviors and the prevalence of obesity and asthma among youth and young adults. The Youth Risk Behavior Surveillance System includes a national school-based survey that is conducted by the CDC. State, territorial, tribal, and district surveys exist that are conducted by state, territorial, and local education and health agencies and tribal governments.

APPLICATION ACTIVITIES

1. Brainstorm a list of reasons why a needs assessment and asset analysis would be necessary as an early step in developing or advancing WSCC in a school district. Then generate a list of possible needs and assets that might surface from the school district assessment and analysis. Write up your results and share them with the class.
2. Conduct a presentation for your peers on program evaluation. Explain the steps in the CDC framework for program evaluation through a 10-minute PowerPoint presentation. Use a WSCC example with the outcome of improved health or academic performance.
3. As a member of a district health council, you are involved in developing an evaluation plan for your district. Fill in the missing pieces of the table to develop an evaluation plan methods grid (for process and outcome evaluation) for the following evaluation question: Are the district's current efforts to communicate the district wellness policy with local families working as planned?

Evaluation question	Indicators or performance measure	Methods of data collection	Data sources	Frequency	Whose responsibility?
Process evaluation					
Outcome evaluation					

REFERENCES

ASCD. (2023). *ASCD Whole Child School Improvement Tool.* https://sitool.ascd.org/Default.aspx?ReturnUrl=%2f

Baldwin, S., & Ventresca, A.R.C. (2020). Every school healthy: An urban school case study. *Journal of School Health, 90*(12), 1045-1055.

Center for Community Health and Development. (2023a). *Chapter 2, section 2: PRECEDE/PROCEED.* Community Tool Box. https://ctb.ku.edu/en/table-contents/overview/other-models-promoting-community-health-and-development/preceder-proceder/main

Center for Community Health and Development. (2023b). *Chapter 3, section 6: Conducting focus groups.* Community Tool Box. https://ctb.ku.edu/en/table-of-contents/assessment/assessing-community-needs-and-resources/conduct-focus-groups/main

Center for Community Health and Development. (2023c). *Chapter 3, section 12: Conducting interviews.* Community Tool Box. https://ctb.ku.edu/en/table-of-contents/assessment/assessing-community-needs-and-resources/conduct-interviews/main

Center for Community Health and Development. (2023d). *Chapter 3, section 21: Windshield and walking surveys.* Community Tool Box. https://ctb.ku.edu/en/table-of-contents/assessment/assessing-community-needs-and-resources/windshield-walking-surveys/main

Center for Community Health and Development. (2023e). *Chapter 36, section 1: A framework for program evaluation: A gateway to tools.* Community Tool Box. https://ctb.ku.edu/en/table-of-contents/evaluate/evaluation/framework-for-evaluation/main

Center for Community Health and Development. (2023f). *Chapter 37, section 1: Choosing questions and planning the evaluation*. Community Tool Box. https://ctb.ku.edu/en/table-of-contents/evaluate/evaluate-community-interventions/choose-evaluation-questions/main

Center for Community Health and Development. (2023g). *Chapter 37, section 5: Collecting and analyzing data*. Community Tool Box. https://ctb.ku.edu/en/table-of-contents/evaluate/evaluate-community-interventions/collect-analyze-data/main

Centers for Disease Control and Prevention. (2011). *Developing an effective evaluation plan*. https://www.cdc.gov/obesity/downloads/cdc-evaluation-workbook-508.pdf

Centers for Disease Control and Prevention. (2017). *Office of Policy Performance and Evaluation: A framework for program evaluation*. www.cdc.gov/evaluation/framework/index.htm

Centers for Disease Control and Prevention. (2018). *Health related quality of life (HRQOL)*. www.cdc.gov/hrqol/wellbeing.htm

Centers for Disease Control and Prevention. (2019a). *Healthy schools: School Health Index*. www.cdc.gov/healthyschools/shi/index.htm

Centers for Disease Control and Prevention. (2019b). *School Health Index guide*. www.cdc.gov/healthyschools/shi/pdf/FINAL_School-Health-Index-Guide-112619_revd-120319_508tag.pdf

Centers for Disease Control and Prevention. (2023a). *Adolescent and school health: Data and statistics*. www.cdc.gov/healthyyouth/data/index.htm

Centers for Disease Control and Prevention. (2023b). *Program evaluation*. www.cdc.gov/evaluation/index.htm

Centers for Disease Control and Prevention. (2023c). *Youth Risk Behavior Surveillance System*. www.cdc.gov/healthyyouth/data/yrbs/index.htm

Food Research and Action Center. (2022). *Child nutrition and reauthorization (NCR)*. https://frac.org/action/child-nutrition-reauthorization-cnr

Green, L., & Kreuter, M. (2005). *Health program planning: An ecological and educational approach*. (4th ed.). McGraw-Hill.

Hodges, B.C., & Videto, D.M. (2011). *Assessment and planning in health programs* (2nd ed.). Jones & Bartlett Learning.

Hunt, P., Barrios, L., Tellijohann, S.K., & Mazyck, D. (2015). A whole school approach: Collaborative development of school health policies, processes, and practices. *Journal of School Health, 88*(11), 802-809.

Kennedy-Shaffer, L., Qiu, X., & Hanage, W.P. (2021). Snowball sampling study design for serosurveys early in disease outbreaks. *American Journal of Epidemiology, 190*(9), 1918-1927.

Kentucky Department of Education. (2020). *Kentucky Healthy Schools year 1 evaluation*. https://education.ky.gov/districts/enrol/Documents/Kentucky%20Healthy%20Schools%20Evaluation%20Year%201%20One-Pager.pdf

National Association of County and City Health Officials. (2022). *Community health assessments and improvement planning*. www.naccho.org/programs/public-health-infrastructure/performance-improvement/community-health-assessment

National Healthy Schools Collaborative. (2022). *District and school: Priorities, opportunities, and case studies*. The Roadmap. www.healthyschoolsroadmap.org/district-and-school

National School Climate Center. (2021). *School climate survey*. https://schoolclimate.org/services/measuring-school-climate-csci/

Rooney, L.E., Videto, D.M., & Birch, D.A. (2015). Using the Whole School, Whole Community, Whole Child model: Implications for practice. *Journal of School Health, 85*(11), 817-823.

Rudd Center. (2021). *WellSAT 3.0 wellness school assessment tool*. www.wellsat.org/about_the_WellSAT.aspx

U.S. Department of Education. (2023). *Learn About ED School Climate Surveys*. National Center on Safe Supportive Learning Environments (NCSSLE). https://safesupportivelearning.ed.gov/edscls

University of Connecticut. (n.d.). *Institute for Collaboration on Health, Intervention and Policy*. WellSAT Suite. https://wellsatsuite.chip.uconn.edu/wellsat-3-0

Videto, D.M., & Dake, J.A. (2019). Promoting health literacy through defining and measuring quality school health education. *Health Promotion Practice, 20*(6), 824-833.

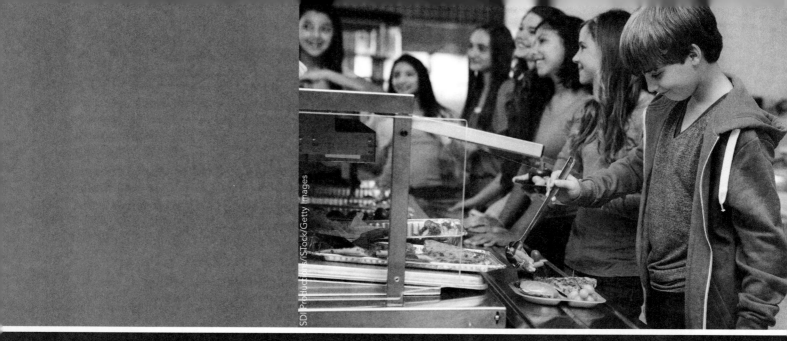

CHAPTER 8

Implementing WSCC

Donna M. Videto • Hannah P. Catalano • David A. Birch

LEARNING OBJECTIVES

1. Describe the application of the 10 steps for implementing the Whole School, Whole Community, Whole Child (WSCC) model.
2. Present the rationale for the need for the school health coordinator, district health council, and school health teams in supporting WSCC implementation.
3. Identify potential health champions in the local community that would support WSCC efforts.
4. Describe the benefits of an action plan for successful implementation of a WSCC action.

KEY TERMS

Health disparity
Infrastructure
Institutionalization
Mission statement

School health advisory council (SHAC)
School health coordinator
School health improvement plan

In 2014, ASCD and the Centers for Disease Control and Prevention (CDC) developed the Whole School, Whole Community, Whole Child (WSCC) model, which serves as an important avenue for improving the academic performance and well-being of youth (ASCD, 2014; CDC, 2021). To implement the WSCC model effectively, schools and school districts need programs, policies, and processes in place to support this approach. Implementing the WSCC model includes identifying important supportive personnel and resources, analyzing initial academic and WSCC assessment data, and creating a clear action plan to provide direction for the development of interventions designed to promote health and wellness while positively influencing academic success (CDC, 2021). Note that when addressing the planning and implementation of supportive structures, the school or district should include the community, families, parents, guardians, caregivers, school administrators, faculty, staff, and youth (CDC, 2022; National Association of Chronic Disease Directors, 2017). Including representatives from across the WSCC components will assist in providing the supportive personnel necessary for a successful approach (CDC, 2022).

Program implementation involves systematically carrying out the activities that make up an intervention while working toward the achievement of program objectives and ultimately program goals (Hodges & Videto, 2011; Rooney et al., 2015). The 10-step process described here needs to take place prior to and during implementation for effective programming. The following steps (adapted from Hunt et al., 2015; Mann et al., 2018; RMC Health, 2022; Rooney et al., 2015) were designed to create the necessary **infrastructure** and processes for successful implementation:

1. Establish leadership with a designated school health coordinator
2. Secure administrative support and develop a district-level school health council and school health teams
3. Identify available resources in the school, district, and community
4. After reviewing the initial data, determine the outcomes of greatest priority
5. Create an action plan based on realistic goals and objectives agreed upon by partners
6. Establish a realistic timeline for implementing strategies from the action plan
7. Implement the plan and strategies
8. Review and implement the evaluation plan
9. Provide professional development for faculty and staff
10. Communicate steps and successes

To better understand the implementation of WSCC, it is necessary to examine how these 10 recommended steps fit in with planning, implementation, and evaluation (see figure 8.1).

Some of the content in this chapter includes strategies conducted during the initial planning stage as well as during the evaluation of the programming efforts (see chapter 7). Steps 1 to 4 may have been established during planning and may need to be reviewed and possibly revised early in the implementation process. Those steps are addressed in this chapter because of their importance in setting the stage for a successful WSCC implementation.

Step 1: Establish Leadership With a Designated School Health Coordinator

Once a school or district decides to implement or expand WSCC efforts, a critical initial strategy is to identify a **school health coordinator** to support the development of the necessary infrastructure and to ensure that the action plan and evaluation move forward (Videto & Dennis, 2021). A full-time or part-time school health coordinator is important for the successful implementation of WSCC. Before program implementation begins, data need to be collected to develop a clear picture of existing policies and programs related to school

FIGURE 8.1 INTEGRATED STEPS FOR IMPLEMENTING WSCC

Creating District Infrastructure and Preparing for Implementation

- Identify a school health coordinator (step 1)
  - Coordinator collects data and oversees planning, implementation, and evaluation processes
- Build administrative support, identify key leaders and community partners, and assemble districtwide and schoolwide teams (step 2)
  - Establish collaborative relationships and mutual understandings
- Identify existing data sources and collect data for a comprehensive view of programs, policies, and processes (step 3)
- Review needs assessment data to determine priorities for action (step 4)
  - Set and agree on goals and objectives
- Develop an action plan (step 5)
- Establish a timeline and evaluation plan (step 6)

Implementation

- Implement the plan (step 7)
  - Implement strategies and evaluation
- Provide professional development (step 9)
- Communicate steps to all partners and stakeholders (step 10)

Evaluation

- Monitor progress and adjust strategies and evaluation as needed (step 8)
- Evaluate results and celebrate successes (addressed in step 10)
- Communicate findings to the district and community (step 10)

Adapted from Hodges (2013); Rooney et al. (2015).

---

health, current gaps, and considerations for new policy and program development (see chapter 7 for more on this process). One role of the school health coordinator is to oversee this initial data collection process. To conduct this baseline assessment, districts and schools can use a number of available tools. See chapter 7 for descriptions of the School Health Index (SHI) and a variety of other tools and strategies that can be used to assess WSCC (e.g., the WellSAT 3.0, ASCD School Improvement Tool, U.S. Department of Education's School Climate Survey).

The role of the school health coordinator includes helping to maintain active school health councils and facilitate health programming between schools in the district and the community (Videto & Dennis, 2021). Videto and Hodges (2009) assessed the level of **institutionalization** of action plans resulting from SHI assessments in school districts throughout upstate and central New York along with the factors that assisted in that process. Findings from this study reinforced the importance of school health coordinators in ensuring successful institutionalization of WSCC plans. A school district may identify a school health educator, school administrator, education administrator, school nurse, food service coordinator, physical educator, or other school health stakeholder as a possible candidate for the role of school health coordinator. In some cases, a community consultant or a university partner may serve in this position. Regardless of who is selected for the role, the school health coordinator needs training in effective leadership, advocacy, grant writing and fund-raising, collaboration, and promotion of the whole child. In addition to this training, the school health coordinator needs to have a solid understanding of the

WSCC model and its link to academic performance (Mann et al., 2018).

The job of the school health coordinator is important to successful implementation of WSCC. For more details on this position, see the American School Health Association's (2018) position statement on the role of the school health coordinator in figure 8.2.

The role of the school health coordinator does not end when the infrastructure for addressing WSCC is in place. Providing ongoing support to committees while overseeing the implementation of an action plan, the resulting interventions, and the evaluation continue to be important as the WSCC efforts move forward. The school health coordinator identifies additional partners for collaborations as needs change and resource requirements shift. Successful implementation of steps 2 to 10 listed earlier requires the oversight and involvement of a competent school health coordinator.

FIGURE 8.2 AMERICAN SCHOOL HEALTH ASSOCIATION'S POSITION STATEMENT ON THE ROLE OF THE SCHOOL HEALTH COORDINATOR

The School Health Coordinator ensures that all local education agency health initiatives, services, and programs, [sic] are aligned, complementary, and effective. As part of this leadership role, the School Health Coordinator:

1. Strengthens and implements school health policies that align with federal and state laws as well as regulations and best practices. Staying abreast of the numerous federal laws and programs that support student health and safety, including but not limited to the Every Student Succeeds Act, [U.S. Department of Agriculture's] Local Wellness Policy, and Safe and Drug Free Schools, [is] essential to this role.

2. Serves as a liaison to community health and safety programs. The coordinator builds bridges, acts as a facilitator and specializes in collaboration, partnership-building, data collection, and advocating for the health, safety, and wellness of students and staff.

3. Communicates school health and safety priorities to district administrators, building principals, staff, parents/families, community organizations and students using a variety of tools. The coordinator skillfully engages all these stakeholders to support the connection between health and learning.

4. Conducts assessments of student health needs and evaluates school health policies, activities and programs. The coordinator researches funding opportunities; uses data to develop funding proposals to support programs, services, and special initiatives; implements funded proposals; develops and manages a school health budget; and uses best practices to evaluate activities.

5. Provides professional development for local education agencies and school-based personnel on policies and the implementation of health-related programming.

6. Establishes and maintains a Health Advisory Committee whose members are subject matter experts for the various components of the WSCC model [and provides] cultural insight on behalf of the community. [Members of a] functional committee can assist the local education agency in ensuring that community values are reflected in health education instruction. Additionally, they can help districts meet performance goals and alleviate financial constraints through their volunteer efforts.

American School Health Association

Step 2: Secure Administrative Support and Develop a District-Level School Health Council and School Health Teams

Ongoing administrative support and involvement along with the development of a districtwide health council and school health teams make up critical infrastructure for implementing the WSCC model.

Gain Administrative Support and Commitment

If the school district has not already secured administrative support, then that needs to happen. During implementation it is critical to ensure that administrative assistance and commitment are maintained and continued throughout the entire process. Critical strategies for WSCC implementation and program maintenance include gaining the superintendent's support at the district level and principals' and assistant principals' support at the school level. Making school health a priority and creating an environment supportive of the whole child, faculty, staff, families, parents, guardians, caregivers, and the community are critical to setting the stage for WSCC. The CDC (2021) suggests that school administrators can create a foundation for WSCC by engaging in the following efforts:

- Incorporating health into the district's or school's vision and mission statements, including incorporating health goals into the school's improvement plan
- Appointing a qualified individual or individuals to oversee school health and WSCC
- Allocating resources, including a WSCC budget for teams
- Initiating completion of WSCC-related assessments and action plan
- Serving as champions and advocates for wellness events while communicating the importance of wellness to students, staff, families, parents, guardians, and caregivers (Children's Hospital of Wisconsin, n.d.)

Develop a District-Level School Health Advisory Council and School Health Teams

Successful planning and implementation of WSCC efforts involve convening a districtwide school health council, also referred to as a **school health advisory council (SHAC)**, as well as designating school health coordinators to oversee school health processes, programs, and policies (RMC Health, 2022; Videto & Dennis, 2021). Establishing a SHAC and a school health team is important for the implementation process and as a critical part of the WSCC infrastructure (CDC, 2021; Videto & Dennis, 2021). A planning team may have been utilized in the early stages of assessment and planning (see chapter 7), and that team, if representative of the community and WSCC, may or may not make up the SHAC or the school health team at a school that moves forward to support implementation and evaluation.

The SHAC consists of a group of teachers, administrators, staff, students, parents, and community members who act collectively to provide input regarding the planning, implementation, and evaluation of policies, programs, and services of the Whole School, Whole Community, Whole Child (WSCC) model in a school or school district. Again, the SHAC may also be referred to as a School Health or Wellness Council. (U.S. Department of Agriculture, n.d., as cited in Videto & Dennis, 2021, p. 16)

Ideally, the district-level SHAC includes at least one representative from each of the 10 WSCC components. It should also include school administrators, parents, students, and community representatives involved in and supportive of the health and well-being of students (CDC, 2021). Table 8.1 provides a list of potential representatives of the 10 components of WSCC for a SHAC. Note that individuals may represent more than one component and that some components may have multiple representatives.

Representatives to the SHAC also need to reflect the demographic composition of the school community. To be truly representative and relatable, the committee should reflect the diversity of the community. The CDC urges that the membership of such committees be as broad and diverse as possible, because this can help to enhance the conversation and assist in the acceptance of proposed activities (CDC, 2019).

The school health team usually consists of administrators, teachers, staff, students, parents, guardians, caregivers, and community members reflective of the components at the district level. The school health team remains focused on implementing work for advancing WSCC, is often constituted at the individual school level, and may inform the work of the districtwide SHAC (CDC, 2021; Videto & Dennis, 2021).

After the council and teams are established, time should be devoted to making sure all representatives understand the goals of WSCC and are aware of the evidence linking academic success and healthy youth. California School Boards Association (CSBA) and Cities Counties Schools Partnership (2009) described the importance of addressing values that the mem-

TABLE 8.1 Possible Representatives to the District SHAC

WSCC component	Possible representatives
Health education	Health coordinator, health teacher, director of curriculum and instruction, student health club representative, family and consumer sciences teacher, district health education consultant, health department health educator
Physical education and physical activity	Physical education coordinator, physical education teacher, district physical therapist, student teachers from local colleges and universities, grant-funded physical activity program investigators
Nutrition environment and services	District dietitian, food service manager or other personnel (business administrator), cafeteria support staff, healthy heart representative from health department
Health services	District medical consultant, school nurse, health department representative, speech therapists, special services personnel for students with special needs
Counseling, psychological, and social services	School psychologist, guidance counselor, social worker, teacher support aide
Social and emotional climate	Administrators such as a principal or vice principal, student representatives, school psychologists, guidance counselors, social workers
Physical environment	Administrators, buildings and grounds administrator, custodian, local law enforcement
Employee wellness	Elementary and secondary-level teachers, staff wellness coordinator, faculty or staff with a passion for wellness, community representative from worksite health
Family engagement	Representatives from parent groups (parents guild, parent–teacher organization, parent–teacher association, issue-related parent groups), youth groups
Community involvement	Representatives from the chamber of commerce, Rotary club, health agencies, government agencies, volunteer associations, colleges and universities; neighborhood and community champions and leaders

bers share because this effort will help establish group cohesiveness. The council and teams should allow the development of a common awareness, review how WSCC has been implemented in other districts, and come to an understanding of what the WSCC approach means and its potential effect on students. Sharing a common understanding of WSCC across the SHAC and school health teams is important to successful implementation.

WSCC IN PRACTICE
Tips for Implementing WSCC at the District Level

A New York school district was highlighted for its work in the component of nutrition environment and services. Six factors were reported as keys to the success of the district:

1. Stakeholders had a vision of being committed to a model such as WSCC.
2. Leadership was demonstrated through administrative support from the board of education, superintendent, and principals of the schools in the district.
3. Collaboration was shown through partnerships established with community agencies, staff, parents, and students.
4. There was teamwork in each building as well as districtwide.
5. Baseline data were collected to demonstrate improvements after repeated assessments, which were then conducted every two to three years.
6. Financial support was apparent in the use of mini-grants offered through state and national organizations.

The former health education and wellness coordinator of the school district offered five suggestions for implementing WSCC programs and policies:

1. Districts need to obtain administrative support for WSCC activities and send out consistent messages.
2. Broad involvement is needed, including support from parents, school staff, and community members. Strong advocates are needed to assist in getting the vision and goals of coordinated school health converted into actual programs and policy. Administrators may respond more positively to general staff and parents than to the typical school health champion, who is generally the health educator or school health coordinator.
3. The most critical WSCC priorities need to be converted into policy. Such a policy will help ensure that work or effort in that area will continue after the champions leave or have moved on to other initiatives because the policy itself will still exist.
4. Each school needs to have a school health coordinator to drive the team and pull its work together. The schools and the district need someone with a real passion for WSCC. WSCC functions best when someone with continuity who believes in what is being done is there to oversee the actions. A school health coordinator helps develop the structure for the work to happen.
5. A healthy school team is needed for every school building, along with a separate district team. The accomplishments in individual schools were made because each school building had its own team to work with and someone to make the program or initiative happen at the school level. It is critical that school principals be members of the school health team. This network needs to be in place to share ideas and to develop and implement districtwide policies (Dippo, J., personal communication, 2014).

Step 3: Identify Available Resources in the School, District, and Community

As an initial step in the implementation process, the SHAC and school health team should conduct another review of the available resources and determine what documents, policies, finances, processes, and staff already exist with potential programming efforts in mind. This process should include a review of the district or school vision statement to determine the extent to which it reflects the guiding principles of WSCC. This activity might have the team or committee reworking the statement by defining the terms that could go into a vision statement reflective of WSCC and then making recommendations for such adjustments to their administrators. Terms such as *healthy school environment*, *active lifestyle*, or *supportive of the whole child* are possibilities (CSBA and Cities Counties Schools Partnership, 2009). The CSBA and Cities Counties Schools Partnership (2009) report *Building Healthy Communities: A School Leader's Guide to Collaboration and Community Engagement* suggests that the planning team develop a vision aligned with common values and community priorities. In the University of Kansas' (2022) Community Toolbox, an organization's vision is described as "your dream . . . the ideal conditions for your community" (p. 6). The vision statement is further described as the "hopes for the future" (p. 6). Characteristics and examples adapted from the Community Toolbox are presented in figure 8.3 (University of Kansas, 2022). The American School Health Association (2010) recommends that the vision statement include information about the importance of the health and well-being of students and staff as a foundation for school improvement and academic success.

FIGURE 8.3   CHARACTERISTICS OF VISION STATEMENTS AND EXAMPLE TERMS

Characteristics of Vision Statements

Understood and shared by members of the community

Broad and inclusive enough to address a diverse variety of local perspectives

Include terms reflective of health and its link to academic success

Inspiring and uplifting to everyone involved

Easy to communicate, generally short enough to fit on a T-shirt

Examples of Vision Statement Terms

Caring communities

Healthy children

Safe streets, safe neighborhoods

Every house a home

Education for all

Lifelong learning

Supportive of social-emotional learning

Fostering resilience

Social justice

Namaste Charter School, near Chicago, is directly founded on the Whole Child principle as demonstrated through its vision statement: "Our vision is to empower the whole child to thrive in a complex, interconnected and changing world" (Namaste Charter School, n.d.).

After a vision statement is established based on WSCC, the SHAC or committee should encourage the development of a **mission statement** that incorporates WSCC. Including terms such as *health*, *wellness*, and *the whole child* or other WSCC principles in a district's mission statement has been encouraged as a way to help move the actions of a district toward the implementation of health-enhancing policies and programs.

The WSCC-founded mission or purpose of Namaste Charter School to support its vision statement states the following:

> *Namaste is a pioneer. Our ground-breaking work to promote equity by addressing the nutrition, health, and wellness needs of our students remains at the forefront; yet, as we grow in our understanding of brain science, mental health, and technology, we recognize improved academic outcomes for our students are a critical focus. (Namaste Charter School, n.d.)*

This statement makes clear to the school community the value of a healthy child and the role that being healthy plays in the school and in the academic success of that child. In some districts, the vision and mission statements may be one and the same.

After the vision and mission statements, with strong WSCC vocabulary, are accepted by administrators and the school board, decisions need to be made regarding sharing them with the greater community. See implementation step 10 for ideas on communicating new or revised statements and policies. After the vision and mission statements are shared, the SHAC and the school health teams need to determine how those statements will drive and determine future efforts in the school or district (University of Kansas, 2022).

The initial assessment of community assets and needs conducted in the planning stage (see chapter 7) will have identified what additional policies and programming are available to support WSCC activities. The assessment team needs to determine existing policies, programming, or processes that will enhance or support a healthy school environment or other components of WSCC that could benefit efforts. Once policies, programming, and processes are determined, potential school district leaders as well as collaborations and partners in the community with staffing and other resources to address existing district gaps and needs should be identified (Mann et al., 2018). Leaders might be individuals known for their interest in health and wellness from their behaviors both in and outside the workplace. A school department chair or director who volunteers with a local health agency, a vice or assistant principal who participates in local races, or a parent who teaches nutrition at a local college are examples of potential leaders and collaborators to be pursued for WSCC support and implementation.

Step 4: After Reviewing the Initial Data, Determine the Outcomes of Greatest Priority

The results of the baseline assessment will help to provide the district or school with guidance for identifying the priority areas to which to direct their efforts. In addition to data on the components and tenets of WSCC, data on academic issues (such as graduation rates), health issues and behaviors, and policies and processes related to health and wellness should have been obtained in the assessment process. It is important to use the data to identify critical areas in need of change and those that have potential for change.

As the data and trends are examined it is important to look beyond the overall trends to determine whether there are **health dispar-**

ities between subgroups or populations. For example, the high school graduation rates for children living in poverty might be lower than the average graduation rate for the district, just as the percentage of students who visit a dentist might differ by gender. Age, race and ethnicity, income, gender, disability, geographic location, religion, national origin, family background, and sexual orientation are subgroups within the population in which **health disparities** are known to exist (CDC, 2023; CSBA, 2019).

While reviewing the data for determining school or district needs it is important to consider students' health-risk behaviors. The CDC (2020) has identified six categories of priority health-risk behaviors linked to the leading causes of death and disability for youth in the United States:

1. Behaviors that contribute to unintentional injuries and violence
2. Tobacco use
3. Alcohol and other drug use
4. Sexual behaviors that contribute to unintended pregnancy and sexually transmitted diseases, including HIV infection
5. Unhealthy dietary behaviors
6. Inadequate physical activity

Schools can assess health-risk behaviors among young people in these six categories as well as how they relate to general health status, asthma, and obesity and in areas such as sexual identity through formal surveys such as the Youth Risk Behavior Survey (YRBS; CDC, 2022). The YRBS, which is available through the CDC, is a national school-based survey that can provide the school and district with behavioral data for 9th through 12th graders and an additional survey for middle school students (CDC, 2022). Data resulting from the surveys can be used to track behavioral trends at the local level for establishing priorities and for monitoring the success of programs and policies. In addition, the local data can be compared to state, regional, and national data available on the CDC's YRBS website. For example, if a school district discovers that the proportion of its students who participate in at least 60 minutes of physical activity per day is lower than the same proportions of students at the state and national levels, the district may decide that it needs to prioritize that issue. This could mean changing the academic schedule and requirements to include daily physical education, training teachers to incorporate physical activity into the classroom, allowing fit breaks throughout the day, or instituting a walk-to-school program. This example demonstrates how data from the YRBS system can be helpful for informing programming and policies as a district tries to improve the health and well-being of students and staff.

After conducting the initial assessment and reviewing the resulting data, the SHAC and school health teams then work to identify the priority areas for driving their programming efforts. With a focus on the priority areas, goals and objects will be established that will shape the content of the action plan. Many nationally available assessment tools, such as the SHI, facilitate steps in the development of an action plan, including establishing priorities and determining implementation steps and strategies based on those priorities (ASCD, 2022; CDC, 2020).

Step 5: Create an Action Plan Based on Realistic Goals and Objectives Agreed Upon by Partners

Once the top priorities to be addressed are selected, then goals and objectives are created, which should result in the generation of an action plan for developing programs, policies, or processes to affect those priorities. While developing the action plan, consider what is important to address as well as what is possible or achievable (Alliance for a Healthier Generation, 2018).

In describing a systematic process for putting the WSCC model into action, Hunt et al. (2015) stated the importance of creating an action plan that is concrete, with all actions or strategies assigned to individuals responsible for implementation and progress monitoring. The CDC stressed the need to base action plans on realistic goals and measurable objectives. Following the format of CDC SMART goal development (SMART represents specific, measurable, attainable, relevant, and time-based) will help to establish goals that are realistic and measurable with a built-in timeline for their achievement (CDC, 2017c). The CDC uses the acronym SMART to help refine short-term and long-term goals and define what is intended to be achieved through a program or policy (CDC, 2017c). A short-term goal might be to implement an anti-bullying policy in all seven schools in a district by the end of the academic year. A long-term goal might be to reduce the number of reported incidences of bullying throughout the district by 25 percent over the next three years.

Again, schools need to identify sufficient resources to help their plans succeed. These resources might include regular use of assessment tools such as the SHI (CDC, 2017a) and the WellSAT 3.0 (Rudd Center, 2021) as well as funding for activities, shared resources, and experience and expertise needed for the successful implementation and maintenance of programs and systems.

After an assessment of the WSCC components with the SHI is completed, the results are often channeled into a series of steps that the district takes to improve or expand its efforts (CDC, 2019). The CDC (2019) recommends completing the following series of steps after assessing the programs and policies related to the 10 WSCC components:

1. *Complete the overall score card for the SHI*
2. *Review the score cards for each module of the SHI*
3. *Discuss the identified strengths and weaknesses*
4. *Discuss the recommended actions in each module*
5. *Review the overall score card*
6. *Have all participants work together to identify the top priority actions for the entire school*
7. *Complete the school health improvement plan*
8. *Discuss how the participants will monitor progress and when the team will meet again*

The **school health improvement plan** (step 7 in the list) is focused on improving some aspect of WSCC efforts. In the SHI assessment, the school health improvement plan comes in the form of a worksheet-based document. The SHI version was developed for writing down actions agreed upon by the assessment team after identifying three to five priority actions and considering the resources needed to address the actions. The steps that could be taken to achieve these actions are described, and the person or persons responsible for their implementation and a target date for achieving the desired outcome are identified. The team then needs to figure out how to present the plan to the school leadership and the community (CDC, 2019).

Figure 8.4 shows an example of part of the SHI school health improvement plan completed for one action resulting from a question in SHI Module 1, School Health and Environment, in the area of nutrition outside regular school hours (CDC, 2019).

Often appearing on school health improvement plans is the need to develop or to revise existing health-related policies, as was addressed earlier in regard to the vision and mission statements in Step 3: Identify Available Resources in the School, District, and Community. Implementing policies has the potential to affect multiple WSCC components because the outreach tends to be broader. Policy review and development often appears on the school improvement plan (not to be confused with the school health improvement plan). School

FIGURE 8.4 SCHOOL HEALTH IMPROVEMENT PLAN EXAMPLE

Action	Steps	By whom and when
1. Develop healthier fund-raising options	a. Revise wellness policy to address fund-raising b. Seek out healthier options to share with groups c. Meet with parent and student groups to address fund-raising options and revised wellness policy d. Communicate on school website the revised wellness policy and highlight fund-raising changes	a. District health council under the leadership of health coordinator Meg D., September b. Subcommittee of district health council under the leadership of health coordinator, September and October c. Principals at each school along with coordinator and health teachers, October and November d. Technology representative Shelia G., September and November

Adapted from Centers for Disease Control and Prevention (n.d.).

improvement plans, which were once required by law for low-performing schools, are usually locally developed documents that keep a school on track as staff work throughout the school year toward overall improvement and academic success for every student (Office of Elementary and Secondary Education, 2020). The Alliance for a Healthier Generation (2014) defines school improvement plans as comprehensive plans that describe long-range improvement goals for the school, which include improving academic performance, professional development, and school facilities. School improvement plans can also include specific goals that pertain to staff and student health and wellness (Alliance for a Healthier Generation, 2014; National Association of Chronic Disease Directors, 2016).

Policies or efforts in school improvement plans should support school health and the development of healthy student behaviors. A review of existing policies might uncover opportunities for revision where new wording is introduced that would create opportunities for an environment conducive to healthy and successful youth (Healthy Schools Campaign, 2016).

A public school posted the following policy to promote respect in schools:

Respect denotes both a positive feeling of esteem for a person and also specific actions and conduct representative of that esteem. Respect can be defined as allowing yourself and others to do and be their best. It is the goal of [this school] to [create] a mutual[ly] respectful atmosphere between all individuals involved within our school including administrators, teachers, staff members, students, parents, and visitors. (Jennings Public Schools, 2021, p. 16)

Jennings Public Schools' policy to promote respect in schools can be rewritten to place a stronger focus on health promotion by using language clearly linked to healthy development and the whole child. It might then look like this:

An environment supportive of the mental, emotional, physical, intellectual, and social health of the whole child includes showing respect for each other. Respect can be defined as allowing yourself to do and be your best and supporting others in doing the same. It is the goal of [this school] to create a healthy, safe, challenging, supportive, and engaging environment based on mutual respect between all individuals involved within our school, including administrators, teachers, staff members, students, parents, and visitors.

Moving the final action plan forward may require the school or district to face the challenge of identifying or developing relevant policies as well as programs with the potential to address district or school needs. Research-based programming that can reduce risk behaviors (as identified in step 4) has been identified in the literature, and information is available through Registries of Programs Effective in Reducing Youth Risk Behaviors on the CDC website as well as through similar sites (CDC, 2018). Identifying programming that has been shown to be effective is important to the success of school- or district-level WSCC efforts.

Step 6: Establish a Realistic Timeline for Implementing Strategies From the Action Plan

Regarding the timeline for the action plan, the SHI includes a question about how much time and effort it will take to complete an action. Possible responses to this question range from "little time and effort" to "very great time and effort" (CDC, 2017a). If an action addresses a high-priority item, then putting in the time and effort will be worth it. Regardless of how much time it might take to implement a policy or program, the assessment team needs to have an understanding of what it might actually take to complete that action in the school or district. It is necessary to take into account challenges to the academic calendar, including interruptions such as school breaks, weather delays or school cancelations, and professional development days or other days when staff may need to devote their complete attention to a different event or project. For example, many school districts went virtual because of COVID-19, and some vacillated between face-to-face and virtual schooling as cases increased or decreased. This type of change to the day-to-day schedule would certainly wreak havoc on a timeline for implementing WSCC activities.

As state and national initiatives change, this too may have an impact on a WSCC programming implementation schedule. If the WSCC action does not align with new mandates or requirements, this could result in a loss of administrative support. Keep in mind that faculty may meet in the spring to develop their priorities and schedules for the following fall, whereas administrators may meet in the summer to do the same. Action plans may be developed for one academic year, one full year, or more and depend on the process decided on by the developers. If the plan is developed for more than one year, conduct an annual reassessment to make potential adjustments to the timeline. Once the WSCC action plan is developed, it is important to make sure the content of the plan is communicated to both faculty and administrators and taken into consideration at the appropriate time for their dedication and involvement (see step 10 for more on the communication of efforts).

Step 7: Implement the Plan and Strategies

Putting the plan into place consists of implementing the school health action plan, which usually involves adopting new or revised policies or programs. When implementing the plan, districts need to direct the focus of school health efforts to meeting the learning and health needs of students (CDC, 2021). Providing opportunities for students to be meaningfully engaged in the process will also serve to encourage the team to direct its attention toward the students. Meaningful student engagement in programming and policies can give youth the chance to develop and exercise leadership abilities, build skills, form positive relationships with caring adults, and contribute to their school and greater community (CDC, 2021).

The CDC (2021) suggests that students can promote a healthy and safe school and community through opportunities such as involvement in peer education, peer advocacy, or cross-age mentoring programs. Other opportunities include involving young people in service-learning avenues and participating on school health teams, advisory committees, and boards that address health and wellness, education, and youth-related issues (CDC, 2021).

The CDC suggests that when moving into the taking-action phase of program and policy implementation districts or schools implement multiple strategies through multiple WSCC components. A variety of efforts are needed to have an effect on one school health component. Because the WSCC components are often overlapping and dependent on one another, addressing multiple if not all components is recommended for achieving the positive health and learning outcomes desired (CDC, 2021). Many possibilities exist for advancing each of the WSCC components, and examples of possible policies and programming efforts can be discovered in any of the WSCC assessment tools or criteria (see table 8.2 for possible strategies for improvement). The CDC's SHI and the ASCD School Improvement Tool are some of the better known and more commonly used tools. Any strategies being pursued should be based on an assessment conducted at the school or district level. During the development of the action plan, evaluation strategies for each identified action need to be identified and described

TABLE 8.2 WSCC Components and Possible Strategies for Improvement

WSCC component	Strategies
Health education	The district requires that all elementary schools teach health education in kindergarten through fifth grade. After an extensive review, an elementary health curriculum is selected and teacher training for implementation is conducted.
Physical education and physical activity	A new district mandate will require all students to participate in a minimum of 150 minutes of physical education per week.
Nutrition environment and services	The breakfast program at the junior high and high school will now offer at least one fruit other than juice at breakfast.
Health services	Each school is now required to have at least one full-time registered school nurse responsible for health services all day, every day.
Counseling, psychological, and social services	The counseling staff will now provide small-group and classroom-based health promotion and prevention activities in each classroom on a regular basis in addition to one-on-one counseling sessions.
Social and emotional climate	Staff receive training on how to foster the emotional growth and development of the elementary school child through guided social skill instruction.
Physical environment	Each school is required to make drinking water available to students free of charge throughout the day by installing additional water coolers when possible, making water available, and providing opportunities to take water breaks as needed.
Employee wellness	Each school is required to evaluate the employee wellness program annually and provide the district wellness coordinator with a report of the findings. These findings will be used to establish yearly staff wellness goals and help shape programming efforts.
Family engagement	People are available during parent meetings and events to help translate into the language understood by a group of refugees who recently relocated into the district.
Community involvement	The district allows a community agency access to school facilities to provide services (mental health services, preventive care) to students and their families.

Adapted from Alliance for a Healthier Generation (2014); Centers for Disease Control and Prevention (n.d.).

so the evaluation plan can be put into place once implementation begins.

Step 8: Review and Implement the Evaluation Plan

When programs and policies have been identified and implementation is underway, all efforts must be monitored to determine how well they are functioning and what impact they are having. Monitoring the progress and effect of policies and programming in terms of achieving objectives provides opportunities to perform needed adjustments as a way to make continuous improvements (Videto & Dake, 2019). After the outcome results are in, and the determination is made about whether the program or policy has achieved its goal, any successes should be celebrated, and findings communicated to the district and the greater community (CDC, 2017b). Chapter 7 provides details about the various types of evaluation that can be conducted with WSCC programming and strategies for conducting those evaluations. Evaluating both implementation (through process evaluation) and the attainment of objectives and goals (through outcome evaluation) is important for achieving desired outcomes and making adjustments along the way (CDC, 2017b; Rooney et al., 2015).

Step 9: Provide Professional Development for Faculty and Staff

Districts need to work to bring faculty and staff on board with WSCC efforts for successful implementation. Professional development opportunities are important for helping faculty and staff see the value of a large-scale collaborative approach and the relationship between health and academics. With proper training, teachers, staff, and school leaders can become important health champions to support and reinforce the efforts of the school health coordinator or administrator (CDC, 2022; Mann & Lohrman, 2019). Identifying professional development needs during the assessment process and then using those data to shape offerings for faculty and staff is important for customizing the process at the local level.

In the 2018 document *A Framework for Safe and Successful Schools*, it was recommended that professional development for school staff and community partners address school climate and safety; positive behavior; and crisis prevention, preparedness, and response (National Association of School Psychologists, 2018). As part of professional development, teachers and school leaders need to be provided with the information and resources they need to address student health issues and support a healthy

WSCC IN PRACTICE
Professional Development Addressing Mental Health Issues

From the CDC Healthy Schools Stories of Achievement related to WSCC, the following example shows how school district personnel worked together to receive training for addressing mental health issues:

> *The Green River Regional Education Cooperative (GRREC), located in south central and central Kentucky, is one of eight educational cooperatives in Kentucky. In response to the mental health issues arising from the COVID-19 pandemic, GRREC trained 689 people in Youth Mental Health First Aid (YMHFA). These teachers, administrators, school nurses, food service personnel, custodians, and others represented 76 schools and central offices in 30 school districts.*
>
> *YMHFA is a course that focuses on how to identify, understand, and respond to signs of mental illnesses and substance use disorders. GRREC identified the need for this training by surveying member districts on what they thought their social and emotional learning needs would be for the 2020-2021 school year. (CDC, 2022, paras. 1-2)*

school environment. Professional development might involve helping teachers to become aware of state-level health education regulations and requirements for health instruction so those issues can be addressed outside the health education classroom and integrated into other subjects to reinforce health-promoting concepts (Healthy Schools Campaign, 2012). Having more teachers and school leaders take on the role of school health champion and work to support health concepts and health policies facilitates moving the district toward a more unified WSCC effort. Table 8.3 provides examples of how all teachers and school lead-

TABLE 8.3 Teachers and School Leaders as Champions of WSCC

WSCC component	Role of teachers	Role of school leader
Health education	Reinforce messages and lessons from health education specialists and promote healthy classroom rewards and celebrations	Support regular health education and support healthy school fundraisers
Physical education and physical activity	Integrate physical activity into lesson plans and model behaviors that promote a healthy, active lifestyle	Support daily physical education and model behaviors that promote a healthy, active lifestyle
Nutrition environment and services	Model healthy behaviors by eating healthy meals and eating school lunches	Eat school lunch, provide students with adequate time to eat lunch, provide students with easy access to breakfast, and incorporate food service workers into the school wellness team
Health services	Provide the school nurse with information about students' health (e.g., vision or hearing issues or symptoms of chronic illness), and provide the school nurse with information about students' family situation (e.g., abuse)	Incorporate the school nurse into the school wellness team; develop a plan for meeting the needs of uninsured students; and offer vision, oral, and hearing screenings
Counseling, psychological, and social services	Support student connectedness and learn how to identify depression and suicidal tendencies	Support school connectedness and develop a plan for assisting students with mental health issues
Social and emotional climate	Create an atmosphere in which all children can thrive and feel accepted by developing a classroom of respect for all	Support a bully-free school and policies that foster acceptance and address harassment of all kinds
Physical environment	Practice good indoor air quality management in the classroom and report problems related to the quality of indoor air in the classroom (e.g., mold)	Organize and support an indoor air quality team and implement a no-idling policy for buses and cars
Employee wellness	Participate in a staff wellness program and be a health role model	Encourage and support a staff wellness program and participate in the events
Family engagement	Encourage and support family participation in a healthy school environment	Encourage and support family participation in a healthy school environment (e.g., open school facilities for family health and wellness events)
Community involvement	Provide administrators with information on needs of students that might hinder health and academic success	Identify opportunities to work with community agencies as a way to address student and family needs

Adapted from Healthy Schools Campaign (2012).

ers can support WSCC through each of the 10 components.

Step 10: Communicate Steps and Successes

Ongoing communication through a variety of modalities and channels must be utilized to ensure all partners and stakeholders are aware of efforts and outcomes. This process will assist in avoiding the duplication of efforts as well as provide a foundation for developing and maintaining trust (Rooney et al., 2015). The coordinator along with the teams and committees need to share changes in policies, new programs, and new processes developed to enhance or expand the WSCC model in the school or district. In addition to WSCC efforts being shared, any resulting outcomes, such as academic or health improvements, need to be communicated to all involved parties. To develop and maintain trust, strong communication efforts must be a continuous priority (Rooney et al., 2015). Consider the strategies offered in figure 8.5 for communicating WSCC-related changes.

Most important is to share positive outcomes of WSCC efforts. Partners, leaders, and administrators are more likely to continue to work on future projects when they know their work has been successful.

Summary

The focus of this chapter was on implementing, or carrying out, WSCC activities to achieve the objectives and ultimately the goal identified by the school district and community partners. WSCC program implementation, like any other process, requires the program planner to follow best practices for creating successful programs and policies whenever possible. The literature includes a great deal of information about planning and implementation steps for school districts and their partners to follow. ASCD and the CDC provide strategies to assist in creating WSCC infrastructure, planning for WSCC implementation, and implementing WSCC policies and programs. These strategies include establishing leadership by appointing a school health coordinator; securing admin-

---

FIGURE 8.5 STRATEGIES FOR COMMUNICATING WSCC-RELATED CHANGES OR OUTCOMES TO STUDENTS, FACULTY, ADMINISTRATORS, PARENTS, AND COMMUNITY PARTNERS

Ensure that partners and administrators absent from meetings receive meeting minutes as soon as possible to keep them informed.

Develop communications in the languages understood by the student and family populations in the district.

Provide information where stakeholders might view it, such as at building entrances and in school gathering places such as restrooms, conference rooms, faculty rooms, and stairwells.

Post announcements on district and school websites, including the athletic schedule page and the school calendar. Create a special section on the district website to be the central location for all WSCC information.

Announce new or changing policies or programs at teacher and parent meetings, athletic events, school concerts, and plays.

Ask students, staff, and community volunteers to assist in distributing informational flyers at school-related events.

Avoid using only one avenue for communication. Limiting communication to social media or to flyers or memos will limit the number of families or stakeholders who receive the intended message.

Adapted from RMC Health (n.d.).

istrative support; developing a district-level SHAC and school health teams; identifying available resources in the school, district, and community; and, after reviewing the initial data, determining the outcomes of greatest priority. Once priorities are identified, school districts and their partners collaborate to create an action plan based on realistic goals and objectives agreed upon by all partners, establish a realistic timeline for the implementation of strategies from the action plan, and implement and review an evaluation plan. Once implementation is underway, districts provide professional development for faculty and staff and, finally, communicate steps and successes to all.

LEARNING AIDS

GLOSSARY

health disparity—A higher burden of illness, injury, disability, or mortality experienced by one group of the population because of disadvantage, oppression, or racism.

infrastructure—Elements necessary for the successful implementation of a system such as coordinated school health or the WSCC approach. Elements such as a council at the district level, committees at each school, a coordinator to oversee the process, and administrator support are considered necessary infrastructure for a coordinated approach to school health.

institutionalization—The embedding of a program or policy in an organization so that it continues after the initial effort ends.

mission statement—A statement used to present the idea, direction, and philosophy of a program. Often broad in nature, it may include the program vision and desired outcome.

school health advisory council (SHAC)—"A group of teachers, administrators, staff, students, parents, and community members who act collectively to provide input regarding the planning, implementation, and evaluation of policies, programs, and services of the Whole School, Whole Community, Whole Child (WSCC) model in a school or school district. The council also may be referred to as a School Health, or Wellness Council/Committee/Team" (U.S. Department of Agriculture, n.d. as cited in Videto & Dennis, 2021, p. 14).

school health coordinator—A person charged with overseeing all efforts toward the achievement of WSCC. The coordinator maintains active school health committees and the districtwide SHAC while facilitating health programming in the district and school and between the school and community. The coordinator organizes the components of school health and facilitates actions to achieve a successful, coordinated system, including policies, programs, activities, and resources.

school health improvement plan—A comprehensive and specific plan that includes goals to be achieved and actions to be taken to move a school district toward implementation or improvement of WSCC. Generally included in the plan is a desired outcome, a description of steps to be taken, a timeline of when those steps will be conducted, and a list of those who are responsible for taking and overseeing those steps.

APPLICATION ACTIVITIES

1. Prepare a presentation on the 10 steps for implementing WSCC with a focus on the value of each step for ensuring successful implementation of a program or policy that would enhance the model in a school or district.
2. Create a job description for a school health coordinator that includes the importance of the position to WSCC as well as a list of skills needed in the position. Include in the job description reasons why the hiring school or district would be a strong potential employer.
3. Develop a presentation for a school board meeting that includes a description of the value of creating a district SHAC and school health teams for each school in the district. Provide a list of suggested representatives for the district-level and school-level groups along with the purposes and possible responsibilities of the council and teams.

REFERENCES

Alliance for a Healthier Generation. (2014). *Healthy schools program framework: Criteria for developing a healthier school environment*. https://schools.healthiergeneration.org/_asset/l062yk/Healthy-Schools-Program-Framework.pdf

Alliance for a Healthier Generation. (2018). *Healthy school program: Framework of best practices*. https://api.healthiergeneration.org/resource/11

American School Health Association. (2010). *What school administrators can do to enhance student learning by supporting a coordinated approach to health*. https://www.oregon.gov/ode/educator-resources/standards/health/Documents/administratorscoordinatedapproachsupport.pdf

American School Health Association. (2018). *ASHA position statement: The role of the school health coordinator*. www.ashaweb.org/wp-content/uploads/2018/06/ASHA-Position-Paper-School-Health-Coordinator-June2018Revision.pdf

ASCD. (2014). *Whole School, Whole Community, Whole Child*. www.ascd.org/whole-child

ASCD. (2022). *ASCD School Improvement Tool*. https://sitool.ascd.org/Default.aspx?ReturnUrl=%2f

California School Board Association. (2019). *Governance and Policy Resources*. https://www.csba.org/GovernanceAndPolicyResources/EducationalEquity

California School Boards Association and Cities Counties Schools Partnership. (2009). *Building healthy communities: A school leader's guide to collaboration and community engagement*. California School Boards Association.

Centers for Disease Control and Prevention. (n.d.). *School Health Index—Middle school/high school, sample school health improvement plan*. Retrieved January 25, 2023, from www.cdc.gov/healthyschools/shi/pdf/training-manual/planning-handout-shi-plan.pdf

Centers for Disease Control and Prevention. (2017a). *CDC Healthy Schools: School Health Index*. www.cdc.gov/healthyschools/shi/index.htm

Centers for Disease Control and Prevention. (2017b). *Program evaluation*. www.cdc.gov/evaluation/framework/index.htm

Centers for Disease Control and Prevention. (2017c). *Writing SMART objectives*. www.cdc.gov/dhdsp/evaluation_resources/guides/writing-smart-objectives.htm

Centers for Disease Control and Prevention. (2018). *Registries of programs effective in reducing youth risk behaviors*. www.cdc.gov/healthyyouth/adolescenthealth/registries.htm

Centers for Disease Control and Prevention. (2019). *Your guide to using the School Health Index*. www.cdc.gov/healthyschools/shi/instructions.htm

Centers for Disease Control and Prevention. (2020). *Youth Risk Behavior Surveillance System (YRBSS)*. www.cdc.gov/healthyyouth/data/yrbs/index.htm

Centers for Disease Control and Prevention. (2021). *CDC Healthy Schools: Whole School, Whole Community, Whole Child (WSCC)*. www.cdc.gov/healthyschools/wscc/index.htm

Centers for Disease Control and Prevention. (2022). *CDC Healthy Schools: Kentucky*. www.cdc.gov/healthyschools/achievement_stories/kentucky.htm

Centers for Disease Control and Prevention. (2023). *Adolescent and school health: Health disparities* www.cdc.gov/healthyyouth/disparities/index.htm

Children's Hospital of Wisconsin. (n.d.). *Secure and maintain administrative support*. Retrieved January 25, 2023, from www.healthykidslearnmore.com/Healthy-Kids-Learn-More1/Documents/wscc/WSCCAdministrativeSupport_WEB.pdf

Healthy Schools Campaign. (2016). *How to include health and wellness in school improvement plans*. https://healthyschoolscampaign.org/blog/include-health-wellness-school-improvement-plans/

Healthy Schools Campaign, Trust for America's Health. (2012). *Health in mind: Improving education through wellness, preparing teachers and school leaders as health champions* [Handout].

Hodges, B.C. (2013). *The changing name of school health* [Webinar].

Hodges, B.C., & Videto, D.M. (2011). *Assessment and planning in health programs* (2nd ed.). Jones & Bartlett Learning.

Hunt, P.H., Barrios, L., Telljohann, S.K., & Mazyck, D. (2015). A whole school approach: Collaborative development of school health policies, processes, and practices. *Journal of School Health*, *85*(11), 802-809. https://doi.org/10.1111/josh.12305

Jennings Public Schools. (2021). *Jennings Public Schools handbook*. https://s3.amazonaws.com/scschoolfiles/86/jennings_21-22_handbook.pdf

Mann, M.J., Kristjansson, A.L., Smith, M.L., Daily, S.M., Thomas, S., & Murray, S. (2018). From tactics to strategy: Creating and sustaining social conditions that demand and deliver effective school health programs. *Journal of School Health*, *88*, 333-336. https://doi.org/10.1111/josh.12614

Mann, M.J., & Lohrman, D.K. (2019). Addressing challenges to the reliable, large-scale implementation of effective school health education. *Health Promotion Practice*, *20*(6), 834-844. https://doi.org/10.1177/1524839919870196

Namaste Charter School. (n.d.). *Vision and purpose—Namaste Charter School*. www.namastecharterschool.org/visionpurpose

National Association of Chronic Disease Directors. (2016). *A guide for incorporating health and wellness into schools*. https://healthyschoolscampaign.org/dev/wp-content/uploads/2020/02/NACDD_SIP_Guide_2016.pdf

National Association of Chronic Disease Directors. (2017). *The Whole School, Whole Community, Whole Child model: A guide to implementation*. www.ashaweb.org/wp-content/uploads/2017/10/NACDD_WSCC_Guide_Final.pdf

National Association of School Psychologists. (2018). *A framework for safe and successful schools*. www.nasponline.org/

Office of Elementary and Secondary Education. (2020). *Plans that work: Tools for supporting school improvement planning*. https://oese.ed.gov/resources/oese-technical-assistance-centers/state-support-network/resources/plans-work-tools-supporting-school-improvement-planning/

RMC Health. (n.d.). *Communication tips: Get the word out about your tobacco-free schools policy*. www.rmc.org/resources-tools/

RMC Health. (2022). *Infrastructure for district and school health*. www.rmc.org/what-we-do/training-expertise-to-create-healthy-schools/infrastructure-for-district-and-school-health/

Rooney, L.E., Videto, D.M., & Birch, D.A. (2015). Using the Whole School, Whole Community, Whole Child model: Implications for practice. *Journal of School Health*, *85*(11), 817-823. https://doi.org/10.1111/josh.12304

Rudd Center. (2021). *WellSAT: 3.0 Wellness School Assessment Tool*. www.wellsat.org/

University of Kansas. (2022). *Section 2. Proclaiming your dream: Developing vision and mission statements*. http://ctb.ku.edu/en/table-of-contents/structure/strategic-planning/vision-mission-statements/main

Videto, D.M., & Dake, J.A. (2019). Promoting health literacy through defining and measuring quality school health education. *Health Promotion Practice*, *20*(6), 824-833. https://doi.org/10.1177/1524839919870194

Videto, D.M., & Dennis, D.L. (2021). Report of the 2020 Joint Committee on Health Education and Promotion Terminology. *The Health Educator*, *53*(1), 4-21.

Videto, D.M., & Hodges, B.C. (2009). Use of university/school partnerships for the institutionalization of the coordinated school health program. *American Journal of Health Education*, *40*(4), 212-219.

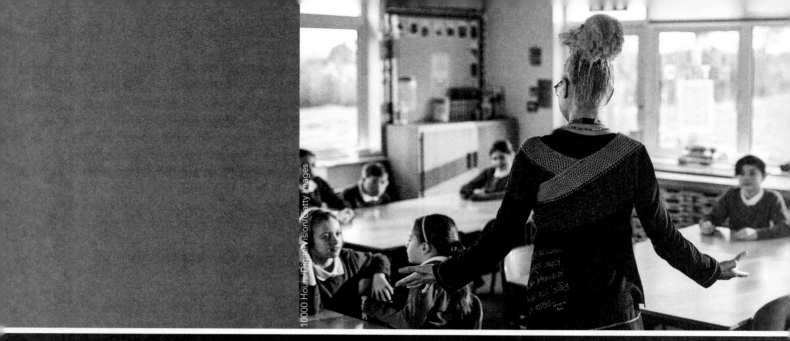

CHAPTER 9

Considerations for WSCC in Practice

Chapters 9 provides five perspectives on considerations related to the Whole School, Whole Community, Whole Child (WSCC) model in practice. The authors are leaders in school health with experience in providing leadership in the application of WSCC at the local, state, national, and international levels.

In this chapter, you will find the following contributions:

- A Perspective on the Role of State Education Agencies in Promoting WSCC—Rosemary Reilly-Chammat
- Every School Healthy: An Urban School Case Study—Sue Baldwin and Assunta R. Ventresca
- A Synopsis of International Efforts to Improve School Health Programs—Lloyd J. Kolbe
- Teacher Education: Preparing Educators for WSCC Engagement—Elisa Beth McNeill
- The Importance of Professional Development—Lori Paisley

LEARNING OBJECTIVES

1. Analyze the role of state departments of education and the Buffalo (NY) School District, an urban school district, in promoting and supporting the implementation of the WSCC model in schools.
2. Compare the WSCC model to other national and international models and initiatives for promoting and supporting health-promoting schools.
3. Identify important considerations in preparing education professionals and school staff, family, and community stakeholders.

A Perspective on the Role of State Education Agencies in Promoting WSCC

Rosemary Reilly-Chammat

State departments of education, which are formally known as state education agencies (SEAs), along with local school districts or local education agencies (LEAs) have a primary role in leading education initiatives in the United States. The significance of this role is underscored as our collective society moves through the endemic phase of the SARS-CoV-2 virus. The National Center for the Improvement of Educational Assessment produced the report *COVID-19 Academic Impact in Rhode Island*, which projected a recovery from the pandemic of 3 to 5 years (Bettebenner & Van Iwaarden, 2022). The Rhode Island Department of Education commissioned this report to understand the academic impact of the pandemic using state assessment scores. This type of impact assessment report can help SEAs determine how to address the health, safety, academic, social, emotional, and behavioral needs of students. It is also useful in considering systemic supports such as organizational structures, professional learning, and other supports for educators. The pandemic also underscored the inequities in our society. SEAs must champion efforts that address health equity and social justice. Schools influence both education and health, thereby influencing the well-being of whole populations. The reciprocal relationship between health and education has long been established in the literature. This perspective explores the role of SEAs in supporting health by identifying frameworks such as the Whole School, Whole Community, Whole Child (WSCC) model and the multitiered system of supports (MTSS) framework, fulfilling health requirements, promoting health and social justice, and addressing inequities in schools.

The Role of the Federal Government in Education

Although the federal government has a smaller role in education than the individual states, it plays a significant role in assisting the states in creating safe, healthy, and supportive environments for students. The Elementary and Secondary Education Act of 1965 codified the role of the federal government in education to ensure that all children have what they need to succeed. This act was updated in 2002 with the passage of the No Child Left Behind Act.

The reauthorization of the Elementary and Secondary Education Act in 2015, the Every Student Succeeds Act (ESSA), repealed the No Child Left Behind Act. ESSA includes specific references to the links between health and education, specifically in Title VI, Part A. The breadth and specificity of language related to health within the statute are unprecedented. ESSA's definition of a well-rounded education goes beyond traditional core academic areas such as English language arts, mathematics, science, and social studies to include the arts, health education, and physical education (U.S. Department of Education [USDOE], 2015). Skills-based instructional practices that support communication and relationship-building skills are emphasized. The intention is to improve health and safety through content on physical activity, nutrition, tobacco (including e-cigarettes), alcohol, substance abuse, chronic disease management, bullying, harassment, and suicide prevention. ESSA recognizes the value of providing school mentoring and school counseling to all students. This is especially important for students at risk for academic challenges, dropping out of school, and associated health-risk behaviors (USDOE, 2015).

State departments of education use ESSA's kindergarten through grade 12 education policy statutory language to guide state plans, allocate resources, and support statewide efforts to continuously improve how districts can support students' health and academic achievement. State departments of education are required to submit proposals to the USDOE that include data on current needs, goals, objectives, and an implementation plan within the statutory framework and evaluation measures and protocols. The implementation plan is available to the public. In a similar way, state departments of education use these plans to define a framework and planning process for LEAs.

ESSA also underscores the need for school-based mental health services including both group and individual services. It also emphasizes the need for community partnerships to support the needs of youth and families that go beyond what the school can provide. These partnerships take time to develop. The partnerships must result in initiatives and services that are in alignment with school expectations for student success. In addition, all initiatives and services must be evidence-based and grounded in trauma-informed policies, practices, and protocols (USDOE, 2015).

The Healthy People 2030 health objectives for the United States provide an example of the relationship between education and health. They include objectives for both reading and math achievement for children in fourth grade. Fourth grade is a pivotal time for the development of reading skills. Children learn to read through third grade. In fourth grade, children are expected to comprehend what they read, making reading a critical skill for learning.

Children with poor reading skills are more likely to struggle in school and to take part in risky behaviors as adolescents. There are significant disparities in reading skills among 4th-graders by race/ethnicity, school type, and eligibility for the National School Lunch Program. Early interventions to develop reading skills can improve school performance, which is linked to healthy behaviors. (U.S. Department of Health and Human Services, 2022, "Summary")

Prior to and in response to the COVID-19 pandemic, federal agencies, including the USDOE and Substance Abuse and Mental Health Services Administration, created substantive funding opportunities directed toward SEAs that clearly connect health and mental health with improved school outcomes. Grant forecasting from the Centers for Disease Control and Prevention (CDC) includes equity-focused opportunities to support student health, academics, well-being, and sexual health, among other relevant topics, directed at SEAs and LEAs. Collectively, these federal funding opportunities are essential for building state-level capacity to support health and education outcomes.

The Role of the States in Education

The United States has not developed centralized bureaucracies with direct control over education like in some countries in Europe. Yet policymakers, advocates for school reform, and other stakeholders expect that state education departments will play an important role in education reform including students' health, especially in this phase of endemic COVID-19. A key priority for SEAs is to develop the administrative capacity to guide and support local school health efforts. Timar (1997) asserted that large-scale education reform is "unlikely in the absence of an institutional center to shape policy, aggregate interests and control and channel conflict" (p. 235). This underscores the unique role of SEAs.

The role of SEAs in comprehensive health efforts and overall education reform is tenuous. The Education Commission of the States identified different governance structures in SEAs; the structures differed in terms of elected officials, appointed officials, and the role of the governor in education. It is important to understand governance structures and decision-making authority to effectively advance education goals (Railey, 2017). Furthermore, research supported by the Education Commission of the States revealed that every state except for the District of Columbia and Hawaii have statutes that define the authority of local school boards (Evans et al., 2020). Research from the Education Commission of the States (M. McCann, personal communication, November 17, 2022) revealed the following:

- *Twenty-five states have outlined a formal constitutional role for their governors specific to education.*
- *Every state has constitutional language detailing the authority and duties of state legislatures in education, and 40 states give their legislatures some role in appointing or confirming the chief state school officer or members of the state board of education.*
- *Thirty chief state school officers have a formal constitutional role in state government. In addition, how they are selected for office varies: 21 are appointed by state boards of education, 16 are appointed by the governor, 12 are elected, and 1 is appointed by the state executive-level secretary. In Oregon, the governor is the superintendent of education.*
- *The authority and duties of state boards of education are also detailed in state constitutions and statutes. Twenty-three states include state boards in their constitutions, and 26 state boards have only statutory powers and duties. Only Minnesota and Wisconsin do not have state boards, and New Mexico's public education commission serves in an advisory capacity only.*
- *Thirty-four states have some variation of an executive-level secretary. Such positions may mean additional formal duties for chief state school officers, or they may be individually appointed positions designated to serve the state board of education or work in some other capacity.*

A more defined and aligned role among state departments of education would assist in the development of a comprehensive education and school health agenda for the United States. Sharing best practices across states is a starting point.

Leadership by State Education Agencies in School Health

SEAs are charged with capacity building to support multidisciplinary approaches such as the WSCC approach. According to the Education Commission of the States policy tracker, 12 SEAs (Alaska, Arizona, Colorado, Connecticut, Kentucky, Louisiana, Massachusetts, Michigan, New Jersey, New Mexico, Pennsylvania, and Utah) reference the WSCC approach on their webpages. Eight states (Arkansas, Mississippi, Nebraska, North Carolina, Oklahoma, Texas, Vermont, and Wisconsin) have adopted, aligned, or integrated a Whole Child model into their coordinated school health program. Six states (California, Delaware, Hawaii, Maine, Montana, and Ohio) have created a state-specific WSCC approach or framework (M. McCann, personal communication, November 17, 2022). The use of the WSCC framework can facilitate robust planning for health and education efforts.

Rhode Island has incorporated the WSCC framework into its health education framework and other grant-funded efforts. The Rhode Island Department of Elementary and Secondary Education convenes a state-level school health advisory council. This council assists the department in guiding the work of various federal grants. It provides a forum for connecting LEAs, other state departments, community-based organizations, and stakeholders. Through both formal and informal communication, members of the school health advisory council develop mutually supportive relationships and bidirectional communication to support both state and local efforts. Capacity building also includes participation in professional associations that help connect staff in similar roles with local and national supports.

SEAs can assemble partners and stakeholders to plan state and local efforts to address health equity and set the conditions for a health-in-all-policies approach. SEAs can also connect LEAs with tools and resources that support communities in addressing their stated needs and priorities. Astute SEA leaders and staff assist local leaders in utilizing tools to build a shared understanding of community needs and consensus around goals and objectives to address health concerns. SEAs can also provide access to professional development and technical assistance to this end. Collectively, these efforts empower communities to address key social justice issues and address systemic causes of disparities specific to the community.

Priorities may change at the federal level; therefore, SEA leaders must frame opportunities to address current contexts. For example, in the early days of the HIV/AIDS epidemic, the CDC provided funding for all states to build capacity for HIV/AIDS and sexual health education and support for adolescents. As HIV/AIDS became more treatable, priorities shifted, and the CDC had less funds. States had to compete for funds to support their work. Then the CDC made a policy decision to shift the focus of the work from SEAs to LEAs (CDC, 2018). Some states were able to continue to support their work through state funds, but others had to find new sources of support. It is an ongoing challenge for SEAs to support the breadth and depth of school health when dedicated funding is exclusively for specific health concerns rather than comprehensive efforts.

SEAs also help build the capacity of LEAs to support the health of school-age children. They promulgate regulations and enforce state statutes concerning health in schools. SEAs can also inform the development of legislation that can further enhance the work. Regulations can help ensure that health concerns such as vision problems, asthma management, teen pregnancy, aggression and violence, lack of physical activity, access to breakfast, and inattention and hyperactivity are reflected in school reform agendas (Basch, 2010). SEAs can implement statewide school climate surveys to gauge the experiences of students, parents, and staff in schools. These school-level data are valuable for assessing strengths and challenges. In addition to providing academic data, school climate surveys can aid in the identification of disparities in experiences across subpopulations in the school community. This is especially important for meeting the academic and behavioral health needs of students with different abilities and multilingual learners.

SEAs partner with the CDC on the Youth Risk Behavior Survey and the School Health Profiles. The Youth Risk Behavior Surveillance System (YRBSS) assists in the identification of statewide trends in health risks among middle school and high school students. The YRBSS includes a national data sample, statewide data samples, and data from large urban districts. The School Health Profiles is a system of surveys assessing school health policies and practices in states, large urban school districts, and territories. Together these surveys help SEAs connect the health risks of youth to the capacity of systems in schools to support them. Collectively, these data assist SEAs in engaging in education and advocacy efforts on behalf of students and the adults who support them.

SEAs work with other state department employees in similar roles across the United States through engagement in professional associations and specific convening around grant funding. These opportunities are essential for information sharing, camaraderie, and problem-solving on our most pressing school health concerns and challenges. Often, these employees are in roles supporting health education and physical education. The WSCC model can aid in the identification of other relevant roles, collaborators, and colleagues within SEAs.

School health efforts can be enhanced or hindered by the expectations of other state departments. Focusing on one issue without recognizing the interconnections among various health topics means missing opportunities to construct a more comprehensive approach. There are also challenges around communicating complex issues and approaches. For example, adverse childhood experiences are widely recognized as the root cause of unhealthy behaviors. The causes of adverse childhood experiences, by their nature, are varied and complex and can include experiencing and witnessing traumas. There is a growing body of research on the impact of adverse childhood experiences on long-term health outcomes and, even more important, protective factors. This research has built a body of evidence that healthy outcomes are achievable even though people experience traumatic life events (CDC, 2019). A South Carolina–based study on strategies for communicating complex issues to legislators made the following suggestions: Frame the issue within the context of current public health issues (e.g., the opioid crisis, climate change); consider the mode of communication, including the use of stories and data to frame concerns; and provide access to credible data along with suggestions on how to identify misinformation. The study was based on semi-structured interviews with state legislators who had served at least one term in office (Srivastav et al., 2020). Most important, school health can provide opportunities to explore, align, and integrate education and public health systems (Institute of Medicine, 2015; Kim, 2018; Kolbe, 2019). A multisystem approach is required to build equity, because disparities do not exist in silos. Education affects health through multiple pathways. More schooling is linked to better health outcomes. Social determinants of health are affected by education. Income from a well-paying and stable job allows access to safe neighborhoods and other resources to support healthy lifestyles (Zajacova & Lawrence, 2018). Beyond school and consistent with the WSCC approach, education affects each level of the socioecological model, including individual, community, and social contexts and policies that influence and may perpetuate health disparities (Zimmerman et al., 2015). The World Health Organization (2011, p.2) asserted

Education is a human right. It enhances people's capacities to have decent jobs and fulfilling lives. Article 26 of the Universal Declaration of Human Rights stipulates that "everyone has the right to education" and that "education shall be free, at least in the elementary and fundamental stages" [United Nations, 1948]. Education is critical for human and economic development and cohesive societies.

The business of education, including school health efforts, takes place within a political environment of often competing interests. It is therefore the work of SEAs to promote research and evidence-based practices, align policies to facilitate change, advance equity, and provide information and education for necessary statutes that strengthen the education system overall by convening stakeholders to inform and support these efforts.

Frameworks to Support the Work: WSCC and the Multitiered System of Supports Framework

Frameworks or models can be useful tools for state agency administrators to consider when building capacity for health both within SEAs and among the LEAs they serve. The WSCC model is a powerful framework because it is child-centered with a focus on keeping children healthy, safe, engaged, supported, and challenged. This model illustrates how health can affect the academic success of students. The WSCC model was developed by the CDC and ASCD to align the common goals of the health and education sectors. Each one of the model's components emphasizes the engagement of schools with people who have certain expertise related to the health of school-age children. This inclusion is a way to identify potential partners in schools for health-related efforts. It is heartening to note how each one of the components is reflected in ESSA.

Another framework applicable to education and health is MTSS. ESSA defines MTSS as "a comprehensive continuum of evidence-based, systemic practices to support a rapid response to students' needs, with regular observation to facilitate data-based instructional decision-making" (Office of Elementary and Secondary Education, 2020, Part A, section 8101[33]). An MTSS framework connects tiered academic, social-emotional, and behavioral health interventions (see figure 9.1). This framework can relate to efforts supported through Individuals with Disabilities Education Act funding and interventions to support multilingual learners. Tier 1 of the framework includes access to the core curriculum with a whole-school focus on safe, supportive, and predictable environments. Tier 2 of the framework is focused on small-group interventions for students who may be struggling academically, behaviorally, or in both realms. Tier 3 focuses on struggling students who may need individualized attention. Sometimes the needs of children and families go beyond what the school can provide. Addressing them necessitates the formation of partnerships with community-based providers. The framework underscores that no matter the level of service a child might need at any given time, all children must have access to tier 1. It is interesting that if more than 10 percent of the school population is identified as being in need of tier 3 interventions, it generally means that the school must focus on tier 1. Tier 1 processes, practices, and protocols may be the hardest to implement because all adults in the building must be aligned in providing a core curriculum within a safe, supportive, and predictable environment. In this way, the MTSS framework is similar to the WSCC model. Aligning the MTSS and WSCC models can help provide additional support and expertise across all members of the school community, which is foundational to the implementation of policies and programs that guide equitable practices to support all students.

Frameworks such as WSCC and MTSS can assist SEA and LEA leaders in thinking broadly about health systems to enhance educational success. Efforts that focus on one health issue, such as obesity or bullying, or the

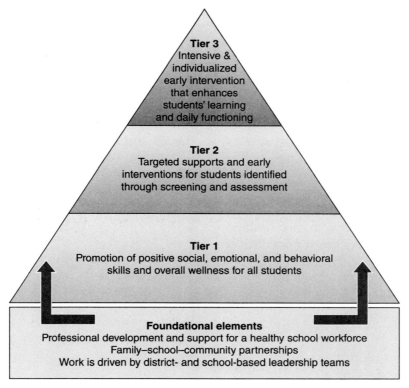

FIGURE 9.1 MTSS.
From Rhode Island Department of Education (2021).

use of disciplinary exclusion practices can be implemented in a silo without recognition of interconnections. Efforts that focus on content without the skills to practice health will fall short of intended outcomes. Similarly, laws and policies are often fragmented and focused on a single issue. It is imperative that SEA leaders assist LEAs and communities as well as state lawmakers in connecting efforts with the larger picture (Solomon et al., 2018; Van Dusen, 2020).

The CDC has long been a champion of substantive and meaningful outcomes that can be realized when the health and education sectors align initiatives. Public health and public education often share concerns about the same children and families. Both systems were created to service all children. Both WSCC and MTSS allow for nuanced implementation to address specific needs of schools and districts. Frameworks can be used bidirectionally. Social, emotional, and mental health was found to be a key priority area among stakeholder groups interested in healthy schools. Social and emotional skills are necessary for adopting healthy behaviors and are foundational to all health education skills. There is a growing awareness of the need to address the wellness of educators and school staff to implement schoolwide approaches. The trauma, both real and existential through the endemic, cannot be ignored. Both the WSCC model and MTSS frameworks can accommodate this approach (Solomon et al., 2018). These frameworks assist in incorporating health considerations across sectors, leading to a health-in-all-policies approach.

Future Opportunities

The role of SEAs will always involve balancing state priorities and existing opportunities to support the work. This involves holding a long-term vision for the work while working on short-term, time-limited objectives. It is imperative that SEA staff remain competitive to acquire federal funds that build state capacity for the work. Accessing federal funds keeps SEAs on the cutting edge of current health issues. Continued work to move from reactionary efforts to proactive, comprehensive ones can assist in a health in all policies, programs, and practices approach. LEAs count on SEA staff to provide support for the field. SEA staff are the best advocates for supporting needs at the school level. This also involves navigating change. For example, current efforts in secondary school reform will likely have an impact on how physical education and health education are taught in schools. By implementing the WSCC model, LEAs can adopt innovative approaches aligned with health education and physical education standards. The presence of standards from WSCC-related professional associations (e.g., school counselors, school social workers, school psychologists, and school nurses) can result in broad and comprehensive efforts across a school community. State-level support in navigating this change within the field is essential. This support helps people feel that they are part of an exciting change rather than having a change imposed on them. Implementing comprehensive approaches to systems change such as the WSCC model and the MTSS framework will ensure that we are meeting the needs and challenges of our time. It is vital for achieving equity. This is the new hope. Our students and all adults connected to schools and in our communities deserve nothing less.

REFERENCES

Basch, C.E. (2010). *Healthier students are better learners: A missing link in school reforms to close the achievement gap* (ED523998). ERIC. https://files.eric.ed.gov/fulltext/ED523998.pdf

Bettebenner, D.W., & Van Iwaarden, A. (2022). *COVID-19 academic impact in Rhode Island*. National Center for the Improvement of Educational Assessment. www.ride.ri.gov/Portals/0/Uploads/Documents/News/Rhode_Island_Academic_Impact_Report_FINAL.pdf?ver=2022-04-27-173245-260

Centers for Disease Control and Prevention, Division of Adolescent and School Health. (2018). *CDC-RFA-PS18-1807: Promoting adolescent health through school-based HIV prevention*. www.cdc.gov/healthyyouth/about/nofo.htm

Centers for Disease Control and Prevention, Division of Injury Prevention and Control. (2019). *We can prevent adverse childhood experiences*. www.cdc.gov/injury/features/adverse-childhood-experiences/index.html#:~:text=Adverse%20Childhood%20Experiences%20%28ACEs%29%20are%20potentially%20traumatic%20events,a%20family%20member%20attempt%20or%20die%20by%20suicide

Evans, A., Erwin, B., Syverson, E., & Whinnery, E. (2020). *50 state comparison: K-12 statewide governance*. Education Commission of the States. www.ecs.org/50-state-comparison-k-12-governance/

Institute of Medicine. (2015). *Exploring opportunities for collaboration between health and education to improve population health: Workshop summary*. www.ncbi.nlm.nih.gov/books/NBK316101/pdf/Bookshelf_NBK316101.pdf

Kim, J.Y. (2018). Eliminating poverty in the 21st century: The role of health and human capital. *Journal of the American Medical Association, 320*(14), 1427-1428. https://doi.org/10.1001/jama.2018.13709

Kolbe, L.J. (2019). School health as a strategy to improve both public health and education. *Annual Review of Public Health, 40*, 443-446. https://doi.org/10.1146/annurev-publhealth-040218-043727

Office of Elementary and Secondary Education. (2020). *Title VIII general provisions*. https://oese.ed.gov/offices/office-of-formula-grants/school-support-and-accountability/essa-legislation-table-contents/title-viii-general-provisions/

Railey, H. (2017, December 19). *Who makes ed policy in your state?* EdNote. https://ednote.ecs.org/who-makes-ed-policy-in-your-state/

Rhode Island Department of Education. (2021). *Universal screening guidance: Mental health, social, emotional, and behavioral health*. https://ride.ri.gov/sites/g/files/xkgbur806/files/Portals/0/Uploads/Documents/Students-and-Families-Great-Schools/Health-Safety/Mental-Wellness/Universal-Screening-Guidance.pdf?ver=2021-12-20-120814-030

Solomon, B., Katz, E., Steed, H., & Temkin, D. (2018). *Creating policies to support healthy schools: Policymaker, educator, and student perspectives*. Child Trends. https://cms.childtrends.org/wp-content/uploads/2018/10/healthyschoolstakeholderreport_ChildTrends_October2018.pdf

Srivastav, A., Spencer, M., Thrasher, J.F., Strompolis, M., Crouch, E., & Davis, R.E. (2020). Addressing health and well-being through state policy: Understanding barriers and opportunities for policy making to prevent adverse childhood experiences (ACES) in South Carolina. *American Journal of Health Promotion, 34*(2), 189-197. https://doi.org/10.1177/0890117119878068

Timar, T.B. (1997). The institutional role of state education departments: A historical perspective. *American Journal of Education, 105*(3), 231-260.

United Nations. (1948). *Universal Declaration of Human Rights*. Retrieved from https://www.un.org/en/about-us/universal-declaration-of-human-rights

U.S. Department of Education. (2015). *Every Student Succeeds Act*. Retrieved December 31, 2022, from www.ed.gov/essa?src%3Drn

U.S. Department of Health and Human Services. (2022). *Increase the proportion of 4th-graders with reading skills at or above the proficient level—AH-05*. Healthy People 2030. https://health.gov/healthypeople/objectives-and-data/browse-objectives/schools/increase-proportion-4th-graders-reading-skills-or-above-proficient-level-ah-05

Van Dusen, D. (2020). *When are we going to teach health? Let's teach health as if each child's life depends on it—Because it does*. Lioncrest.

World Health Organization. (2011). *Education: Shared interests in well-being and development* (Social Determinants of Health Sectoral Briefing 2). www.who.int/publications/i/item/9789241502498

Zajacova, A., & Lawrence, E.M. (2018). The relationship between education and health: Reducing disparities through a contextual approach. *Annual Review of Public Health, 39*, 273-289. https://doi.org/10.1146/annurev-publhealth-031816-044628

Zimmerman, E.B., Woolf, S.H., & Haley, A. (2015). Understanding the relationship between education and health: A review of evidence and an examination of community perspectives. In R.M. Kaplan, M.L. Spittel, & D.H. David (Eds.), *Population health— Behavioral and social science insights* (AHRQ Publication No. 15-0002, pp. 347-384). Agency for Healthcare Research and Quality and Office of Behavioral and Social Sciences Research.

Every School Healthy: An Urban School Case Study

Sue Baldwin • Assunta R. Ventresca

Buffalo Public Schools makes up the second largest school district in New York State. Demographic data from the U.S. Census Bureau showed that in 2018 almost half of the district's children lived in poverty, which reflects Buffalo's rank as the fourth most impoverished city among the nation's major cities (Buffalo Public Schools, 2019). As of 2018, the district supported 33,415 students, of whom 35 percent were English language learners and 21 percent were students with disabilities. Approximately 77 percent of the district population was considered economically disadvantaged, and 96 percent were classified as Title I. The racial distribution of the population was 45 percent Black, 21 percent Hispanic, 20 percent White, 10 percent Asian, and 4 percent other. More than 82 different languages were spoken by students in this district. For the 2017-2018 school year, the district's four-year graduation rate was 64 percent (Buffalo Public Schools, 2019). These demographics led the Whole Child Advisory Board into discussion and concerted efforts to ensure equity in the development of wellness policies.

In this district, the Whole Child Advisory Board, Whole Child district health committees, and school-level Whole Child well-being teams are managed by the Office of Whole Child Initiatives, which is led by a seasoned district wellness coordinator, as illustrated in the Whole School, Whole Community, Whole Child (WSCC) organizational chart (figure 9.2). (All district and school Whole Child well-being committees and teams begin their names with "Whole Child." For reader ease and readability, we have omitted "Whole Child" from their titles for the remainder of this perspective.) This district wellness coordinator assesses, plans, and evaluates the implementation and reported progress on the wellness policy titled *Making Health Academic*. The district wellness coordinator directs the administration, collection, analysis, and reporting of the Youth Risk Behavior Survey (YRBS) and the School Health Index (SHI) data across the district. The coordinator annually leads all 60 school well-being teams, 13 district health committees, and the Whole Child Advisory Board. All teams and committees use YRBS and SHI data to create specific, measurable, attainable, realistic, and timely committee goals to decrease student health-risk behaviors. The WSCC vision, mission, roles, responsibilities, and organizational chart (see figure 9.2) and the wellness policy form the infrastructure of the WSCC model and foster its sustainability (Murray et al., 2015). The coordinator ensures fidelity of implementation of the WSCC model across the district and all its schools.

There are 60 schools in the district: elementary schools supporting students in prekindergarten through grade 8, a few schools with students in grades 5 to 12, and 19 high schools that accommodate students in grades 9 to 12. Unlike many school districts, the district is fortunate to have a full-time nurse in each building. Nearly all schools have a full-time school psychologist, counselor, and social worker based on school enrollment and need.

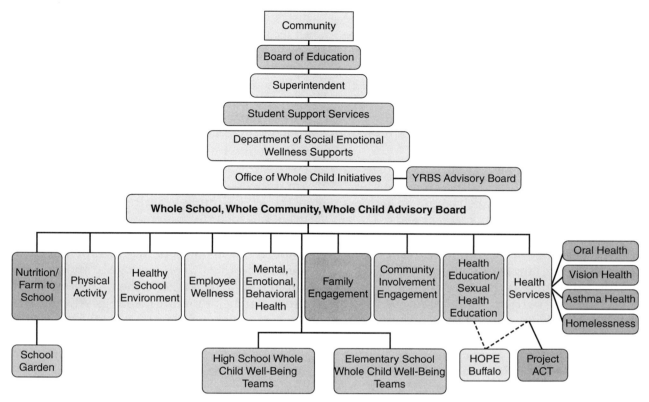

FIGURE 9.2 Buffalo Public School District Office of Whole Child Initiatives: WSCC organizational chart. Adapted from Baldwin and Ventresca (2020).

Needs Assessment and District Response

This section focuses on the impact of the district's wellness policy, the data that drove changes, and continual professional development across WSCC components. The Buffalo Public School District wellness policy plays an important role in the presence and implementation of the WSCC model in the district. The strength of the wellness policy is driven by the leadership of the district wellness coordinator and the fact that the policy is implemented across all WSCC model components (i.e., parent and community engagement, school guidance, school psychology and social work, health-related services, health education, and physical education). Not only does the wellness policy stress coordination, collaboration, and communication (3Cs) among all district policies, programs, and practices (3Ps), but it was created through the continual use of the 3Cs and 3Ps. This approach has become the district's standard of practice. We recognize through our years of experience that school districts can be successful in creating, adopting, and implementing a WSCC-based wellness policy with these essential elements: administrative support, a wellness champion, and engaged parent and community partners who have a passion for, vision for, and experience with health promotion. A district wellness champion can be a physical educator, health teacher, nurse, school administrator, parent, or anyone who has a passion to create a healthier school environment (Steckler & Goodman, 1989). Data are an important component and can drive action. This case study occurred over a period of seven years, and the work continues to become institutionalized across the district and city. Research indicates that schools in districts with strong policies are more likely to implement the policy and associated practices

(Boehm et al., 2020; Schwartz et al., 2012). The strength of the policy lies in strong language to indicate that action is required, including words such as *shall*, *will*, *must*, *require*, *all*, *comply*, and *enforce* (Schwartz et al., 2012). The policy has clearly stated goals that can be enforced via the district wellness coordinator, district health committees, and all 60 school well-being teams.

The district wellness coordinator fostered trusting relationships with parent leaders, including parents of English language learners and other students with special needs. These parents have been a driving force for strengthening wellness policy development and implementation. The language in the wellness policy addressed students with disabilities and those with language barriers. The continuous use of the 3Cs, with more than 275 community partners, led to the development of a data-driven wellness policy that was coordinated with a variety of partners. It took a year to redesign the policy around the WSCC model using the WellSAT 3.0 (Rudd Center, 2019a).

Creating a wellness policy using the WSCC model formalized the development of specific committees. School district departments took leadership roles on these committees. For example, the Department of Food Service became highly engaged in addressing obesity in our district, the Parent Engagement Office integrated WSCC language into its department policies, and the Department of Health and Physical Education formed the Comprehensive Health Education Committee to implement a stronger health curriculum and address risky sexual health behaviors. Once all WSCC components were assessed for clarity, language, and comprehensiveness, the district health committee leaders then worked with their committees and used the assessment results to revise their designated WSCC domain of the policy. Many parent, student, and large community partner meetings were held to provide opportunities for feedback on each WSCC domain of the policy. All school well-being teams completed a wellness policy feedback activity in their school at a faculty meeting to seek feedback from all school-level staff. The Whole Child Advisory Board, composed of district and community partner coleaders from all 16 district health committees, reviewed and edited the feedback from all stakeholders on all components to finalize the policy.

The finalized policy was unanimously adopted by the board of education. Every school had a well-being team, received its own YRBS school report, and participated in and obtained its own SHI needs assessment. The district advisory board and district health committees (each representing the components of the WSCC model; figure 9.2) consistently strived to include students, parents, teachers, school administrators, partners in higher education, research partners, members of the board of education, health professionals, appropriate community partners, and the district medical director in their monthly meetings. All committees and teams utilized data from the YRBS, the SHI, school climate surveys, and county and state health reports and any other pertinent health or educational data (i.e., attendance rates, suspension rates, bullying rates) to create district and school action plans. These action plans were incorporated into the state-mandated school improvement plan as part of each school's work to improve students' academic and health outcomes (U.S. Department of Agriculture, 2016). The wellness policy mandated the development of a districtwide plan, progress monitoring, and reporting on the implementation of the WSCC-based policy to the board of education and community.

In 2019, the district responded to a U.S. Department of Agriculture (2016) requirement to update the wellness policy. A more robust policy continued to evolve utilizing the Rudd Institute's WellSAT WSCC assessment. The WellSAT WSCC tool was used to examine the strength of the wording in and comprehensiveness of the policy around all components of the WSCC model (Rudd Center, 2019b).

Key Stakeholder Engagement

One example of the impact of stakeholder involvement was the work of the School Health and Wellness Collaborative. The collaborative was formed to promote communication, collaboration, information sharing, shared decision-making, and continued research on best practices for family engagement in school sexual health education. It included parents and students trained by community health workers, including parents of students with special needs and English language learners. These families attended various community forums organized by the school district in order to advocate for a comprehensive sexual health education curriculum and the adoption of a condom availability policy. Community health workers attended, participated in, or led school-based well-being teams and participated on the district Comprehensive Health Education Committee. Community health workers were also engaged in advocating for comprehensive sexual health education. Parents and students have been highly involved in decision-making and empowered to participate in meaningful, open dialogue. The district also recognized that parents and students have direct knowledge of the diverse family- and community-level assets and challenges that affect them around sexual health. Research has shown that parents who are involved in school health activities affect not only their children's health behaviors but also their academic achievement (Basch, 2011; Centers for Disease Control and Prevention, 2023).

Professional Development

Community involvement was evident in the Buffalo Public Schools' efforts through stakeholder engagement in professional development related to sexual health. The SHI, which was completed in all schools, revealed that students were not receiving appropriate comprehensive sexual health education and that teachers had not received professional development to teach sexual health education. Community partners who were members of the Comprehensive Health Education Committee helped address this gap, engaged in advocacy, and contributed to successful sexual health outcomes. The Genesee Valley Educational Partnership provided professional development for teachers on the adopted sexual health curriculum, including adaptations for students with special needs and students for whom English was a new language. Teachers received training on the Centers for Disease Control and Prevention's characteristics of effective health education and health instruction that incorporated the use of HealthSmart, Reducing the Risk, and the condom availability program (Centers for Disease Control and Prevention, 2015). Professional development also included skill development on how to utilize school YRBS data to prioritize district health education pacing guides for buildings.

Sexual health community partners from Genesee Valley Educational Partnership, Planned Parenthood of Western New York, Native American Community Services, the Erie County Department of Health, and the Federation of Neighborhood Centers collaborated to supplement sexual health education instruction in seventh- and ninth-grade health courses. These partners assisted the committee in the creation and implementation of the condom availability policy and provided professional development to all district health teachers on how to incorporate the condom availability policy into the sexual health curriculum.

The Erie County Department of Health provided professional training for all district nurses on the condom availability program as it related to the Reducing the Risk sexual health curriculum. Another example of the use of the 3Cs with the Erie County Department of Health, Cicatelli Associates, and the district resulted in federal funding of a grant for teen pregnancy and prevention. This $10 million grant fostered the establishment of H.O.P.E. Buffalo. H.O.P.E. Buffalo is a community-wide pledge for teen health—a youth- and community-led collaborative of diverse stakeholders, teens, and adults working together to promote equitable access to high-quality and comprehensive sexuality education and reproductive health services. H.O.P.E. Buffalo supported student visits to community sexual health agencies and created the *H.O.P.E. Buffalo Pocket Guide*, a student-friendly resource for sexual health services. H.O.P.E. Buffalo funds were used to purchase Be Proud, Be Responsible, the district's seventh-grade evidence-based sexual health curriculum. The grant also funded Raising Healthy Children, an evidence-based youth development curriculum targeting students in grades one through six that seeks to reduce childhood risk behaviors, including sexual health behaviors. Professional development on this curriculum is being provided to appropriate grade-level teachers.

Say Yes to Education Buffalo, a district-contracted partner organization, supported 28 district community schools and aimed to increase rates of completion of high school and postsecondary education. Say Yes school facilitators participated on school well-being teams, received professional development on WSCC implementation, and utilized YRBS data to guide their community school programming. The school facilitators assisted with the implementation of the wellness policy, built relationships with students, and linked students to appropriate sexual health service providers by promoting the *H.O.P.E. Buffalo Pocket Guide*.

Implications for School Health

Implementing a comprehensive wellness policy in a large urban setting with more than 6,000 employees and 34,000 students is challenging. By having a strong written district wellness policy with clear action-oriented language, we increased implementation across the district and its schools (Boehm et al., 2020; Schwartz et al., 2012).

Ongoing use of the 3Cs when it comes to policy development and implementation through school well-being teams, district health committees, families, and community partners can be realized with a knowledgeable district wellness coordinator. Our experience suggests that a coordinator should be a certified district employee with training in educational leadership and education in public, community, and school health. Districts should dedicate fiscal resources to funding this position.

Districts should intentionally plan to develop strong partnerships and relationships across numerous WSCC components, including relationships with parents, students, and community partners, that are fostered through trust and transparency. Trust takes time to develop. We met parents where they were—at churches, in community centers, at parent-sponsored meetings—and created nonthreatening spaces across the community to hear parents' voices.

Districts should provide continuing professional development for implementing and sustaining the WSCC model. We strongly encourage schools to administer the YRBS in their district, because data drive policy actions: In schools, what gets measured gets done.

This case study illustrated how a strong wellness policy, YRBS and SHI data, ongoing professional development, and the use of the 3Ps and 3Cs had a positive impact on parent and student engagement, community involvement, and health services (services provided by counselors, psychologists, and social workers). The WSCC organizational structure provides numerous channels for the communication and coordination of district and community resources so every student will have the health knowledge, attitudes, skills, and behaviors to be healthy.

REFERENCES

Baldwin, S., & Ventresca, A.R.C. (2020). Every school healthy: An urban school case study. *Journal of School Health, 90(12)*, 1045–1055. https://doi.org/10.1111/josh.12965

Basch, C.E. (2011). Healthier students are better learners: A missing link in school reforms to close the achievement gap. *Journal of School Health, 81*(10), 593-598.

Boehm, R., Schwartz, M.B., Lowenfels, A., Brissett, I., & Ren, J. (2020). The relationship between written district policies and school practices among high-need districts in New York State. *Journal of School Health, 90*(6), 465-473.

Buffalo Public Schools. (2019). *Buffalo Public Schools at a glance 2018-2019*. Retrieved May 1, 2020, from www.buffaloschools.org/site/Default.aspx?PageID=234

Centers for Disease Control and Prevention. (2015). *Characteristics of effective health education*. Retrieved June 5, 2020, from www.cdc.gov/healthyschools/sher/characteristics/index.htm

Centers for Disease Control and Prevention. (2023). *Parent engagement in schools*. Retrieved July 17, 2023, from www.cdc.gov/healthyyouth/protective/parent_engagement.htm

Murray, S.D., Hurley, J., & Ahmed, S.R. (2015). Supporting the whole child through coordinated policies, processes, and practices. *Journal of School Health, 85*(11), 795-801.

Rudd Center for Food Policy & Obesity. (2019a). *WellSAT 3.0 Wellness School Assessment Tool*. Retrieved May 1, 2020, from www.wellsat.org/about_the_WellSAT.aspx

Rudd Center for Food Policy & Obesity. (2019b). *WellSAT WSCC*. Retrieved May 1, 2020, from https://csch.uconn.edu/wellsat-wscc/#

Schwartz, M.B., Henderson, K.E., Fable, J., Novak, S.A., Wharton, C.M., Long, M.W., O'Connell, M.L., & Fiore, S.S. (2012). Strength and comprehensiveness of district school wellness policies predict policy implementation at the school level. *Journal of School Health, 82*(6), 262-265.

Steckler, A., & Goodman, R.M. (1989). How to institutionalize health promotion programs. *American Journal of Health Promotion, 3*(4), 34-43.

U.S. Department of Agriculture, Food and Nutrition Services. (2016). *Local school wellness policy implementation under the Healthy, Hunger-Free Kids Act of 2010*. Retrieved May 29, 2020, from www.federalregister.gov/documents/2016/07/29/2016-17230/local-school-wellness-policy-implementation-under-the-healthy-hunger-free-kids-act-of-2010

A Synopsis of International Efforts to Improve School Health Programs

Lloyd J. Kolbe

The Need for International Efforts to Improve School Health Programs

Within and across nations, populations increasingly are experiencing the synergistic effects of economic inequities, environmental degradation, climate change, natural disasters, food and water shortages, emerging and reemerging communicable and noncommunicable diseases and pandemics, armed conflict and violence, and failing governance. These conditions are weakening the well-being and stability of every nation, especially low- and middle-income nations, and have spawned significant population anxiety, depression, and mass migrations. To effectively mitigate these threats, individuals and organizations will need to work together within and across nations, perhaps now more than ever before. Each nation may not have the same resources, but each has the same incentives: a national interest in protecting its own residents from increasing threats to their health and well-being; the obligation to enable healthy individuals, families, and communities everywhere to live more productive and fulfilling lives; and a broader mission to reduce poverty, build stronger economies, promote peace, increase national security, and strengthen its own image in the world. Governmental and nongovernmental organizations, universities, philanthropies, and commercial entities could take concerted actions to improve health within their own nations and internationally (globally) by working collaboratively with partners around the world to build better international relationships, to collaboratively generate and share knowledge, and to expand effective and promising new interventions (Assefa et al., 2022; Chen et al., 2020; Institute of Medicine, 2009; National Academies of Sciences, Engineering, and Medicine, 2017; United Nations Development Program, 2022; World Health Organization [WHO], 2022a, 2022b; Yiu et al., 2020).

In this context, more than 1.5 billion young people worldwide attend primary and secondary schools every school day (United Nations Educational, Scientific, and Cultural Organization [UNESCO], n.d.c). The COVID-19 pandemic has severely eroded the capacity of the world's schools and thus the learning, mental health, and economic productivity of their students, who consequently may lose $17 trillion in lifetime earnings, or the equivalent of 14 percent of the global gross domestic product (Azevedo et al., 2021; World Bank et al., 2021). Because schools materially influence the interdependent health, education, and economic productivity of each nation, and of humankind more broadly, the world's schools must be part of strategic national and international efforts to improve the well-being of populations in the 21st century (Kolbe, 2019; Kolbe et al., 2022; St. Leger et al., 2007). No single nation uses the only, or the best, efforts to help its schools improve the well-being of generations. Each nation could learn much from and with other nations, especially by collaborating with those in other nations and international organizations who are working to improve such programs. By working together, nations could demonstrate that the world's young people, no matter in which nation they live, are our young people—the hope and the future of each nation and of humankind collectively.

U.S. and International School Health Program Frameworks

Modern, multicomponent school health programs could become one of the most effective means available to improve the health, education, and economic productivity of nations. These programs have been called variously child-friendly schools; coordinated school health programs; health-promoting schools; healthy schools; school health promotion programs; schools for health; thriving schools; and Whole School, Whole Community, Whole Child (WSCC) programs (Kolbe, 2019).

The WSCC Framework

During the mid-1980s, the U.S. Centers for Disease Control and Prevention used a multicomponent school health program framework, which in 2014 evolved into the WSCC framework depicted in figure 3.1 on p. 33 (ASCD, 2014; Centers for Disease Control and Prevention, n.d.; Hunt, 2015).

As described more fully in previous chapters, the WSCC framework identifies 10 integrated components (depicted in the outer ring) that can be implemented by coordinating respective policies, processes, and practices to improve learning and health (as depicted by the middle ring) to ensure that students are healthy, safe, engaged, supported, and challenged (as depicted by the inner ring). This framework focuses in more detail on the 10 components than on the coordinating of policies, processes, and practices to implement these components. More than 100 national organizations in the United States are involved in implementing one or more of these 10 components (Kolbe, 2015).

The Health-Promoting Schools Framework

In 2021, WHO and UNESCO jointly developed a health-promoting schools framework by establishing the System of Eight Global Standards for Health-Promoting Schools depicted in figure 9.3 (WHO & UNESCO, 2021a, 2021b, 2021c).

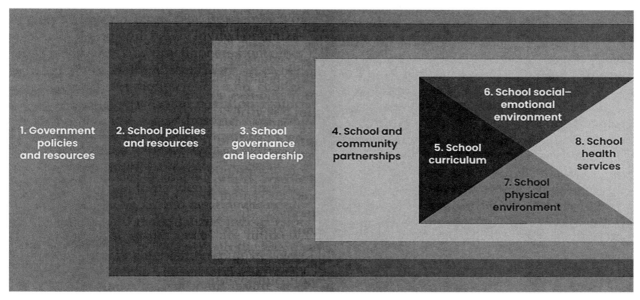

FIGURE 9.3 Health-promoting schools framework.
Reprinted by permission from WHO and UNESCO (2021a); WHO and UNESCO (2021b); WHO and UNESCO (2021c).

These standards include

1. Government policies and resources
2. School policies and resources
3. School governance and leadership
4. School and community partnerships
5. School curriculum
6. School social-emotional environment
7. School physical environment
8. School health services

Compared to the WSCC framework, the health-promoting schools framework focuses in more detail on the policies, processes, and practices (in standards 1-4) used to implement program components (in standards 5-8) than on the components themselves. Neither framework is better; each may complement the other.

FRESH—A Multisector International School Health Partnership

In 1997, WHO published *Promoting Health Through Schools: Report of a WHO Expert Committee on Comprehensive School Health Education and Promotion*. The purpose of the report was to offer and substantiate recommendations for policies and actions that WHO, other United Nations (UN) agencies, national governments, and nongovernmental organizations could implement to help schools improve the health of students, school staff, families, and community members.

In 2000, WHO, UNESCO, the United Nations Children's Fund (UNICEF), and the World Bank jointly established a multisector global partnership called FRESH (Focusing Resources on Effective School Health) that would enable these agencies to work together to improve school health programs (FRESH Partners, n.d.a; World Bank, 2003). These four agencies subsequently have been joined by other UN agencies, international nongovernmental organizations, networks, and donors that are collaborating as FRESH Partners. It is important to note that FRESH provides a mechanism for these organizations to collaboratively address the UN's Sustainable Development Goals (SDGs) for 2030, especially SDG3 (good health and well-being) and SDG4 (quality education; FRESH Partners, n.d.b; UN, n.d.b). The collaborating agencies developed *Monitoring and Evaluation Guidance for School Health Programs* to help organizations and nations assess their school health programs. The first part of *Guidance* focuses on eight core indicators to help assess the extent to which a nation and its schools have implemented the four FRESH pillars of school health programs:

1. Equitable school health policies
2. Safe learning environment
3. Skills-based health education
4. School-based health and nutrition services

The second part of *Guidance* focuses on thematic indicators to help assess the extent to which individual schools are implementing programs to address 15 themes, such as food and nutrition, physical activity, sexual and reproductive health, immunization, and disaster risk reduction (FRESH Partners, 2014a, 2014b).

International Organizations Working to Improve School Health Programs

Of course, as highlighted briefly here, vital international organizations also work independently or collaboratively outside the FRESH partnership to improve school health programs.

World Health Organization

The WHO headquarters in Geneva, Switzerland, its six regional offices, and its 150 country offices long have helped schools improve health. In 1995, the WHO headquarters launched its Global School Health Initiative to mobilize and strengthen international, regional, national, and local efforts to improve school health programs (WHO, n.d.b). The WHO headquarters helps nations conduct the Global School-Based Student Health Survey to monitor critical health-risk behaviors among students, establish school health programs that can reduce those risks, and compare the impact of risk reduction efforts within and across countries over time (Abdalmaleki et al., 2022; WHO, n.d.a). Moreover, in 2019 the WHO Regional Office for Europe convened the Fifth European Conference on Health Promoting Schools, during which participants from 40 nations developed 23 recommendations and calls for action to improve school health programs in Europe (Dadaczynski et al., 2020; WHO Regional Office for Europe, 2020).

United Nations Educational, Scientific, and Cultural Organization

UNESCO addresses a broad range of school health issues, such as providing education on HIV and sexuality and reducing school violence and bullying (UNESCO, n.d.a, n.d.b, 2022). UNESCO and other international organizations collaboratively prepared the report *Ready to Learn and Thrive: School Health and Nutrition Around the World*, which (1) describes the extent to which countries have implemented school health and nutrition policies and programs and (2) encourages efforts to monitor and improve such policies and programs (UNESCO et al., 2022).

United Nations Children's Fund

UNICEF has characterized the COVID-19 pandemic as the greatest threat to the world's children in its 75-year history. The pandemic threatens children by increasing the number who are hungry, out of school, abused, living in poverty, or forced into marriage and decreasing the number who are vaccinated and have access to food, health care, and other essential services. UNICEF has proposed that governments urgently implement five RAPID actions for education recovery:

- Reach every child and retain them in school
- Assess current learning levels
- Prioritize fundamentals
- Increase catch-up learning
- Develop student psychosocial health and well-being (UNICEF, 2021; UNICEF et al., 2022; World Bank et al., 2022)

World Bank

The World Bank is the largest financier of education in the developing world. It uses a systems approach to strengthen those national education system elements that most influence learning, including education policies, institutions, governance, financing, and school management. As part of this approach, in 2011 the World Bank established the Systems Approach for Better Education Results (SABER), which enables national education reform efforts to analyze comparative national data on 13 essential education system elements that matter most to improve learning. One example of the World Bank's efforts to address elements that are important to the improvement of school health programs was its analysis of national data on school health and school feeding (World Bank, n.d.a, n.d.b, 2011, 2016, 2020).

International School Health Network

The International School Health Network is an informal network of practitioners and researchers who work within and across nations and international organizations to help schools implement policies, programs, and practices that improve health, education, and other forms of human development. This network provides ongoing information about international developments in school health; prepares reports; and convenes online international school health working meetings, consultations, webinars, and symposia (International School Health Network, n.d.).

Save the Children

Save the Children School Health and Nutrition programs are active in 30 nations in Africa, Asia, Latin America, and the Middle East. Save the Children has developed the *School Health and Nutrition Health Education Manual*, which includes lesson plans for 23 topics that make up its comprehensive school health and nutrition curriculum (Save the Children, n.d.a, n.d.b).

Schools for Health in Europe Network Foundation

Supported by the European Union and the WHO Regional Office for Europe, the Schools for Health in Europe Network (SHE) is a network of professionals from 40 countries in Europe and Central Asia who work together to improve school health programs in their nations. For example, each year it convenes an international SHE Academy of leading scholars and experts to improve school health program research and practice (SHE, n.d.a, n.d.b).

Research Consortium for School Health and Nutrition

The Research Consortium for School Health and Nutrition is a global partnership of academic, scientific, and technical institutions that conducts research on the health, nutrition, well-being, education, and development of school-age children and adolescents. In one of its activities, consortium researchers found the benefit-to-cost ratio of school feeding programs in 14 nations across four sectors (health and nutrition, education, social protection, and local agriculture) ranged from $7 to $35 for each dollar invested (Research Consortium for School Health and Nutrition, n.d.; Verguet et al., 2020).

Journals of School Health

Academic journals provide an essential means by which modern societies systematically build scientific disciplines, professions, and practices to improve the lives of their people. Such journals provide the means for experts in a discipline to systematically identify, communicate, and archive carefully reviewed information that can be used by researchers, policymakers, practitioners, and the public. Journals thus enable a discipline to iteratively develop and evolve over time (Kolbe, 2022). Many academic journals may include important articles on school health; however, the following four journals specifically focus on building the scientific discipline of school health.

Chinese Journal of School Health (CJSH)

Established in 1980, the *Chinese Journal of School Health* is sponsored by the Chinese Preventive Medicine Association and supervised by the National Health Commission of the People's Republic of China (CJSH, n.d.).

International Journal of School Health (IJSH)

The *International Journal of School Health* is published by the Health Policy Research Center, Shiraz University of Medical Sciences, in Iran (IJSH, n.d.).

Japanese Journal of School Health (JJSH)

The *Japanese Journal of School Health* is a publication of the Japanese School Health Association (JJSH, n.d.).

Journal of School Health (JOSH)

Established in 1930, the *Journal of School Health* is a publication of the American School Health Association (JOSH, n.d.).

The Future of National and International Efforts to Improve School Health Programs

Too often, those who address school health programs in nations do so ethnocentrically—often more through the lens of public health than through the lens of education and, perhaps understandably, more through the lens of their respective national circumstances than through the lens of our collective global condition.

In 2021, a report of the International Commission on the Futures of Education observed the following:

> *We [humans] face an existential choice: continue on an unsustainable path or radically change course. To continue on the current path is to accept unconscionable inequalities and exploitation, the spiralling of multiple forms of violence, the erosion of social cohesion and human freedoms, continued environmental destruction, and dangerous and perhaps catastrophic biodiversity loss. To continue on the current path is to fail to anticipate and address the risks that accompany the technological and digital transformations of our societies.*
>
> *We urgently need to reimagine our futures together and take action to realize them. Knowledge and learning are the basis for renewal and transformation. But ... education is not doing what it could to help us shape peaceful, just, and sustainable futures.* (UNESCO, 2021, p. 7)

The commission reported that "vast numbers of people—children, youth and adults—are keenly aware that *we are connected* on this shared planet and that it is imperative that *we work together*" (p. 1, emphasis in the original). The report called for forging a new social contract for education by refocusing research and innovation, establishing international cooperation and global solidarity, and actively engaging universities and other vital stakeholders in building the new social contract.

To begin the international building process, the UN Secretary-General convened the Transforming Education Summit during the 2022 World Health Assembly as a means of mobilizing national and global actions to recover from pandemic-related learning losses, to attain UN SDG4 (quality education), and to reimagine and improve the world's education systems (UN, n.d.a). At the summit, the UN Secretary-General offered a vision statement (UN, 2022a) as a political manifesto for urgent collective action and as a platform for a proposed 2024 UN Summit of the Future. The Secretary-General noted that education systems no longer equip young people with the knowledge, skills, or values needed to thrive in a rapidly changing world and suggested that transformative education must enable learners to learn to learn, learn to live together, learn to do, and learn to be—including by "developing every student's disposition for leading a healthy life" (UN, 2022a, p. 4).

The Transforming Education Summit included five thematic tracks. The first three tracks, which are outlined here, have direct implications for the future of school health programs. Action Track 4—Digital Learning and Transformation and Action Track 5—Financing of Education have indirect implications.

Action Track 1—Inclusive, Equitable, Safe, and Healthy Schools

The discussion on inclusive, equitable, safe, and healthy schools (UN, 2022b), in part addressing school health programs, noted, "COVID-19, violence, armed conflict, refugee and internal displacement, natural hazards including climate-induced disasters and associated economic migration, and a growing backlash against gender equality and women's rights are reversing progress and widening inequalities in many contexts" (p. 1). Discussants proposed that "inclusive, transformative education must ensure that all learners have unhindered access to and participation in quality education, that they are safe and healthy, free from violence and discrimination, and are supported with comprehensive care services within school settings" (p. 3). To achieve this transformation, key recommendations called for governments and their partners to do the following:

- Protect rights and change mindsets (e.g., ending bans on pregnant girls and young mothers)
- Invest in those furthest behind (e.g., poor people and marginalized individuals)
- Ensure visibility of the least visible
- Empower teachers to empower learners
- Build the foundations for learning to live together

- Create safe learning spaces to thrive
- Nourish healthy bodies and healthy minds
- Realize the idiom "It takes a village"

Action Track 2—Learning and Skills for Life, Work, and Sustainable Development

The discussion on learning and skills for life, work, and sustainable development (UN, 2022c), in part addressing school health education, noted the following:

> Education that lays a solid foundation for life needs to address an increasingly complex and interconnected world faced with the real existential threat of climate change, mass loss of biodiversity, natural disasters, pandemics, extreme poverty and inequalities, rapid technological change, violent ideologies and conflicts, structural discrimination and marginalization, and democratic backsliding, among others. (p. 5)

Discussants suggested the following:

> Education [must be] about balancing learning to be *and* learning to live together *with our current preoccupation on* learning to know *and* learning to do. [Education must be] about learning from the past for the present and for anticipating and shaping a better future. (p. 6, emphasis in the original)

Discussants suggested that the key to transformation is to "empower learners for well-being, the future of work, and planetary sustainability by mainstreaming education for sustainable development" (p. 9). Key action areas called for every country to do the following:

- Empower learners for human and planetary sustainability by mainstreaming education for sustainable development
- Build and implement robust lifelong learning policies and systems
- Promote a whole-institution approach to learning
- Address evolving skills demands in changing economies and transition to green and digital economies
- Ensure inclusion, equity, and justice
- Strengthen governance and financing

Across these six key action areas, 16 more detailed recommendations were listed.

Action Track 3—Teachers, Teaching, and the Teaching Profession

The discussion on teachers, teaching, and the teaching profession (UN, 2022d), in part addressing the health of teaching personnel, noted that teachers are the most influential variable in achieving learning outcomes and stated the following:

> Currently, education systems are confronted by four major challenges related to the education workforce: personnel shortages; difficulties in ensuring adequate qualifications, skills and professional development needs of teaching personnel; low status and working conditions, and lack of opportunities to develop teacher leadership, autonomy, and innovation. (p. 1)

Discussants identified 10 strategies to create an effective education workforce and recommended three initiatives for future global action and national commitments (pp. 11-12):

1. Accelerate efforts to improve the status of teachers and their working conditions to make the teaching profession more attractive through robust social dialogue and teacher participation in educational decision making.
2. Accelerate the pace and improve the quality of teacher professional development through the adoption of comprehensive national policies for teacher and teaching personnel.
3. Improve the financing for teachers through integrated national reform strategies and effective functional governance and dedicated financial strategies.

Summary

The success of the many international efforts to improve school health programs, as outlined in this chapter, could markedly improve the health, education, economic productivity, and well-being of future generations. However, this will require a greater commitment to strengthen the quality of school health programs in each of our own nations as well as in other nations.

REFERENCES

Abdalmaleki, E., Abdi, Z., Isfahani, S.R., Safarpoor, S., Haghdoost, B., Sazgarneijad, S., & Ahmadnezhad, E. (2022). Global school-based student health survey: Country profiles and survey results in the eastern Mediterranean region countries. *BMC Public Health, 22*, Article 130. https://doi.org/10.1186/s12889-022-12502-8

ASCD. (2014). *Whole School, Whole Community, Whole Child: A collaborative approach to learning and health.* https://files.ascd.org/staticfiles/ascd/pdf/siteASCD/publications/wholechild/wscc-a-collaborative-approach.pdf

Assefa, Y., Woldeyohannes, S., Cullerton, K., Gilks, C.F., Reid, S., & Van Damme, W. (2022). Attributes of national governance for an effective response to public health emergencies: Lessons from the response to the COVID-19 pandemic. *Journal of Global Health, 12*, Article 05021. https://doi.org/10.7189/jogh.12.05021

Azevedo, J.P., Montoya, S., Akmal, M., Wong, Y.N., Gregory, L., Koen Geven, K.M., Cloutier, M., Iqbal, S.A., Imhof, A.G., De Andrade Falcao, N., Kouame, C.S., Dahal, M., Gebre, T.Z., & Vargas Mancera, M.J. (2021). *Learning poverty updates and revisions: What's new?* World Bank. https://openknowledge.worldbank.org/handle/10986/36082

Centers for Disease Control and Prevention. (n.d.). *Whole School, Whole Community, Whole Child.* Retrieved January 8, 2023, from www.cdc.gov/healthyschools/wscc/index.htm

Chen, X., Li, H., Lucero-Prisno, D.E., III, Abdullah, A.S., Huang, J., Laurence, C., Liang, X., Ma, Z., Mao, Z., Ren, R., Wu, S., Wang, N., Wang, P., Wang, T., Yan, H., & Zou, Y. (2020). What is global health? Key concepts and clarification of misperceptions: Report of the 2019 GHRP editorial meeting. *Global Health Research and Policy, 5*, Article 14. https://doi.org/10.1186/s41256-020-00142-7

Chinese Journal of School Health. (n.d.). Accessed January 8, 2023, from http://www.cjsh.org.cn/

Dadaczynski, K., Jensen, B., Viig, N., Sormunen, M., von Seelen, J., Kuchma, V., & Vilaça, T. (2020). Health, well-being and education: Building a sustainable future. The Moscow statement on health promoting schools. *Health Education, 120*(1), 11-19. https://doi.org/10.1108/HE-12-2019-0058

FRESH Partners. (n.d.a). *FRESH Partners website.* Retrieved January 8, 2023, from www.fresh-partners.org/

FRESH Partners. (n.d.b). *Schools, the FRESH framework, and achieving the UN goals: An overview.* Retrieved January 8, 2023, from www.fresh-partners.org/overview-schools-fresh--un-goals.html

FRESH Partners. (2014a). *Monitoring and evaluation guidance for school health programs—Eight core indicators to support FRESH.* Retrieved January 8, 2023, from https://drive.google.com/file/d/0B76Y7Zl6A-eBcnRfc2tpLUd-6VUk/view?resourcekey=0-ObXpszNERMbqK-zdH-qo_7A

FRESH Partners. (2014b). *Monitoring and evaluation guidance for school health programs—Thematic indicators supporting FRESH.* Retrieved January 8, 2023, from https://drive.google.com/file/d/0B76Y7Zl6A-eBejVPQUd2dlJrLTA/view?resourcekey=0-RaB_PAwlao8_kBRddPosFA

Hunt, H. (Ed.). (2015). The Whole School, Whole Community, Whole Child model [Special issue]. *Journal of School Health, 85*(11). https://onlinelibrary.wiley.com/toc/17461561/2015/85/11

Institute of Medicine. (2009). *The U.S. commitment to global health: Recommendations for the public and private sectors.* National Academies Press. Retrieved January 8, 2023, from https://doi.org/10.17226/12642

International Journal of School Health. (n.d.). Accessed January 8, 2023, from https://intjsh.sums.ac.ir/

International School Health Network. (n.d.). *International School Health Network website.* Retrieved January 8, 2023, from www.internationalschoolhealth.org/

Japanese Journal of School Health. (n.d.). Accessed January 8, 2023, from https://www.jstage.jst.go.jp/browse/jpnjschhealth/-char/en

Journal of School Health. (n.d.). Accessed January 8, 2023, from. https://www.ashaweb.org/resources/journal-of-school-health/

Kolbe, L.J. (2015). On national strategies to improve both education and health—An open letter. *Journal of School Health, 85*(1), 1-7. https://doi.org/10.1111/josh.12223

Kolbe, L.J. (2019). School health as a strategy to improve both public health and education. *Annual Review of Public Health, 40*, 443-463. https://doi.org/10.1146/annurev-publhealth-040218-043727

Kolbe, L.J. (2022). The journal and scientific discipline of school health. *Journal of School Health, 92*(8), 822. https://doi.org/10.1111/josh.13161

Kolbe, L.J., Hunt, H., & Ben Abdelaziz, F. (2022). Chapter 12: Planning efforts to help schools prevent noncommunicable diseases—Integrating local, state, national, and international resources. In L.W. Green, A.C. Gielen, J.M. Ottoson, D.V. Peterson, & M.W. Kreuter (Eds.), *Health program planning, implementation, and evaluation: Creating behavioral, environmental, and policy change* (pp. 322-360). Johns Hopkins University Press.

National Academies of Sciences, Engineering, and Medicine. (2017). *Global health and the future role of the United States*. National Academies Press. https://doi.org/10.17226/24737

Research Consortium for School Health and Nutrition. (n.d.). *RCSHN website*. Retrieved January 8, 2023, from www.lshtm.ac.uk/research/centres-projects-groups/research-consortium-for-school-health-and-nutrition

Save the Children. (n.d.a). *School health and nutrition health education manual*. www.savethechildren.org/content/dam/global/reports/education-and-child-protection/health-ed-man.pdf

Save the Children. (n.d.b). *School health and nutrition website*. Retrieved January 8, 2023, from www.savethechildren.org/us/what-we-do/education/school-health-and-nutrition#:~:text=Save%20the%20Children's%20School%20Health,micronutrient%20supplementation%20and%20healthy%20environment

Schools for Health in Europe Network. (n.d.a). *Schools for Health in Europe Academy*. Retrieved January 8, 2023, from www.schoolsforhealth.org/she-academy

Schools for Health in Europe Network. (n.d.b). *Schools for Health in Europe website*. Retrieved January 8, 2023, from www.schoolsforhealth.org/

St. Leger, L., Kolbe, L.J., Lee, A., McCall, D.S., & Young, I.M. (2007). School health promotion. In D.V. McQueen & C.M. Jones (Eds.), *Global perspectives on health promotion effectiveness* (pp. 107-124). Springer. https://doi.org/10.1007/978-0-387-70974-1_8

United Nations. (n.d.a). *Transforming education summit website*. www.un.org/en/transforming-education-summit

United Nations. (n.d.b). *UN sustainable development goals website*. Retrieved January 8, 2023, from https://sdgs.un.org/goals

United Nations. (2022a). *Transforming education: An urgent political imperative for our collective future—Vision statement of the secretary-general on transforming education*. www.un.org/sites/un2.un.org/files/2022/09/sg_vision_statement_on_transforming_education.pdf

United Nations. (2022b). *Transforming education summit—Action track 1 discussion paper: Inclusive, equitable, safe and healthy schools*. https://transformingeducationsummit.sdg4education2030.org/system/files/2022-07/AT1%20Discussion%20Paper_15%20July%202022%20%28With%20Annex%29.pdf

United Nations. (2022c). *Transforming education summit—Action track 2 discussion paper: Learning and skills for life, work, and sustainable development*. https://transformingeducationsummit.sdg4education2030.org/system/files/2022-07/Digital%20AT2%20dicussion%20paper%20July%202022.pdf

United Nations. (2022d). *Transforming education summit—Action track 3 discussion paper: Teachers, teaching and the teaching profession*. https://transformingeducationsummit.sdg4education2030.org/system/files/2022-07/Thematic%20Action%20Track%203%20teachers%20discussion%20paper%20July%202022.pdf

United Nations Children's Fund. (2021). *Preventing a lost decade: Urgent action to reverse the devastating impact of COVID-19 on children and young people*. www.unicef.org/media/112891/file/UNICEF%2075%20report.pdf

United Nations Children's Fund, United Nations Educational, Scientific, and Cultural Organization, & World Bank. (2022). *Where are we on educational recovery?* www.unicef.org/media/117626/file/Where%20are%20we%20in%20Education%20Recovery

United Nations Development Program. (2022). *Human development report 2021/2022: Uncertain times, unsettled lives—Shaping our future in a transforming world*. Retrieved September 8, 2023, from https://hdr.undp.org/system/files/documents/global-report-document/hdr2021-22pdf_1.pdf

United Nations Educational, Scientific, and Cultural Organization. (n.d.a). *Education for health and well-being website*. Retrieved July 15, 2022, from https://en.unesco.org/themes/education-health-and-well-being

United Nations Educational, Scientific, and Cultural Organization. (n.d.b). *Health and education resource center website—Building healthy lives through education*. Retrieved January 8, 2023, from https://healtheducationresources.unesco.org/

United Nations Educational, Scientific, and Cultural Organization. (n.d.c). *UNESCO Institute for Statistics website: Education—Primary and Secondary School Enrolled Numbers (Both Sexes)*. http://data.uis.unesco.org/

United Nations Educational, Scientific, and Cultural Organization. (2021). *Reimagining our futures together: A new social contract for education—Report from the International Commission on the Futures of Education*. https://unesdoc.unesco.org/ark:/48223/pf0000379707

United Nations Educational, Scientific, and Cultural Organization. (2022). *UNESCO strategy on education for health and well-being*. https://unesdoc.unesco.org/ark:/48223/pf0000381728

United Nations Educational, Scientific, and Cultural Organization, United Nations Children's Fund, & World Food Program. (2022). *Ready to learn and thrive: School health and nutrition around the world—Highlights*. https://unesdoc.unesco.org/ark:/48223/pf0000381965

Verguet, S., Limasalle, P., Chakrabarti, A., Husain, A., Burbano, C., Drake, L., & Bundy, D. (2020). The broader economic value of school feeding programs in low- and middle-income countries: Estimating the multi-sectoral returns to public health, human capital, social protection, and the local economy. *Frontiers in Public Health, 8*, Article 587046. https://doi.org/10.3389/fpubh.2020.587046

World Bank. (n.d.a). *Education website*. Retrieved January 8, 2023, from www.worldbank.org/en/topic/education

World Bank. (n.d.b). *Systems approach for better education results (SABER) website*. Retrieved January 8, 2023, from www.worldbank.org/en/topic/education/brief/systems-approach-for-better-education-results-saber

World Bank. (2003). *Public health at a glance—School health*. http://web.worldbank.org/archive/website01213/WEB/0__C-102.HTM

World Bank. (2011). *Rethinking school health: A key component of education for all*. https://openknowledge.worldbank.org/bitstream/handle/10986/2267/600390PUB0ID171Health09780821379073.pdf?sequence=1&isAllowed=y

World Bank. (2016). *Systems approach for better education results (SABER): School health and school feeding*. https://documents1.worldbank.org/curated/en/239141496301589942/pdf/Systems-Approach-for-Better-Education-Results-SABER-school-health-and-school-feeding.pdf

World Bank. (2020). *Learning for all: Investing in people's knowledge and skills to promote development*. https://openknowledge.worldbank.org/bitstream/handle/10986/27790/649590WP0REPLA00WB0EdStrategy0final.pdf?sequence=1&isAllowed=y

World Bank, Bill & Melinda Gates Foundation, Foreign, Commonwealth, and Development Office, United Nations Educational, Scientific, and Cultural Organization, United Nations Children's Fund, & United States Agency for International Development. (2022). *Guide for learning recovery and acceleration: Using the RAPID framework to address COVID-19 learning losses and build forward better*. Retrieved January 8, 2023, from www.worldbank.org/en/topic/education/publication/the-rapid-framework-and-a-guide-for-learning-recovery-and-acceleration

World Bank, United Nations Educational, Scientific, and Cultural Organization, & United Nations Children's Fund. (2021). *The state of the global education crisis: A path to recovery*. Retrieved January 8, 2023, from www.unicef.org/media/111621/file/%20The%20State%20of%20the%20Global%20Education%20Crisis.pdf%20.pdf

World Health Organization. (n.d.a). *Global school-based student health survey website*. Retrieved January 8, 2023, from www.who.int/teams/noncommunicable-diseases/surveillance/systems-tools/global-school-based-student-health-survey

World Health Organization. (n.d.b). *Health promoting schools website*. Retrieved January 8, 2023, from www.who.int/health-topics/health-promoting-schools#tab=tab_1

World Health Organization. (1997). *Promoting health through schools: Report of a WHO expert committee on comprehensive school health education and promotion*. https://apps.who.int/iris/handle/10665/41987

World Health Organization. (2022a). *World health statistics 2022: Monitoring health for the SDGs: Sustainable development goals*. Retrieved January 8, 2023, from www.who.int/data/gho/publications/world-health-statistics

World Health Organization. (2022b). *World mental health report: Transforming mental health for all: Executive summary*. Retrieved January 8, 2023, from www.who.int/publications/i/item/9789240049338

World Health Organization Regional Office for Europe. (2020). *Health, well-being, and education: Building a sustainable future*. www.schoolsforhealth.org/sites/default/files/editor/conference%20statements/moscow-conference-who-report.pdf

World Health Organization & United Nations Educational, Scientific, and Cultural Organization. (2021a). *Making every school a health-promoting school: Volume 1—Global standards and indicators for health-promoting schools and systems*. Retrieved January 8, 2023, from www.who.int/publications/i/item/9789240025059

World Health Organization & United Nations Educational, Scientific, and Cultural Organization. (2021b). *Making every school a health-promoting school: Volume 2—Implementation guidance*. Retrieved January 8, 2023, from www.who.int/publications/i/item/9789240025073

World Health Organization & United Nations Educational, Scientific, and Cultural Organization. (2021c). *Making every school a health-promoting school: Volume 3—Country case studies*. Retrieved January 8, 2023, from www.who.int/publications/i/item/9789240025431

Yiu, K.C., Solum, E.M., DiLiberto, D.D., & Torp, S. (2020). Comparing approaches to research in global and international health: An exploratory study. *Annals of Global Health, 86*(1), Article 47. https://doi.org/10.5334/aogh.2799

Teacher Education: Preparing Educators for WSCC Engagement

Elisa Beth McNeill

An important determinant of the effectiveness of the Whole School, Whole Community, Whole Child (WSCC) model is the quality of the professional preparation and professional development received by the individuals responsible for implementing the model. It is essential that these individuals have a clear understanding of the model and its connection to education and health outcomes. In an ideal world, a commitment to developing the whole child would be a universal foundation of every teacher preparation program. Murray et al. (2015) suggested the following:

> Colleges of education at institutions of higher education are encouraged to embed health-promoting and learning practices into all aspects of teacher and administrator preparation programs. Future teachers and administrators, regardless of subject matter expertise or professional focus, will play a role in implementing the WSCC framework. Teacher and administrative candidates should be prepared to view student health outcomes as integral to all aspects of learning and the school environment. (p. 800)

For most teacher education programs the primary role of preparation is to facilitate the acquisition of pedagogical knowledge and skills by students. However, it has become evident that many 21st-century prekindergarten through grade 12 (preK-12) learners require more social and emotional support to thrive. Current trends in teacher preparation are dedicated to equipping prospective educators with the knowledge and skills to promote positive teacher–student relationships. The goal is to create a culture that supports students' social-emotional well-being through connectedness. The framework of the WSCC model promotes the development of a schoolwide infrastructure that enhances positive teacher–student relationships. Multiple studies suggest that positive teacher–student relationships are associated with fewer behavioral issues, improved working memory, better academic outcomes, improved graduation rates, fewer mental health issues, and improved emotional and social development (Burns, 2020; Clements-Nolle & Waddington, 2019; Cook et al., 2018; Sabol & Pianta, 2012). These types of positive outcomes are desirable for all academic disciplines. Thus, there is a need for interdisciplinary teacher education instruction on the utilization of the WSCC model to support the needs of the whole child.

Unfortunately, most professional preparation programs for general educators have yet to embrace their potential role in promoting the WSCC model as a resource for developing the whole child. When professional preparation practices prepare educators according to categories of learners—such as bilingual, special education, or English language learners—or prepare them as content-specific specialists, it reinforces the notion that different groups of teachers have sole responsibility for addressing specific learner needs (Blanton et al., 2011). "The notion that some children 'are not my job' has built silos in the preparation of teachers and specialists, as well as in the delivery of services in [preK-12] schools" (Blanton et al.,

2011, p. 29). This specialization perspective contributes to the notion that implementation of the WSCC model falls to educators who specialize in health. Training on the WSCC model is frequently reserved for individuals who are specializing in majors or certifications focused on school health education and promotion. This approach is problematic because there are fewer opportunities to earn a degree in school health education than in other areas of teacher education. Changes in higher education and state certification requirements have resulted in a reduction in the number of school health education preparation programs. The National Commission for Health Education Credentialing maintains the Health Education and Promotion Program Directory as a resource on its website. This directory lists programs that offer coursework that enables students to become qualified to sit the Certified Health Education Specialist (CHES) credential. The CHES certificate attests that an individual possesses the knowledge and skills deemed necessary to the field of health education as delineated by the profession. Although the Health Education and Promotion Program Directory does not include all professional preparation programs, of the 52 undergraduate programs listed in the directory, only four offer teacher certification in health education (National Commission for Health Education Credentialing, 2018).

Another factor that has an impact on WSCC-related instruction in teacher education programs is the presence of school health education teachers who have become certified in health as a minor or a supporting field instead of having health as a major. Because there are fewer health-related courses in a minor, these individuals have less of an opportunity to be exposed to WSCC-related instruction.

In addition to the limited number of undergraduate programs dedicated to school health education there has been a decrease in the number of higher education faculty who specialize in school health. Although quality WSCC-related research exists, there is a need for an increase in research that cuts across the complete model or, at the very least, involves multiple components of the model (Willgerodt et al., 2021). Because schools and districts are often motivated or mandated to use evidence-based programs, and because there is an absence of empirical data to support WSCC as an effective model (despite research focused on individual elements of the model), the likelihood of the WSCC model being adopted by schools can be limited (Willgerodt et al., 2021). To expand the existing body of research, school health faculty will need to leverage opportunities to participate in interdisciplinary research related to WSCC.

Teacher education programs have the capacity to influence implementation of the WSCC model. Exposure to the WSCC model needs to occur early within teacher education programs in all disciplines, and the model needs to be presented as a foundational framework for creating child-centered schools. The focus on WSCC-related instruction needs to move beyond memorizing the components of the model. Instruction needs to gradually move students from knowledge related to the content and structure of the model to its application in a community and school setting. The Centers for Disease Control and Prevention (CDC; 2022) has developed an online tool, Virtual Healthy School, that models authentic examples of the WSCC components in a school setting. This virtual tool depicts the model within a healthy school and provides resources and downloadable files to help users understand how to incorporate the concepts in an authentic school environment.

Professional organizations dedicated to school health education also provide valuable resources for training prospective and current educators on the model. The Society for Public Health Education (SOPHE) has developed 10 WSCC training modules designed to build, strengthen, and sustain efforts to implement the model (SOPHE, 2022). These one-hour modules can be used by teacher preparation programs to develop skills for using data, build and sustain administrative support, use policy and systems to create change, engage youth, showcase results, and promote health equity in schools (SOPHE, 2022). In addition, many professional organizations provide access to peer-reviewed journal articles describing how schools and districts incorporate the components of the model. Having preservice educators investigate authentic examples of the model in use facilitates their own understanding of the model's capacity to support the whole child.

Because WSCC is an interdisciplinary community- and school-based model, teacher education programs should build skills that enable students to embrace the concepts associated with systems thinking. A systems approach prepares students to evaluate challenges present in an interrelated context. Mind maps and webbing are commonly used methodologies in systems thinking. These strategies are used to identify a central theme and then examine the relationships of other entities to the central theme. When learning about the WSCC model each component can be investigated by students as a central theme. After learners feel confident in their ability to recognize how their assigned components contribute to supporting the whole child, they can then work with other learners to determine how their components might work together to address student needs. For example, a case study approach could be used to provide background information on a student's situation. The learners would be challenged to offer recommendations for how each component of the WSCC model could contribute to support the needs of the child. An abbreviated example is provided in figure 9.4. This webbing technique enables teachers to

FIGURE 9.4 CASE STUDY: USING THE WSCC MODEL TO ADDRESS THE NEEDS OF THE WHOLE CHILD

Aiden, age 14, lost both his parents in a house fire at age 7. He lives in a one-bedroom apartment with his grandmother, who has a physical disability and uses a wheelchair. Their only source of income is his grandmother's monthly Social Security check. Aiden experiences frequent headaches because the prescription in his glasses is outdated. Aiden is bitter about his circumstances and is known to have violent outbursts. His peers avoid contact with him. He has little desire to do well in school and only attends so he can eat.

How might each of the components of the WSCC model be used to support Aiden from a Whole Child perspective?

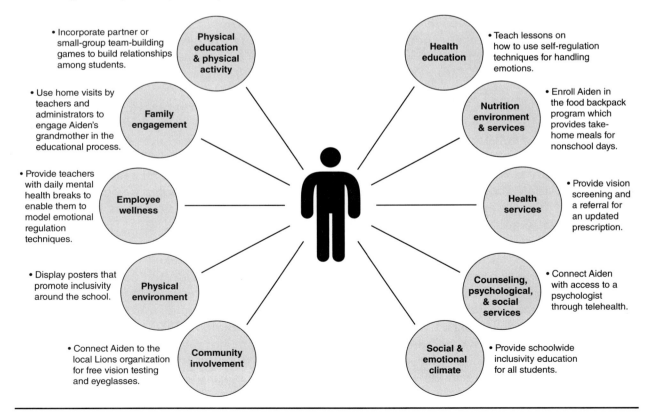

discover potential resources from a variety of sources that otherwise might not be apparent. Once the connections are made to show how each of the components of the model can support the child, prospective teachers can then speculate on how educators from different academic disciplines can also contribute.

The CDC also provides examples of activities or events that facilitate collaboration among the various components of the WSCC framework in one-page summary sheets available on its website. These summaries provide evidence-based strategies and promising practices for using the WSCC framework to promote student health (CDC, 2019). These resources are valuable assets for use in teacher preparation programs and are available for use in presentations, on websites, and as handouts. As preservice educators analyze the positive impact of incorporating the WSCC framework within a school, it helps them to deepen their understanding of the model, which would hopefully encourage them to advocate for its use. An example of a summary sheet is provided in figure 9.5.

It is important to recognize and address the challenges associated with assimilating WSCC if uptake of the model is to be achieved. Health professionals must continue to act as WSCC advocates and work to mitigate barriers to implementation. Taking advantage of opportunities to promote the WSCC model at various levels within the educational system will also facilitate its acceptance.

REFERENCES

Blanton, L.P., Pugach, M.C., & Florian, L. (2011). *Preparing general education teachers to improve outcomes for students with disabilities.* www.ncld.org/wp-content/uploads/2014/11/aacte_ncld_recommendation.pdf

Burns, E.C. (2020). Factors that support high school completion: A longitudinal examination of quality teacher-student relationships and intentions to graduate. *Journal of Adolescence, 84,* 180-189. https://doi.org/10.1016/j.adolescence.2020.09.005

Centers for Disease Control and Prevention. (2019). *Strategies for using the WSCC framework.* www.cdc.gov/healthyschools/wscc/strategies.htm

Centers for Disease Control and Prevention. (2022). *Virtual healthy school.* www.cdc.gov/healthyschools/vhs/index.html

Clements-Nolle, K., & Waddington, R. (2019). Adverse childhood experiences and psychological distress in juvenile offenders: The protective influence of resilience and youth assets. *Journal of Adolescent Health, 64*(1), 49-55. https://doi.org/10.1016/j.jadohealth.2018.09.025

Cook, C.R., Coco, S., Zhang, Y., Fiat, A.E., Duong, M.T., Renshaw, T.L., Long, A.C., Frank, S., & Curby, T. (2018). Cultivating positive teacher-student relationships: Preliminary evaluation of the establish-maintain-restore (EMR) method. *School Psychology Review, 47*(3), 226-243. https://doi.org/10.17105/SPR-2017-0025.V47-3

Murray, S.D., Hurley, J., & Ahmed, S.R. (2015). Supporting the whole child through coordinated policies, processes, and practices. *Journal of School Health, 85,* 795-801.

National Commission for Health Education Credentialing. (2018). *Health Education and Promotion Program Directory.* Retrieved January 19, 2023, from www.healtheddirectory.org/.

Sabol, T.J., & Pianta, R.C. (2012). Recent trends in research on teacher-child relationships. *Attachment & Human Development, 14*(3), 213-231. https://doi.org/10.1080/14616734.2012.672262

Society for Public Health Education. (2022). *WSCC team training modules.* https://elearn.sophe.org/wscc-training-modules

Willgerodt, M.A., Walsh, E., & Maloy, C. (2021). A scoping review of the Whole School, Whole Community, Whole Child model. *Journal of School Nursing, 37*(1), 61-68. https://doi.org/10.1177/1059840520974346

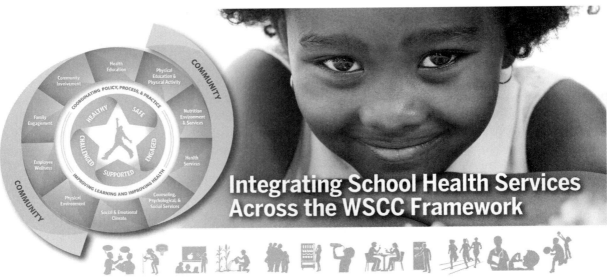

FIGURE 9.5 School health services integrated with the other components of the WSCC model.
Reprinted from CDC (2019).

The Importance of Professional Development

Lori Paisley

Whether you are a veteran or first-year teacher, engaging in professional development ensures professional growth as an educator and can result in improvements in students' learning outcomes. Professional development in education consists of ongoing learning experiences such as advanced education and specific training that assists educators and school staff in improving their professional knowledge and effectiveness. It provides a foundation and structure for increasing educator knowledge and skills, implementing best practices, and promoting positive student outcomes.

Educators who are passionate about their own learning can inspire their students to love learning. Education is an ever-evolving field, and educators, both teachers and administrators, should continuously engage in ongoing, effective professional development that keeps them up to date on emerging research and strategies, new curricula and resources, current educational technology, and relevant societal issues. When school staff participate in quality professional development, their connections with students can be enhanced and even transformed so everyone, schoolwide, will be engaged in learning.

Professional development may include training, coaching, or ongoing follow-up supports and should respond to needs identified by teachers, administrators, and staff. Trainings should be of an appropriate duration to learn and apply new learning. They should be partnered with ongoing support that allows educators not only to learn new strategies but also to identify ways to implement those strategies successfully. All professional development should include ongoing support, such as monitoring of implementation, modeling, peer coaching, and mentoring. In a review of 35 methodologically rigorous professional development programs that demonstrated a positive relationship between teacher professional development, teaching practices, and student outcomes, most or all programs did the following:

- Focused on content
- Incorporated active learning
- Supported collaboration
- Used models of effective practice
- Provided coaching and expert support
- Offered feedback and reflection
- Had a sustained duration (Darling-Hammond et al., 2017)

Students never stop learning, and neither do educators. Professional development in education ensures that school staff are always improving no matter where they are in their careers. Ongoing professional development provides strategies for teachers to adapt to the changing needs of their students and broader changes across education. When professional development is continuous and models effective practices, educators gain techniques to keep up with education's changing priorities.

WSCC Professional Development

As stated earlier, educator professional development is structured professional learning that provides improved educator practices that lead to positive student learning outcomes. In general, educator professional development is content focused and incorporates teaching strategies for specific content and curriculum (Darling-Hammond et al., 2017). Whereas general education professional development focuses on teaching practices, classroom strategies, and teaching methodology, professional development related to the Whole School, Whole Community, Whole Child (WSCC) model focuses on building, strengthening, and sustaining school staff implementation of the WSCC approach. The school staff members who can benefit from WSCC-related professional development include professionals representing all components of the model, including teachers, administrators, school nurses, school counselors, school psychologists, school resource officers, social workers, nutrition professionals, and paraprofessionals. WSCC-specific professional development and training provides a foundation for building knowledge and expertise in aligning and integrating education and health to strengthen academic achievement and health outcomes.

For WSCC to be successful, school staff need to fully understand the connection between health and education. WSCC-related professional development must emphasize the importance of focusing on the needs of students and how those needs are supported through collaboration among schools, families, and communities. For schools, a core starting point is an annual training for faculty and staff that provides an overview of WSCC. This provides both existing and new staff an overview of the essential elements of the WSCC model and affords an opportunity to identify gaps in and resources needed for the WSCC components within the school. An annual training should include the importance of engaging families and community members and organizations along with strategies for strengthening this engagement throughout the school year. Schoolwide WSCC professional development gives faculty and staff an opportunity to identify areas of improvement and evidence-based strategies, curricula, and resources.

One important consideration for WSCC-specific professional development is the need to understand how the 10 WSCC components are interrelated. Ensuring that school staff understand how the components work together to support the whole school, whole community, and whole child is critical. Although the 10 WSCC components are separate elements in the model, their interconnection has the potential to have an important impact on students' health and learning. WSCC-specific professional development should provide information, best practices, and resources on how to improve coordination among the components of the model and further the relationship between health and education within the school and community to support the whole child.

As part of any professional learning activity related to WSCC, school staff should be given the opportunity to assess their school's implementation of each of the 10 components. This ensures that each staff member knows who is leading the work in each component and who has expertise in each component area. Demonstrating the need for collaboration and reinforcing that the whole school must integrate all 10 components is critical to supporting each child. The Centers for Disease Control and Prevention's (CDC) School Health Index is a self-evaluation tool that empowers schools to identify strengths and weaknesses in health policies and programs and use a collaborative approach to make improvements. The *School Health Index Self-Assessment and Planning Guide* includes information, materials, and resources (such as trainings, workshops, and presentations) for implementing the School Health Index in schools (CDC, 2019).

Although integrating all 10 components of the WSCC model is critical, providing professional development for each specific component is essential. Health education should be based on curriculum and instruction that is aligned with the *National Health Education Standards: Model Guidance for Curriculum and Instruction* (3rd ed.; National Consensus for School Health Education, 2022). Professional development can ensure that teachers of health education are trained on the curriculum by modeling lessons, providing skills practice, and providing ongoing follow-up support that will lead to a more engaging learning environment for students. However, professional development in health education should not just engage the educators providing health instruction. It should also involve staff from outside the health education classroom. Providing training to all school staff on state health education standards increases awareness of the knowledge and skills students need to adopt and maintain healthy behaviors throughout their lives. When this awareness of health education is present among all school staff members, the likelihood is increased that health knowledge will be reinforced and students will have opportunities to apply health skills before, during, and after the school day.

Physical education and physical activity professional development should include learning opportunities for all educators, physical education teachers, regular classroom teachers, and administrators. Physical education teachers need annual professional development to ensure that instruction is aligned with state standards and based on best practices. It is also important to provide professional development to regular classroom teachers and administrators on integrating physical activity into the classroom to ensure that students get daily physical activity throughout the school day and not just in physical education class. One way to lead teachers to apply this in their own classrooms is to integrate physical activity into each faculty meeting. This activity can be led by the physical education teacher or teachers and will demonstrate how teachers can do such activity with their students each day. Trainings should also address how physical activity can enhance classroom management and how it can be integrated into other subject areas.

Professional development for school nutrition professionals can provide learning opportunities and exposure to resources that enable them to acquire, enhance, and refine the knowledge and skills needed to provide nutritious school meals to all students in the cafeteria. However, the nutrition environment goes beyond the cafeteria. All school staff can benefit from professional development that focuses on providing students with the opportunity to learn and apply healthy eating habits. Training all school staff on how to incorporate nutrition education throughout the school day and in various locations throughout the school can increase the likelihood that education for healthy eating will take place in the classroom, in morning announcements, at school assemblies, in materials sent home to parents or guardians, and in parent–teacher meetings. School staff can learn about including farm-to-school and school garden learning activities in various subjects and within other school venues and activities to actively engage students in nutrition education.

Investing in professional development for all school staff to support a positive social and emotional climate is imperative. Trainings should be designed to increase awareness among all school staff of how the social and emotional climate of the school and classroom can improve student engagement by ensuring a safe and supportive learning environment. Supporting a positive social and emotional climate should not be seen as an additional task for school staff but should be integrated into the school day. Providing professional development related to the promotion of a positive school climate and culture is an important step in enhancing the school as a center for promoting students' health and learning.

Providing all school staff with professional development focused on instruction designed to promote students' development of skills to be actively engaged in school safety is an opportunity to support the physical environment component. Professional development should provide opportunities for staff to learn how to engage their students in discussion on promoting a healthy and safe physical school environment. Providing teachers with learning opportunities on how to teach their students about preparedness and ways to engage their students in discussion on promoting a healthy and safe physical school environment will lead to educating students on real-world connections to their school, home, and community environments.

School health services personnel can lead professional development for staff-related school district policy. Although qualified professionals such as school nurses must receive annual training and demonstrate competency on specific tasks, school nurses can train unlicensed assistive personnel, such as nursing assistants, health aides, paraprofessionals, and other designated school staff to function in an assistive role to the licensed nurse. Trained unlicensed assistive personnel can administer medications and assist with tasks to support the diverse health care needs of students.

Similar to school nurses, school counselors, school psychologists, and school social workers provide services and support systems for students. These professionals, along with other school-employed mental health professionals, when appropriate, can train teachers in advocating for students and identifying their needs. Community resources can be tapped into to provide professional development to support school staff in addressing the mental, behavioral, and social-emotional health barriers that challenge students.

School staff must be committed to making parents and families feel welcome at school by learning how to transform family engagement. Professional development of administrators, teachers, and all school staff can provide tools and resources to facilitate family engagement that establishes and builds strong partnerships with parents and families. To build capacity and to strengthen family engagement, schools can involve parents in the development of training for teachers, principals, and other educators, which can improve the effectiveness of the training. Professional development on family engagement should focus on the value and contributions of families, how to communicate with and work with families as equal partners, how to implement and coordinate parent programs, and how to build ties between families and schools.

The WSCC model emphasizes the role of the community in supporting schools, and community surrounds the model. Partnerships with the community can generate support for implementation of the WSCC model and provide opportunities for community members to be engaged in the district's school health advisory council and other meaningful activities. Professional development provided to school staff can present strategies for creating partnerships that teachers can use to expand the curriculum beyond the classroom and school. Training school staff on creating a community resource map and toolkit, and involving the community throughout the process, can raise awareness of local student and family needs while promoting collaboration and the sharing of resources.

When planning WSCC-related professional development, it is important to provide annual training on the district and school's health and wellness policies. Policies not perceived to be specific to health—such as those related to school absenteeism, homework, transportation to and from school, discipline, and student representation on decision-making bodies—can also have an impact on a school's efforts to promote student health. Making the connection between all elements of the WSCC model and each policy will strengthen educators' awareness of the connection between education and health. This annual training should focus on not only student policies but staff policies as well. Healthy school staff can model healthy behaviors, and by prioritizing employee wellness school districts and schools can strengthen employees' commitment to healthy students and their learning. Healthy eating and physical activity programs for all school employees can be developed and implemented through professional development for staff. School employee wellness programs should include a library of trainings, tools, and resources to support staff physical, mental, and emotional wellness through quality professional development.

Summary

Educator professional development is focused primarily on teachers learning and refining their methods and practice of teaching. Whereas effective educator professional development leads to increased teacher competency, WSCC-specific professional development builds the capacity of all school staff to implement the WSCC model through collaboration and engagement with partners within and outside the school. Professional development in general education is focused on content to improve education outcomes, but WSCC-specific professional development supports continuous improvement by addressing the needs of the whole child to improve both student health and education outcomes. Important WSCC-related professional development resources are presented in the WSCC Professional Development Resources sidebar.

Supporting WSCC through professional development calls for school health champions to lead the way in providing continuous quality, WSCC-specific professional development at the state, district, and school levels.

WSCC Professional Development Resources

Overall WSCC Model
- American School Health Association
- CDC Healthy Schools
- Healthy Schools Toolkit, Washington University in St. Louis
- National Association of Chronic Disease Directors
- Society for Public Health Education

WSCC Components and Whole Child Tenets
- American School Health Association (health education)
- CDC Division of Adolescent and School Health (health education)
- National Consensus for School Health Education (health education)
- Society for Public Health Education (health education)
- National Association of School Nurses (health services)
- School-Based Health Alliance (health services)
- Society of Health and Physical Educators (physical education and physical activity)
- Institute of Child Nutrition (nutrition environment and services)
- School Nutrition Association (nutrition environment and services)
- American School Counselor Association (counseling, psychological, and social services)
- National Association of School Psychologists (counseling, psychological, and social services)
- School Social Work Association of America (counseling, psychological, and social services)
- National Center for School Mental Health (social and emotional climate)
- National Center on Safe Supportive Learning Environments (social and emotional climate)
- U.S. Department of Health and Human Services, Substance Abuse and Mental Health Services Administration, Project AWARE (social and emotional climate)
- National School Climate Center (social and emotional climate)
- National Network of Partnership Schools (community involvement, family engagement)
- Community Schools (community involvement)
- ASCD Whole Child approach to education (WSCC tenets)

REFERENCES

Centers for Disease Control and Prevention. (2019). *School Health Index*. www.cdc.gov/healthyschools/shi/index.htm

Darling-Hammond, L., Hyler, M.E., & Gardner, M. (2017). *Effective teacher professional development*. Learning Policy Institute. https://doi.org/10.54300/122.311

National Consensus for School Health Education. (2022). *National Health Education Standards: Model guidance for curriculum and instruction* (3rd ed.). www.schoolhealtheducation.org/

LEARNING AIDS

APPLICATION ACTIVITIES

1. Identify multiple state departments of education and review the various ways in which they promote and support health for students. Review each department's website, using the 10 components of the WSCC model as a framework for your assessment. Indicate whether use of the WSCC model is mentioned on the website. Organize your review by what you perceive as strengths and weaknesses and any recommendations you have for the future. Present the review as a written report that will be provided to WSCC stakeholders at the state level.

2. Analyze the international models and initiatives for health-promoting schools presented by Lloyd J. Kolbe in his perspective, A Synopsis of International Efforts to Improve School Health Programs. Based on your analysis, compare and contrast at least two of the models to the WSCC model. Describe common foundational principles and content that are present in both the WSCC and the international models. In addition, describe content that is unique to one or two models that you consider to be important in supporting health-promoting schools. Organize all elements of your review into a PowerPoint presentation for your class. The presentation will serve as a lead-in to a discussion of Kolbe's perspective.

3. You are hired as a consultant to prepare school administrators, teachers, staff, and stakeholders to initiate the WSCC model in both a middle school and a high school in the same school district. You will conduct three two-hour sessions during the spring semester. The initial implementation of WSCC will occur in the fall. Develop a content outline for each of your three sessions. Provide at least one example of an activity for each session that will actively engage participants in learning about WSCC.

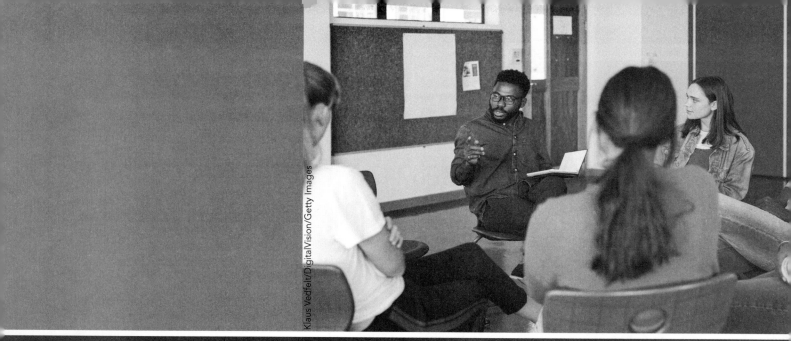

CHAPTER 10

Perspectives on WSCC in Practice

Chapter 10 provides five perspectives on the application of the Whole School, Whole Community, Whole Child (WSCC) model in practice. The authors are leaders in school health with experience in providing leadership in the application of WSCC at the local, state, national, and international levels.

In this chapter, you will find the following contributions:

- The American School Health Association's Perspective on the WSCC Framework—Kayce D. Solari Williams and Randi J. Alter
- Society for Public Health Education: Champion for Quality School Health Education—M. Elaine Auld
- The Whole Campus Model: A WSCC Framework for Health Promotion on College Campuses—Bonni C. Hodges, Donna M. Videto, and Alexis Blavos
- The Need for a WSCC-Based School Health Research Agenda—Michael J. Mann
- WSCC: A Future Perspective—Sean Slade

LEARNING OBJECTIVES

1. Analyze the actions taken by the American School Health Association (ASHA) and Society for Public Health Education (SOPHE) to support and advance the WSCC model.
2. Analyze the rationale, components, and considerations related to the implementation of the WSCC model on a college or university campus.
3. Describe the rationale, potential focal points and research questions, and processes related to the development of a WSCC research agenda.
4. Synthesize future priority actions for supporting and advancing the WSCC model from the perspectives of thought leaders and organizations presented in chapter 10.

The American School Health Association's Perspective on the WSCC Framework

Kayce D. Solari Williams • Randi J. Alter

The Role of the American School Health Association in Advancing the WSCC Framework

The American School Health Association (ASHA), founded in 1927, is a professional association focused on leading efforts to prioritize school-based approaches that promote lifelong health, build a community to support the whole child, and activate champions of school health. With a mission "to transform all schools into places where every student learns and thrives" (ASHA, 2023, para. 1), ASHA supports student-centered, integrated, and collaborative approaches that address the needs of the whole child. This approach aligns with the tenets of the Whole School, Whole Community, Whole Child (WSCC) framework (Centers for Disease Control and Prevention, 2022). This mission is built on the foundation of ASHA's core beliefs (ASHA, 2023), which are as follows:

- Core belief 1. *Health and learning are directly linked and are essential to the development of healthy, resilient citizens. Academic success is an excellent indicator of the overall well-being of youth and a primary predictor of adult health outcomes. This belief addresses the issue of disparities and the achievement gap and offers solutions.*

- Core belief 2. *Schools are uniquely positioned to help students acquire healthy habits for a lifetime. Schools prepare students to be ready for college and a career, which includes being a health-literate adult. Health curricula should be medically and scientifically accurate, aligned with the National Health Education Standards, taught by highly qualified professionals, and focused on healthy living skills.*

- Core belief 3. *The use of a coordinated school health approach is the most effective and efficient means of promoting healthy citizens. A coordinated approach includes stakeholders from all components of a student's environment, creates a system to support student academic achievement, eliminates gaps, and reduces redundancies across initiatives and funding streams through appropriately licensed and certified disciplines.*

- Core belief 4. *School health professionals should be highly qualified and should be able to use current theory and research to select and design effective health and education strategies. The need for undergraduate and graduate training in health education and the need for certified, licensed, or state-endorsed professionals are addressed in this belief and supported by the Healthy People 2030 objectives.*

- Core belief 5. *Schools should be safe, nurturing environments that facilitate learning for all. School climate, school connectedness, and a caring and safe learning environment promote student success and teacher retention through parent and community partnerships, policies, and practices. All students should be healthy, safe, supported, challenged, and engaged.*

The WSCC framework is the best representation of a truly collaborative approach to health and learning and aligns with ASHA's mission and core beliefs. Thus, ASHA centers its work around enhancing the awareness, adoption, implementation, and evaluation of WSCC by schools and the communities that support them.

ASHA raises awareness of the value of the WSCC framework through its professional journal, online communications, annual conference, and webinars around the connection between health and learning and the value of the WSCC framework in strengthening this connection. For example, its *Journal of School Health (JOSH)* is a trove of evidence of the impact of student health on academic success. A 2015 issue of *JOSH* focused on the critical connections between health and learning and discussed each component of the WSCC framework (Hunt, 2015). Also, ASHA utilizes social media and other communication channels to amplify the importance of students' health to their academic success. In addition, it lends its diverse voice through the development of learning opportunities (e.g., webinars, workshops) that highlight the value of the WSCC framework to student success. These professional development opportunities utilize current science to raise awareness of the positive influence of physical and behavioral well-being on student behavior, classroom management, school connectedness, and the school climate.

In addition, ASHA provides support for the adoption of the WSCC framework by highlighting how WSCC can be incorporated into existing initiatives such as school wellness policies or staff wellness initiatives. It provides examples of how WSCC is being implemented in schools around the United States and positive outcomes that have been realized by those schools. Its annual conference features sessions and keynote presentations that share successful implementation of WSCC policies and practices while providing guidance on how to incorporate components into existing efforts. In addition, ASHA's monthly webinar series covers topics such as collaborations with community-based and public health organizations. Finally, ASHA recognizes and celebrates schools and districts that are successfully implementing the WSCC framework. These ASHA WSCC Award recipients represent school–community partnerships that have applied the philosophy associated with the WSCC framework, specifically in terms of the alignment, integration, and collaboration between education and health, to improve each child's cognitive, physical, social, and emotional development.

ASHA supports the implementation of WSCC by highlighting schools and districts that are successfully improving the health of students. In addition, it provides learning opportunities (e.g., webinars and conferences) and *JOSH* articles throughout the year. For example, a 2020 issue of *JOSH* sponsored by the Robert Wood Johnson Foundation focused on the positive outcomes of WSCC-focused policies, engagement strategies, and community-based systems (Howley & Hunt, 2020). ASHA also provides access to vetted and evidence-based resources such as programs, policies, and practices through its website, newsletter, and professional development offerings. Finally, in the spirit of collaboration, it amplifies the work being done by governmental and nongovernmental organizations to support successful implementation of the WSCC framework through social media and its membership network.

JOSH is ASHA's greatest contribution to furthering the evaluation of evidence-based research and best practices in school health. This journal, which is published monthly,

> *communicates current scientific discoveries about how schools, educational systems, and communities can reliably maximize safety, health, learning, growth, and access to opportunity for all [prekindergarten through grade 12] students. Further, JOSH advances knowledge about how to support and enhance the health, wellbeing, and expertise of every professional that serves young people in schools and across the broader educational system. Finally, JOSH supports efforts to better understand the many impacts health promoting schools can make in the communities they serve and to equip advocates for children's health with scientifically sound information they can use to promote school health around the world. (ASHA, n.d., para. 1)*

The *JOSH* editorial board has also developed a set of research priorities that highlights additional areas of need related to the evidence base for specific aspects of the WSCC framework, settings, and populations (Mann, 2022).

Working Across Disciplines for Student Success

ASHA is one of several professional associations in the school health space that serve to provide professional development, networking opportunities, and identity development to practitioners and researchers alike. It holds a unique position within the landscape of professional associations in the school health field in that its work is focused on implementing a multidisciplinary approach to student health with a specific focus on the WSCC framework. ASHA's members are a network of administrators, counselors, dietitians, nutritionists, health educators, physical educators, psychologists, school health coordinators, school nurses, school physicians, and social workers who collaborate in a coordinated fashion to support the whole child. Just as the WSCC framework encourages components within a school community to work together across disciplines to support student health, ASHA models this coordination through its composition, programming, services, events, and collaborations. It works with specialized associations in the school health space to advocate with one voice for the health of students. In collaboration with the Society of State Leaders of Health and Physical Education, ASHA convenes state-level leaders on an annual basis for the School Health Action Congress. Goals of the School Health Action Congress include the following:

1. Better connecting state-level leaders
2. Providing opportunities for attendees to learn from one another
3. Supporting efforts to build strong institutions that prioritize student health and well-being
4. Activating state-level decision-makers to advocate for the health of students

In addition, ASHA partners with the Society for Public Health Education to support the field of health education through the National Committee on the Future of School Health Education in developing recommendations for strengthening school health education programs. ASHA contributes to advocacy efforts through meetings and joint letters to decision-makers and leaders at the national level. Actively engaging in conversations and correspondence fosters collaborations to increase the use of the WSCC framework to address emerging issues facing schools and students. ASHA recognizes the importance of diverse perspectives of nonprofit organizations throughout the school health space as well as its collaborations with other nongovernmental and governmental organizations. For example, it partners with a diverse group of nongovernmental organizations, including Erika's Lighthouse, on Shine Light on Depression, a project funded by Elevance Health Foundation to amplify the conversation around teen depression and suicide. In addition, ASHA serves on the national advisory group for the Center of Excellence for Protected Health Information, a project funded by the Substance Abuse and Mental Health Services Administration to create resources and trainings to ensure that health information is protected when seeking care. ASHA supplements the work of governmental organizations such as the Centers for Disease Control and Prevention to prioritize issues that align with its mission, swiftly adapt and adjust to changing circumstances and conditions, and speak out on issues that may be controversial or difficult for governmental organizations to address. These collaborations not only model the coordinated aspect of the WSCC framework but also help ensure that the WSCC framework can address the future needs of students.

The Role of Associations in Advancing WSCC Into the Future

As ASHA and other associations that serve the multidisciplinary school health community move into the future, it will be critical to fully understand the changing needs of school health professionals, students, and stakeholders. Multiple incidences of racially motivated violence have brought about a renewed focus on diversity, equity, inclusion, and accessibility. This has been amplified by the repercussions of the COVID-19 pandemic and the existing inequities the pandemic exacerbated. Associations must ensure that internal structures, processes, and controls—including the way they spend their funds, the leaders they select, the causes they support, the issues around which they advocate, the services they offer, and the individuals they celebrate—are built on the foundations of diversity, equity, inclusion, and accessibility. In general, associations must devote time, effort, and resources to fostering greater involvement of marginalized communities in WSCC to ensure that all students' needs are met equally and equitably. This includes offering learning and growth opportunities for the next generation of school health professionals, educators, and administrators who are aware of and able to successfully implement the WSCC framework. ASHA has added to its existing university partnerships, including partnerships with Historically Black Colleges and Universities, to continue investing in the long-term sustainability of the profession and the preparation of the next generation of school health professionals across disciplines and backgrounds. This includes providing opportunities for students to participate in conferences, share their research, and gain experience through internships and volunteering. The pandemic, technological advances, and changing demographics have enhanced the desire and ability to connect virtually and lessened the need for colocation (Annie E. Casey Foundation, 2021). This has presented an opportunity for more timely and wider dissemination of innovative research, learning opportunities, and expanded collaborations. Adapting to changing conditions and facilitating new opportunities for engagement will offer school health professionals more accessible research, resources, and skill-building opportunities as they relate to WSCC.

Kolbe et al. (2015) emphasized that schools play a critical collaborative role in meeting the needs of students. This role was exemplified in both the HIV/AIDS epidemic in the 1980s and the COVID-19 pandemic. Despite the tremendous stresses placed on schools and the communities supporting them throughout the COVID-19 pandemic, full implementation of WSCC can alleviate the social, emotional, and physical effects felt by students and school staff. ASHA is committed to continuing to disseminate evidence of the effectiveness of WSCC, provide translational professional development on the implementation of WSCC, and convene leaders to activate systems change that increases the adoption of WSCC with an equity focus. Through coordinated and comprehensive practices, we can ensure that future generations will have the support they need to be healthy, safe, engaged, supported, and successful for years to come.

REFERENCES

American School Health Association. (n.d.). *Mission and scope*. www.ashaweb.org/journal-of-school-health/

American School Health Association. (2023). *Priority areas and core beliefs in action*. Retrieved from www.ashaweb.org/priority-areas-and-core-beliefs-in-action/

Annie E. Casey Foundation. (2021, January 13). *What are the core characteristics of generation Z?* Retrieved November 28, 2022, from www.aecf.org/blog/what-are-the-core-characteristics-of-generation-z

Centers for Disease Control and Prevention. (2022, June 27). *Whole School, Whole Community, Whole Child (WSCC)*. www.cdc.gov/healthyschools/wscc/index.htm

Howley, N., & Hunt, H. (Eds.). (2020). [Special issue]. *Journal of School Health*, 90(12). https://doi.org/10.1111/josh.12774

Hunt, H. (Ed.). (2015). The Whole School, Whole Community, Whole Child model [Special issue]. *Journal of School Health*, 85(11). https://doi.org/10.1111/josh.12310

Kolbe, L.J., Allensworth, D.D., Potts-Datema, W., & White, D.R. (2015). What have we learned from collaborative partnerships to concomitantly improve both education and health? *Journal of School Health*, 85(11), 766-774. https://doi.org/10.1111/josh.12312

Mann, M.J. (2022). *Journal of School Health* editorial transition and research priorities for 2022-2024. *Journal of School Health*, 92(1), 7-10. https://doi.org/10.1111/josh.13098

Society for Public Health Education: Champion for Quality School Health Education

M. Elaine Auld

The Society for Public Health Education (SOPHE) serves as a national voice and advocate for quality school health education so children are healthy and ready to learn. Founded in 1950, SOPHE supports leaders in health education and promotion working in kindergarten through grade 12 (K-12) schools, academia, the government, health care settings, community organizations, and worksites to achieve the vision of a "healthy world through health education" (SOPHE, 2022, "Our Vision"). With its offices in Washington, D.C., SOPHE publishes textbooks and three peer-reviewed scientific journals; provides preservice and in-service professional development and training through conferences and distance education; develops tools and resources for the field; advocates for the public's health and the profession; develops competencies and standards used in credentialing; and partners with numerous public and private organizations to promote and protect the health of individuals, families, and communities.

School health champions avow that children must be healthy to learn and must learn to stay healthy. Given that prekindergarten through grade 12 (preK-12) schools represent one of the most important avenues for improving Americans' health, SOPHE has a long history of being involved in school health education and empowering youth to become health-literate adults. SOPHE's inaugural president, Dr. Clair E. Turner, published the first principles of health education that guided schools in developing and refining their early curricula (Means, 1975). Since that time, many other SOPHE presidents and distinguished award winners have advanced school health theory and practice. Three landmark conferences (i.e., in Birmingham in 1981 and in Dallas in 1996 and 2006) explored strengthening quality assurance in professional preparation and practice, including K-12 schools (Taub et al., 2009). SOPHE's contributions to credentialing firmly established a single set of competencies that undergird the professional preparation and practice of both school and community health educators (Gilmore et al., 2005). Today SOPHE's Children, Adolescents and School Health Education community of practice serves as the nexus and think tank for its programs, policies, professional development, and advocacy related to school health.

The purpose of this perspective is to highlight SOPHE's seminal roles in advancing school health education, including its involvement in developing and promoting the Whole School, Whole Community, Whole Child (WSCC) framework. I conclude by identifying WSCC challenges in a post–COVID-19 era that will need to be addressed with sustained organizational leadership to eliminate health disparities and foster healthy, academically successful children and youth.

The Early Years

In the early decades after its founding, SOPHE focused on developing its infrastructure and expanding its membership. Among its school health members honored as Distinguished Fellows (i.e., SOPHE's highest award to a member who has made significant and lasting contributions to health education) were Sally Jean Lucas (1965), Ruth Grout (1969), Elena Sliepcevich (1972), and Mayhew Derryberry (1970). Dr. Derryberry, SOPHE's second president and a renowned behavioral scientist, was the associate director of one of the first large-scale studies of the health of U.S. schoolchildren (Allegrante et al., 2004). In 1961, SOPHE's board of trustees adopted a resolution to cooperate with the nationwide School Health Education study funded by the Samuel Bronfman Foundation. Taking a leave from her academic post at The Ohio State University, Dr. Sliepcevich directed the investigation, which involved some 1,460 schools and more than 840,000 students in 38 states (Means, 1975). Her report documented major deficiencies in school health instruction in terms of content and time, qualified teachers, facilities, instructional materials, and other areas and called for major school health reforms.

In the 1970s, SOPHE's 21st president, Dr. Scott Simonds, and other SOPHE representatives were appointed to President Richard Nixon's Committee on Health Education. Although not specifically focused on school health, the committee was charged with raising the level of health consumer citizenship; establishing goals, priorities, and immediate and long-term objectives for health education; and developing a plan for implementation (Guinta & Allegrante, 1992). Two major outcomes of the President's committee were the establishment of the federal Bureau of Health Education within what was then called the Center for Disease Control (CDC) and the founding of the private-sector National Center for Health Education (NCHE). The Bureau of Health Education contributed to the first *Surgeon General's Healthy People Report on Disease Prevention and Health Promotion* in 1979, in which three of the five national goals addressed infants, children, and adolescents.

NCHE developed and disseminated Growing Healthy, America's first comprehensive school health education curriculum for children in kindergarten through grade 6. The curriculum was designed to help youth develop the skills and attitudes necessary for health-related problem-solving and informed decision-making. Subsequently, the nonprofit organization launched Starting Healthy, a comprehensive preschool health education program for children ages 3 to 5. Clarence Pearson, Lloyd Kolbe, and many other SOPHE members had key roles in NCHE in administration, research, and providing training to schools that adopted the curriculum (Allegrante & Auld, 2016).

Ramping Up Efforts

With the momentum of new research and federal agency interest in school health education, national guidance on the who, what, where, and why of health instruction for children became increasingly apparent. In 1995, SOPHE provided comments on the first *National Health Education Standards: Achieving Health Literacy*, which was developed by school health experts convened by the American Cancer Society (Joint Committee on National Health Education Standards, 1995). The standards emphasized the need to address functional health information (essential knowledge) and health skills necessary for preK-12 students to adopt, practice, and maintain health-enhancing behaviors. The standards were the first *national* framework for state and local teachers, administrators, and policymakers (who have the responsibility for overseeing education) to use in developing or selecting their curricula, administering instructional resources, and assessing student achievement and progress.

SOPHE provided substantial input into subsequent editions of the National Health Education Standards in 2004 and 2022. It was one of six leading national organizations that formed the National Consensus for School Health Education, which provided support and leadership in the development of the 2022 standards. SOPHE past presidents and luminaries were among the 50 national developers, writers, and reviewers of *National Health Education*

Standards: Model Guidance for Curriculum and Instruction (3rd ed.; National Consensus for School Health Education, 2022).

The early 21st century was also a significant time for SOPHE activism in terms of school health policy efforts (see table 10.1). The board of trustees adopted resolutions on the interrelationship between health and education outcomes, improving graduation rates, and health literacy and called for advocacy on the part of the national office and individual SOPHE chapters. In 1998, SOPHE organized an annual health education advocacy summit that served as a united voice for health education policy issues, including school health (Auld & Dixon-Terry, 1999). The advocacy summit continues to this day as the major focal point for educating students and faculty on effective policy advocacy and meeting with federal policymakers to advocate for school health education and other policy priorities and funding. One example of the impact of the summit actions was the successful advocacy by SOPHE and key groups for congressional passage of the Every Student Succeeds Act (ESSA). The Act was signed into law in December 2015.

Title IV, part A, of the ESSA legislation authorizes three activities (Hampton et al., 2017):

1. Providing students with a well-rounded education (science, technology, engineering, and mathematics; arts; civics; International Baccalaureate and Advanced Placement courses; health and physical education)
2. Supporting safe and healthy students through drug and violence prevention, school mental health, and health and physical education
3. Encouraging the effective use of technology for professional development and blended learning

Senator Tom Udall, a Democrat from New Mexico, was awarded SOPHE's 2018 Honorary Fellow Award, the highest honor to a nonmember, for championing the legislation.

TABLE 10.1 Chronology of SOPHE Milestones in School Health Education

Year	Activity
1950-1970s	Clair E. Turner, leader in school health, served as the first SOPHE president; subsequently many SOPHE leaders made seminal contributions to school health education
1971-1973	Participation in President Nixon's Committee on Health Education, which led to the creation of the Bureau of Health Education in the CDC and the private-sector NCHE
1981	Participation in the first landmark conference on the future of quality assurance in health education in Birmingham, Alabama, which eventually led to the first competencies for school and community health educators affirming that health education is a unified profession with common roles and responsibilities
1995	Input into the first National Health Education Standards specifying functional health information (essential knowledge) and health skills necessary for preK-12 students to adopt, practice, and maintain health-enhancing behaviors
1996	Participation in the Second National Congress for Institutions Preparing Health Educators in Dallas, Texas
2001-2004	Convened with the American Association for Health Education (AAHE) the National Task Force on Accreditation in Health Education, which recommended the National Council for Accreditation of Teacher Education (NCATE) as the preferred accrediting entity to provide a single coordinated accreditation mechanism for school health education programs at the undergraduate and graduate levels; if a dual teacher certification program was in place, health education was to be reviewed as a separate program. (As a new accrediting agency for teacher education, the Teacher Education Accreditation Council [TEAC] was not considered as part of the recommendations)
2001	Adopted *Resolution on Eliminating Health Disparities Based on Sexual Orientation*

Year	Activity
2002	Adopted a resolution on comprehensive sexuality education
2004	Chief executive officer invited to testify before the U.S. House of Representatives Committee on Appropriations Subcommittee on Labor, Health and Human Services, Education, and Related Agencies on the recommended appropriation for the CDC's Coordinated School Health program
2004-2007	Appointed with AAHE the National Transition Task Force on Accreditation in Health Education, which convened the Third National Congress for Institutions Preparing Health Educators: Linking Program Assessment, Accountability and Improvement in Dallas in 2006 to present the recommendations of the Accreditation Task Force and gather input related to other actions and issues associated with a unified accreditation system
2005	Adopted a resolution on coordinated school health
2007	Monitored the work of the American Association of Colleges for Teacher Education to develop a unified national accreditation system in educator preparation, which led to the unification of NCATE and TEAC into the Council for the Accreditation of Educator Preparation (CAEP)
2008	Adopted the resolution *Improving Population Health by Improving Graduation Rates*
2010	Adopted the resolutions *Health Literacy: Gateway to Improving the Public's Health* and *Increasing K-12 Health Education to Improve Health Literacy*
2010	Published a special issue of *Health Promotion Practice* titled "Reducing Health Disparities Among Youth: Promising Strategies" and funded by the CDC's Division of Adolescent and School Health
2015	Advocated for the passage of the federal Every Student Succeeds Act recognizing health education and physical education as core academic subjects; subsequently submitted comments to the U.S. Department of Education on a proposed rule implementing programs under Title I of the Elementary and Secondary Education Act
2016	Comments to the U.S. Department of Education provided nonregulatory guidance to states, school districts, and other stakeholders in understanding and implementing the Every Student Succeeds Act
2016-2020	Convened the School Health Teacher Education Writing Standards Work Group to develop standards for the preparation of school health educators; recognized by CAEP as a Specialized Professional Association in school health education
2016-2021	Convened the National Committee on the Future of School Health Education with the American School Health Association to (1) assess the status of school health education in the United States, (2) identify assets and barriers related to the implementation of quality school health education, and (3) identify strategies designed to enhance the perceived value of school health education and maintain and improve programs
2019	Adopted the Whole School, Whole Community, Whole Child resolution
2019	Published a focus issue of *Health Promotion Practice* addressing school health education with a call to action in five areas to strengthen both the professional preparation and professional development of school health educators
2019-2023	Fulfilled CDC cooperative agreements to strengthen professional preparation in school health and develop presentations, resources, and tools on WSCC, social-emotional health, and staff wellness
2020-2022	Developed and published *National Health Education Standards: Model Guidance for Curriculum and Instruction* (3rd ed.) with five other leading national health education organizations
2021	Adopted the *Resolution on Eliminating Health Inequities for Sexual and Gender Diverse Populations*
2021	Published the National Academy of Medicine paper "Health Literacy and Health Education in Schools: Collaboration for Action"

WSCC Takes Center Stage

Although SOPHE had a long history of key leadership in school health, events at the turn of the 21st century precipitated more attention to breaking down the silos between health and education, leading the way for an emerging WSCC model. The importance of moving beyond individual lifestyle factors and addressing broader social and economic issues (e.g., disadvantaged socioeconomic status, discrimination, racism) took center stage. In a 2008 resolution, SOPHE called for improving graduation rates to reduce health disparities by addressing school and nonschool factors that contributed to lower student achievement (e.g., poverty, hunger, poor nutrition) and urged health departments to collaborate with local education agencies and community organizations to reduce health disparities. A special issue of SOPHE's journal *Health Promotion Practice*, "Reducing Health Disparities Among Youth: Promising Strategies," featured individual, family, and community practice-based programs and environmental modifications to promote health equity.

To further catalyze action, SOPHE President Diane Allensworth organized an expert panel with the education organization ASCD (formerly the Association for Supervision and Curriculum Development) called "Health Disparities Among Youth: Breaking Down the Silos Between Health and Education" (Allensworth, 2011). Many of the discussions and much of the collaboration between these education and health leaders were later reflected in the WSCC framework (Lewallen et al., 2015). The new WSCC model was formally unveiled in a keynote session at SOPHE's 2014 annual meeting in Baltimore by Dr. Eugene Carter, former chief executive officer of ASCD, and Dr. Lloyd Kolbe, former director of the CDC's Division of Adolescent and School Health.

As attention turned to implementing the WSCC model, SOPHE and the American School Health Association launched the National Future of School Health Education Expert Panel (Birch, 2017). The charge to the group was to

a. assess the status of school health education in the United States;

b. identify assets and barriers related to the implementation of quality school health education; and

c. identify strategies designed to enhance the perceived value of school health education and maintain and improve programs. (Birch, 2017, p. 840)

Cochaired by SOPHE's president in 2016, Dr. David Birch, and the president of the American School Health Association, Sharon Murray, the expert panel was later renamed the National Committee on the Future of School Health Education to better reflect its interdisciplinary work. In addition to several surveys of the field, the panel produced a manuscript series outlining persistent school health education problems and recommendations for strengthening professional preparation, in-service education, and programs supporting WSCC (Birch et al., 2019). Four open-access articles were published in *Health Promotion Practice* with support from the CDC's Healthy Schools branch. SOPHE was also involved in producing with the National Academy of Medicine and National Association of State Boards of Education educational briefs and workshops that highlighted the WSCC model (Auld et al., 2020; Goekler et al., 2019).

To strengthen professional preparation related to school health and WSCC, SOPHE convened the seven-member School Health Teacher Education Writing Standards Work Group in 2016 to develop teacher preparation standards for initial teaching licensure programs in school health education, which would meet requirements for SOPHE's recognition as a Specialized Professional Association by the Council for the Accreditation of Educator Preparation (CAEP). SOPHE's standards (SOPHE, 2019) were developed over several years based on scientific literature and with input from health education faculty, K-12 teachers, professional associations, and other stakeholders in the field. The standards aligned with the latest Areas of Responsibility, Competencies, and Sub-competencies in the

Health Education Specialist Practice Analysis II (HESPA II) as well as the latest pedagogical standards of the Interstate Teacher Assessment and Support Consortium. SOPHE was officially recognized as a Specialized Professional Association by CAEP in spring 2020 and as of 2023 reviews school health academic programs applying for CAEP recognition.

SOPHE also received CDC funding for two school health initiatives to continue WSCC implementation. A national environmental scan of higher education programs in school health and recommendations from its expert SOPHE School Health Think Tank (Dombrowski & Mallare, 2020) led to SOPHE developing and conducting a digital Institute for Higher Education Academy. The academy aims to strengthen the capacity of preservice health education faculty to prepare school health education teacher candidates to utilize CDC tools and resources (including WSCC resources) and pedagogical best practices. By the end of the academy, participants are expected to describe the characteristics of high-quality health education curricula for preservice teachers, integrate key CDC Healthy Schools tools and resources within their preservice health education curricula, and develop an action plan to make the needed changes to the curricula. Faculty teams from health education and joint health and physical education programs are invited to participate in several days of presentations, technical assistance, and office hours. On the final day, attendees share their plans for improving the comprehensiveness of their curricula and their plans for using CDC tools and resources as part of this process.

With CDC support, SOPHE has also developed multiple school health tools and resources, such as the WSCC Team Training Modules for CDC-funded state education agencies. Topics addressed in the 10 modules include building administrative support for the WSCC framework, using data to guide WSCC planning and implementation, assessing school health needs, and integrating health equity as part of the WSCC framework. A WSCC fact sheet series and a guide, *Social and Emotional Learning (SEL) and School Health: Addressing SEL Through the Whole School, Whole Community, Whole Child Framework*, have also been developed. In response to the many pressures exposed and exacerbated during the COVID-19 pandemic, SOPHE is developing new culturally appropriate, turnkey tools to promote staff wellness from both personal and school environmental perspectives. Contemporary issues such as Healthy People 2030 objectives, social determinants of health, health equity, school staff mental health, adult social-emotional learning, and risk factors that contribute to chronic disease are addressed within the context of the WSCC framework.

Moving Forward

Despite these and other WSCC implementation efforts, the COVID-19 pandemic significantly slowed progress advancing WSCC. At the preservice level, faculty struggled with pivoting to distance education and university housing policies to limit COVID-19 exposure. State and local school K-12 teachers juggled a patchwork of different policies and procedures that shifted often based on the latest scientific guidance on the virus, the availability of vaccines, misinformation and disinformation in the media, and contentious local politics. Students and school staff in districts with fewer resources experienced the most severe disparities, which led to decreased student academic achievement (Agostinelli et al., 2020).

The impact of COVID-19 on schools and students will be discussed, debated, and researched for decades to come. However, the pandemic not only exacerbated many long-standing challenges in school health education but also resulted in new issues that WSCC champions must confront. SOPHE and other health and education partners must take advantage of this teachable moment to promote the WSCC model by doing the following:

- Emphasizing the long-standing and emerging science on the links between health and academic outcomes and the need to address underlying social factors to improve high school graduation rates

- Advocating for the hiring of faculty and preK-12 teachers who are qualified in health education to help plan and coordinate the 10 components of the WSCC model
- Unifying health and education organizations in advocating to policymakers and the public for funding and implementation of WSCC at the state and local levels
- Stressing the importance of preK-12 schools in producing a health-literate citizenry that empowers students with the necessary knowledge and skills to evaluate health information from multiple sources
- Reengaging parents and families as positive advocates for quality school health education and their role in WSCC and supporting the whole child
- Promoting improved collaboration between public health departments, community organizations, and schools to fully implement WSCC's 10 components
- Supporting school health education studies and evidence-based programs related to WSCC implementation so resources are used most effectively

The WSCC model provides a critical framework in which children who are healthy to learn can also learn to be healthy. Now more than ever in this post-pandemic era, SOPHE must continue working with partners to support WSCC implementation as a vital avenue for realizing its vision of a healthy world through health education.

REFERENCES

Agostinelli, F., Doepke, M., Sorrenti, G., & Zilliboti, F. (2020). *When the great equalizer shuts down: Schools, peers, and parents in pandemic times* (Working Paper No. 28264). National Bureau of Economic Research. www.nber.org/system/files/working_papers/w28264/w28264.pdf

Allegrante, J.P., & Auld, M.E. (2016). Clarence E. Pearson, MPH (1925-2014). *Health Education & Behavior*, 43(3), 359. https://doi.org/10.1177/1090198116648687

Allegrante, J.P., Sleet, D.A., & McGinnis, J.M. (2004). Mayhew Derryberry: Pioneer of health education. *American Journal of Public Health*, 94, 370-371. https://doi.org/10.2105/AJPH.94.3.370

Allensworth, D.D. (2011). Addressing the social determinants of health of children and youth: A role for SOPHE members. *Health Education & Behavior*, 38(4), 331-338. https://doi.org/10.1177/1090198111417709

Auld, M.E., Allen, M., Hampton, C., Montes, J.H., Sherry, C., Mickalide, A.M., Logan, R., Alvarado-Little, W., & Parson, K. (2020). *Health literacy and health education in schools: Collaboration for action*. National Academy of Medicine. https://doi.org/10.31478/202007b

Auld, M.E., & Dixon-Terry, E. (1999). The role of health education associations in advocacy. *The Health Education Monograph Series*, 17(2), 10-14.

Birch, D.A. (2017). Improving schools, improving school health education, improving public health: The role of SOPHE members. *Health Education & Behavior*, 44(6), 839-844.

Birch, D.A., Goekler, S., Auld, M.E., Lohrmann, D.K., & Lyde, A. (2019). Quality assurance in teaching K-12 health education: Paving a new path forward. *Health Promotion Practice*, 20(6), 845-857. https://doi.org/10.1177/1524839919868167

Dombrowski, R.D., & Mallare, J. (2020). *Environmental scan of health education teacher preparation programs 2020*. www.sophe.org/professionalpreparation/teacher-preparation/

Gilmore, G.D., Olsen, L.K., Taub, A., & Connell, D. (2005). Overview of the National Health Educator Competencies Update Project, 1998-2004. *Health Education & Behavior*, 32(6), 725-737. https://doi.org/10.1177/1090198105280757

Goekler, S., Auld, M.E., & Birch, D.A. (2019). The role of health education. *The State Education Standard*, 19(1), 39-43.

Guinta, M.A., & Allegrante, J.P. (1992). The President's Committee on Health Education: A 20-year retrospective on its politics and policy impact. *American Journal of Public Health*, 82, 1033-1041. https://doi.org/10.2105/AJPH.82.7.1033

Hampton, C., Alikhani, A., Auld, M.E., & White, V. (2017). *Advocating for health education in schools* (Policy brief). Society for Public Health Education. www.sophe.org/wp-content/uploads/2017/01/ESSA-Policy-Brief.pdf

Joint Committee on National Health Education Standards. (1995). *National Health Education Standards: Achieving health literacy*. American Cancer Society.

Lewallen, T.C., Hunt, H., Potts-Datema, W., Zaza, S., & Giles, W. (2015). The Whole School, Whole Community, Whole Child model: A new approach for improving educational attainment and healthy development for students. *Journal of School Health, 85*(11), 729-739. https://doi.org/10.1111/josh.12310

Means, R.K. (1975). *Historical perspectives on school health.* Auburn University, Department of Health, Physical Education and Recreation.

National Consensus for School Health Education. (2022). *National Health Education Standards: Model guidance for curriculum and instruction* (3rd ed.). www.schoolhealtheducation.org/wp-content/uploads/2022/10/National_Health_Education_Standards_Guide-10.02.2022.pdf

Society for Public Health Education. (2019). *SOPHE 2019 health education teacher preparation standards: Guidelines for initial licensure programs.*

Society for Public Health Education. (2022). *SOPHE vision statement.* www.sophe.org/about/mission/

Taub, A., Birch, D.A., Auld, M.E., Lysoby, L., & Rasar King, L. (2009). Strengthening quality assurance in health education: Recent milestones and future directions. *Health Promotion Practice, 10*(2), 192-200. https://doi.org/10.1177/1524839908329854

The Whole Campus Model: A WSCC Framework for Health Promotion on College Campuses

Bonni C. Hodges • Donna M. Videto • Alexis Blavos

The National Academy of Sciences report *Mental Health, Substance Use, and Wellbeing in Higher Education: Supporting the Whole Student* (Committee on Mental Health, 2021) recommended coordination and collaboration among and across campus services and offices to build and maintain a culture of well-being as an effective strategy for addressing issues with college student well-being (p. 114). The Whole School, Whole Community, Whole Child (WSCC) model creates a foundation and infrastructure for building and maintaining such a culture of well-being in higher education.

Kindergarten through grade 12 schools, along with colleges and universities, share common goals of positive health and strong academic outcomes for their students. Services for students in higher education contain many components that are similar to the components described in the WSCC model (ASCD, 2022; Centers for Disease Control and Prevention [CDC], 2023b). Thus, the WSCC framework can be adapted to provide a model for health promotion planning to support and enhance the well-being and academic success of college students.

The Whole Campus model proposed here (see figure 10.1) reshapes WSCC to align with tenets and components common to most colleges and universities and can be used to build and support the American College Health Association's (ACHA; 2020) Healthy Campus framework.

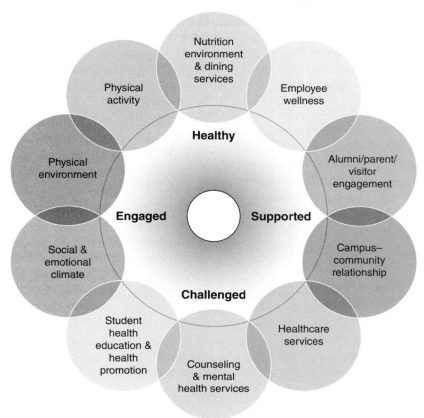

FIGURE 10.1 Whole Campus model.
Adapted from Centers for Disease Control and Prevention (2023b).

The Whole College Student

To support the development of WSCC and the whole child, WSCC tenets and indicators are provided to support school-age youth (ASCD, 2022). Table 10.2 presents the tenets and indicators included with what we are referring to as the "whole college student." The tenets and indicators traditionally used to support the whole child are adapted and described in the table as principles that reflect values and issues related to the ideal role of higher education in fostering and supporting healthy students equipped to engage in lifelong learning, professional development, and personal growth. We revised the ASCD Whole Child tenets and indicators (ASCD, 2022) based on a review of national recommendations for higher education from ACHA's Healthy Campus framework (ACHA, 2021) and the Healthier Campus Initiative through the Partnership for a Healthier America (2022).

TABLE 10.2 Whole College Student Tenets

Tenet	Indicators
Tenet 1: Each college student values and practices a healthy lifestyle.	1. The institutional culture supports and reinforces the health and well-being of students, faculty, and staff. 2. The institution's facilities and environment support and reinforce the health and well-being of students, faculty and staff. 3. The institution facilitates student and staff access to health services. 4. The institution supports, promotes, and reinforces healthy eating patterns and food safety.
Tenet 2: Each college student experiences a supportive environment in which the campus community facilitates personal and professional well-being.	1. The institution's buildings and grounds are secure and meet all established safety and environmental standards. 2. The institution's physical, emotional, academic, and social climate is safe, friendly, and student-centered. 3. Students feel valued, respected, and are motivated to learn. 4. The institution upholds social justice and equity concepts and practices mutual respect for individual differences at all levels of interactions—student to student, faculty/staff to student, and faculty/staff to faculty/staff.
Tenet 3: Each college student is connected to the campus and broader community for active learning, engagement, and growth.	1. Faculty use active learning strategies, such as cooperative learning and project-based learning. 2. The institution offers a range of opportunities for students to contribute to and learn within the community at large, including service-learning, internships, apprenticeships, field experiences, and volunteer projects. 3. Students have access to a range of options and choices for a wide array of extracurricular and cocurricular activities that reflect student interests, goals, and learning profiles. 4. The institution supports, promotes, and reinforces responsible environmental habits through recycling, trash management, sustainable energy, and other efforts.
Tenet 4: Each college student is challenged and prepared for professional success in a global environment.	1. The institution provides opportunities for students to develop critical thinking and reasoning skills, problem-solving competencies, and technological proficiency. 2. The institution's curricula include evidence-based strategies to prepare students for further education, career, and citizenship. 3. The institution provides students with experiences relevant to higher education, career, and citizenship. 4. The institution develops students' global awareness and understanding of cultural competencies.

Adapted from ASCD (2022).

The Whole Campus Model

Attending college challenges the well-being of many students. Reports indicate that long-standing challenges such as substance use remain a concern while student mental health issues are becoming increasingly complex (ACHA, 2021; Committee on Mental Health, 2021). The impact of infectious diseases such as meningitis and COVID-19, along with the measures required to protect students from them, may increase students' stress levels, anxiety, and depression (Wattick et al., 2021). At the same time, issues such as documented food insecurity have been becoming more prevalent for a number of years (ACHA, 2021).

The Whole Campus model provides an adaptable framework to use in guiding actions to foster the whole college student. Working individually and collaboratively, experts can use its components to implement programs, policies, services, and environments that foster a healthy campus community (ASCD, 2022). To create the Whole Campus model we adapted and revised the WSCC model (ASCD, 2022; CDC, 2023b) and its 10 components to reflect the needs of the college student (see table 10.3).

TABLE 10.3 Components of the Whole Campus Model

Component	Description
Nutrition environment and dining services	The campus ensures that all campus food service and dining environments are clean, safe, well maintained, comfortable, and attractive. Food service menus are planned by a registered dietitian and based on current U.S. dietary standards, and all food service locations provide sufficient and appropriate options for vegetarians, vegans, and persons with dietary restrictions. Food service programs plan and implement nutrition education activities. Campus dining services engage in best practices as identified by the National Association of College and University Food Services or other appropriate organizations.
Employee wellness	The campus has established policies and programs that support and assist all its employees in fostering and enhancing physical, mental and emotional, and social well-being. The campus has developed and established programs to prevent and address workplace violence and other emergency situations.
Alumni, parent, and visitor engagement	The campus creates inviting and healthy physical, social, and virtual environments and practices that foster alumni, parent, and visitor engagement with one another and with the institution and its students, faculty, and staff. Advancement, alumni, career services, and other groups on campus actively seek the input and involvement of alumni, parents, and community members to support and enhance all dimensions of student wellness.
Campus–community relationships	The campus and the community work synergistically to promote and support a good quality of life for individuals on campus and in the community. Community groups, organizations, businesses, and individuals work in conjunction with the campus to create and maintain an environment that supports the health and academic success of students, faculty, and staff. Campus groups, organizations, and programs and individual faculty, staff, and students work in conjunction with community groups, organizations, and individuals to contribute positively to the health, economy, and physical and social environments of the community.
Health care services	College or university health care services are designed to provide high-quality, cost-effective health care to support, improve, and promote the health of students. Care is provided by qualified health care professionals such as nurses, nurse practitioners, dentists, physicians, physician assistants, and allied health personnel.
Counseling and mental health services	The campus provides programs and services to foster the personal, academic, and career development of students. Services include psychological, psychoeducational, and psychosocial assessments and direct and indirect interventions to address psychological, academic, and social barriers to learning and career development. Services are delivered by licensed and accredited practitioners and centers.
Student health education and promotion	A robust health education and promotion environment includes programs and policies that promote and support healthy decision-making delivered by credentialed professionals in a variety of formats, locations, and affinity groups.
Social and emotional climate	The campus creates and maintains a social and emotional climate that allows students, faculty, staff, alumni, and visitors to feel safe, secure, supported, and accepted. Campus mission statements explicitly reflect values that foster social justice, equity, and inclusion and provide direction for all students, staff, faculty, alumni, and visitors to actively engage in activities that reflect these values.
Physical environment	Buildings and campus grounds, including athletic facilities, are developed and maintained as safe, accessible, and environmentally friendly. Campuses engage in routine upkeep and maintenance of buildings and grounds, implement and enforce building security mechanisms and policies, implement tobacco-free and weapons-free policies, and seek Leadership in Energy and Environmental Design certification for buildings.
Physical activity	The institution's physical environment, social environment, programming, and facilities motivate and support physical activity among students, faculty, staff, alumni, and visitors.

Adapted from Centers for Disease Control and Prevention (2023b).

The Whole Campus model sits on the foundation of a diverse, equitable, and inclusive environment. Campuses, their components, and their services must intentionally engage in actions and create policies "to decrease bias, reduce harm, and to ensure representation" (Committee on Mental Health, 2021, p. 131) to support the well-being of the whole college student. For the Whole Campus model to be successful, diversity, equity, and inclusion (DEI) must be a driving force that runs through all efforts. Colleges and universities that have taken DEI beyond just using terminology reflective of DEI in their mission statement and policies will plan and deliver programs and policies that include and represent the diverse identities of the student population. When we work toward a campus where all students are encouraged and supported, then we are making a real commitment to DEI.

Nutrition Environment and Dining Services

The nutrition environment on a college or university campus should provide students, faculty, and staff with opportunities for nutrition education and skill development while encouraging the practice of healthy eating through available food and beverage choices, nutrition education, and educational messages about food in the various cafeterias and dining halls and throughout the campus (CDC, 2023b). Students and staff should have access to healthy foods and beverages in a variety of venues, including cafeterias and dining halls, vending machines, grab-and-go kiosks, stores, concession stands, and food trucks. Campuses should make available food pantries for the growing number of students who are food insecure (U.S. Department of Agriculture, n.d.). Food and nutrition professionals should meet minimum education requirements and receive annual professional development and training to ensure that they have the knowledge and skills to provide the necessary services (CDC, 2023b; National Association of College and University Food Services, 2018). Staff can support a healthy campus nutrition environment by marketing and promoting healthier foods and beverages, making nutritional education widely available through traditional and nontraditional avenues (such as peer education), and providing signage encouraging the selection of healthy options in eating establishments. In addition, it is important for healthy snacks to be available at all hours and for students to have access to free and safe drinking water (CDC, 2023b; U.S. Department of Agriculture, n.d.).

Employee Wellness

Fostering employees' physical and mental health protects staff and, by doing so, helps to support college students' health and academic success. Colleges and universities are not only places of higher education but also worksites. Healthy college and university employees are more productive and can serve as powerful role models for college students and one another. Making adequate mental health resources and training available to faculty to "notice, intervene, and refer students and colleagues in distress" (p. 4) supports the notion that all contribute to a healthy campus (American Council on Education, 2020). Campuses should adopt a comprehensive employee wellness approach that includes a coordinated set of programs, policies, benefits, and environmental supports designed to address multiple risk factors (e.g., lack of physical activity, tobacco use) and health conditions (e.g., diabetes, depression) to meet the health and safety needs of all employees (CDC, 2023b). Partnerships between colleges or universities and student health services and employee health insurance providers can help offer resources, including personalized health assessments and vaccinations. Employee wellness programs and healthy work environments can improve a college or university's financial bottom line by decreasing employee health insurance premiums and reducing employee turnover (CDC, 2023b; Employee Assistance Trade Association, 2015).

Alumni, Parent, and Visitor Engagement

Alumni, parent, and visitor engagement with the campus and one another should be encouraged to support the whole college student.

Alumni, parents, and visitors may serve as role models across the dimensions of wellness and provide expertise or financial support for the establishment, growth, or sustainability of health promotion and other programs supporting the whole college student (The NAPA Group, 2018). In the post-pandemic era, engagement such as alumni preparing students for career readiness becomes more important and may affect students' health and success (The NAPA Group, 2021). Programs that include students' families where appropriate can also support the whole college student, because parents and families often continue to play a role after their child becomes a college student. For example, providing resources for families of first-generation college students to support students' academic and social efforts is important for successful retention (Minor, 2016). In the 2021 College Student Mental Health Survey, 80 percent of respondents reported talking to friends and family to reduce stress and anxiety; this shows the continued need to involve families as support agents for college students (American Campus Communities, 2022).

Campus–Community Relationships

Colleges and universities should be engaged in two-way collaborations with the communities in which they are located (Gavazzi, 2017). Higher education institutions have a responsibility to foster the health and well-being of surrounding communities, and engagement with the community can enhance the student, faculty, and staff experience. The campus and the community should work together to achieve a harmonious relationship in which both entities are engaged in shared activities that create contentment and mutual benefit. A harmonious relationship may include enacting and implementing policies and programs that create on- and off-campus environments that are safe and support students' engagement in health-enhancing behaviors; campus–community problem-based learning collaborations that engage students, faculty, and community members in identifying and implementing solutions to local challenges; and regular town–gown meetings, not just meetings in response to a negative event.

Two examples of support for positive college and community relations can be seen at a state college in central New York. First, the Start-Up NY program (Empire State Development, n.d.) provides tax incentives for selected new or expanding businesses that partner with New York colleges and universities to create jobs and enhance the economic development of the colleges' community. In a small city in central New York, three entrepreneurs partnered with a business incubator housed in the local college's economics department. The trio collaborated with college faculty and alumni, provided internship experiences in several disciplines to students, and contributed to the economic growth of the community (SUNY Cortland, 2019). Second, each year, the college participates in The Big Event, sending students, faculty, staff, and alumni volunteers into the surrounding community to engage in a variety of odd jobs and community spring clean-up activities (SUNY Cortland, 2015). The student-organized activity is designed as a community service project to "show how much [the volunteers] appreciate and value the [local] community" (p. 1). The Big Event was pioneered by Texas A&M University and has spread to numerous colleges and universities across the United States.

Health Care Services

Health care services to enhance the college experience and remove barriers to learning should be provided to or accessible to students (ACHA, 2018; National Association of Student Personnel Administrators, 2017). Whether a first aid center, a comprehensive health center with specialty care, or something in between, college health care services should collaborate with other departments on campus to identify the health care needs of students, implement appropriate services, and evaluate these services. This may include linking with applicable health care services in the community. The following services are some of those recommended through the Healthy Campus framework (ACHA, 2021) for developing and sustaining the health and well-being of all college campuses:

- Procedures for addressing sexual and relationship violence on college and university campuses
- Drug education and testing of student-athletes
- HIV pre-exposure prophylaxes
- Guidelines for hiring health promotion professionals in higher education
- Standards for student health insurance coverage
- Trans-inclusive college health programs (ACHA, 2020)

In addition to following recommendations from ACHA and the Healthy Campus framework, health care service centers should seek appropriate accreditation through such organizations as the Accreditation Association for Ambulatory Health Care. This organization provides accreditation to primary care practice settings, including college and university health care centers (Accreditation Association for Ambulatory Health Care, 2022).

Counseling and Mental Health Services

Although college and university counseling and mental health services may be accessible to students, these programs alone are not able to treat all students on campus who are seeking services (ACHA, 2022). Mental health services should use a public health approach by collaborating with other sectors on campus to expand and move beyond treatment services and address socioecological factors to improve the mental, emotional, and social health of all students (The Jed Foundation & Education Development Center, 2017). In one survey, as a result of the COVID-19 pandemic, 85 percent of college students reported being more stressed than in previous years (American Campus Communities, 2020), thus highlighting an even stronger need for this component. Mental health and counseling services should seek accreditation through such organizations as the International Accreditation of Counseling Services (2022) to ensure that mental health services meet a high standard and to increase opportunities to network with other accredited centers.

Student Health Education and Promotion

A diverse and holistic health education and promotion environment on a college or university campus should provide students with a variety of opportunities to learn, grow, and practice healthy lifestyle behaviors and skills across wellness dimensions across a variety of locations and time frames. These efforts may be targeted to affinity groups such as first-year students, intramural and intercollegiate sports teams, Greek organizations, or student clubs and organizations. Requiring multiple health and wellness courses as options for general education coursework provides additional opportunities for students to gain knowledge and skills to maintain a healthy lifestyle. Polacek et al. (2013) found that general education health and wellness courses had a positive effect on the wellness and wellness knowledge of undergraduates both during their college years as well as after graduation.

Colleges and universities should develop and implement policies that create and support a safe and accessible campus. The health education and promotion professionals who are developing and implementing such programs should not only hold a degree appropriate to the work they are performing but also have appropriate certification or licensing, such as the Certified Health Education Specialist national credential (National Commission for Health Education Credentialing, n.d.).

Social and Emotional Climate

The campus should create and maintain a social and emotional climate that allows students, faculty, staff, alumni, and visitors to feel safe, secure, supported, and accepted. The campus environment must be equitable, inclusive, and accessible to all students and the campus to create opportunities for students, faculty, staff, alumni, and community members to engage in skill development to communicate successfully, negotiate conflict, interact effectively with others, and control emotional impulses (American Institutes for Research, 2017). The campus should foster an inclusive environment that encourages students, faculty, and staff to explore ideas that are different from their own in safe spaces. The campus should work with the surrounding community to support an equitable, inclusive, and accessible environment off campus as well. This dimension is reflected in the DEI efforts described earlier.

Physical Environment

Campus physical environments should support the daily needs of students, faculty, and staff and enhance pedagogy. The development and maintenance of safe, accessible, and aesthetically pleasant physical environments across all aspects of a campus contribute to the prevention of intentional and unintentional injuries and minimize exposure to pollutants that can have short- and long-term adverse effects on health (Seabert et al., 2022). The natural and built physical environments of campuses can affect how students build and sustain community, encourage student engagement, and create psychological safe spaces (Strange & Banning, 2021). The physical environment should communicate to students, faculty, staff, and visitors in a way that has potential to affect health-related behaviors (Bandura, 1986; Strange & Banning, 2021). Campuses should strive to create physical environments that provide a sense of security and inclusion, facilitate involvement in educational and extracurricular activities, and foster a sense of community (Strange & Banning, 2021).

Physical Activity

A campus should support engagement in physical activity among all constituents. Physical activity levels contribute to short- and long-term health benefits and the prevention of chronic disease (Office of Disease Prevention and Health Promotion, 2022). Changes should be made to the built environment to encourage and support physical activity, such as maintaining sidewalks and offering bicycle lanes; improving access to fitness facilities at low or no cost for faculty, staff, and students on campus; or collaborating with community facilities on costs and transportation to local recreational and fitness facilities (Small et al., 2013). The following suggestions for improving student activity are adapted from CDC (2023a) recommendations:

1. Promote community plans and policies to design areas around campus to support safe and easy places for people to walk, bike, wheelchair roll, and be physically active.
2. Promote programs and policies that make it safe and easy to walk, bike, wheelchair roll, and be physically active.
3. Provide professionals with ideas on how to promote physical activity.

The following example indicates how two campuses promoted biking communities both on and off campus:

Texas Southmost College and Santa Monica College were recognized as Bicycle Friendly Universities for their work to promote biking. Both schools used [a] variety of resources to make it easier for people in the community to bike to and on campus. These efforts included providing infrastructure such as bike parking, showers and lockers, lighting and cameras, bike repair stations, and bike share options. They also promoted local bicycling events, provided bicycle-related workshops, and gave free bikes to students receiving financial assistance. (CDC, 2023a, "What Other Organizations Are Doing," para. 3)

Summary

The components of the Whole Campus model presented here may appear to be separate and distinct entities; however, we feel there is a great deal of overlap among and between the components, the Whole College Student tenets, and DEI efforts. We contend that a strong holistic foundation for college student well-being can be created by using the Whole Campus model and its tenets within a dynamic DEI framework to guide health promotion programming on college campuses. The Whole Campus model can foster the academic and personal success of college students, similar to what the WSCC model does for youth in prekindergarten through grade 12. Efforts to address the COVID-19 pandemic on campuses show that it is very possible to cooperate and collaborate to improve the health and wellness of college students and the college community. During the pandemic many campuses learned to collaborate efficiently and effectively to address a health challenge and developed strong relationships with state and local public and community health agencies in the process. Campuses need to maintain and continue to build these partnerships and others to optimize the public and community health presence and efforts to address the Whole Campus model. Such efforts will expand the vision of college health promotion and provide support and direction for the collaborations needed for a healthy campus community.

REFERENCES

Accreditation Association for Ambulatory Health Care. (2022). *Accreditation for primary care providers.* www.aaahc.org/accreditation/primary-care/

American Campus Communities. (2020). *College students' perspective on mental health during COVID-19.* www.americancampus.com/assets/about-us/media/ACC-HHAY-Survey-Report-Oct-2020.pdf

American Campus Communities. (2022). *College students are prioritizing mental health and wellness; Stress and anxiety levels declining, new nationwide survey reveals.* https://www.americancampus.com/news-and-insights/college-students-are-prioritizing-mental-wellness-stress-and-anxiety-levels-declining-new

American College Health Association. (2018). *Healthy Campus 2020: The action model.* www.acha.org/HealthyCampus/Implement/About_the_Action_Model/HealthyCampus_Action_Model.aspx?hkey=3d97df9b-41f7-46f3-a0f0-30a4d0890489

American College Health Association. (2020). *The Healthy Campus framework.*

American College Health Association. (2021, Fall). *National College Health Assessment undergraduate student reference group: Reference group.* www.acha.org/documents/ncha/NCHA-III_FALL_2021_UNDERGRADUATE_REFERENCE_GROUP_EXECUTIVE_SUMMARY.pdf

American College Health Association. (2022). *ACHA guidelines: COVID-19 considerations for institutions of higher education, fall 2022.* www.acha.org/documents/Resources/Guidelines/ACHA_COVID_Considerations_for_IHEs_Fall_2022.pdf

American Council on Education. (2020). *Mental health, higher education and COVID-19: Strategies for leaders to support campus well-being.*

American Institutes for Research. (2017). *Social and emotional learning.* www.air.org/topic/social-and-emotional-learning

ASCD. (2022). *Whole child.* https://www1.ascd.org/whole-child

Bandura, A.C. (1986). *Social foundations of thought and action.* Prentice Hall.

Centers for Disease Control and Prevention. (2023a). *Physical activity: What's your role: Education.* www.cdc.gov/physicalactivity/activepeoplehealthynation/everyone-can-be-involved/education.html#:~:text=Colleges%20and%20universities%20can%20promote,that%20encourage%20walking%20and%20biking

Centers for Disease Control and Prevention. (2023b). *Whole School, Whole Community, Whole Child (WSCC): A collaborative approach to learning and health.* www.cdc.gov/healthyschools/wscc/

Committee on Mental Health, Substance Use, and Wellbeing in STEMM Undergraduate and Graduate Education, National Academies of Sciences, Engineering, and Medicine. (2021). Summary. In A.I. Leshner & L.A. Scherer (Eds.), *Mental health, substance use, and wellbeing in higher education: Supporting the whole student.* National Academies of Sciences, Engineering, and Medicine. 111-142

Empire State Development. (n.d.). *START-UP NY program.* https://esd.ny.gov/startup-ny-program

Employee Assistance Trade Association. (2015). *EAP best practices: The value of employee assistance programs.* www.easna.org/wp-content/uploads/2016/02/Value-of-EAP-2015.pdf

Gavazzi, S. (2017). *The optimal town-gown marriage: Taking campus-community outreach and engagement to the next level.* Amazon Digital Services.

International Accreditation of Counseling Services. (2022). *International Accreditation of Counseling Services.* http://iacsinc.org/home.html

Minor, J.T. (2016). *Five things families of first-generation college students need to know.* HuffPost. www.huffpost.com/entry/five-things-families-of-f_b_7959708

National Association of College and University Food Services. (2018). *Best practices: CAS standards.* www.nacufs.org/resources-best-practices/cas-standards/

National Association of Student Personnel Administrators. (2017). *Wellness and health promotion.* www.naspa.org/division/wellness-and-health-promotion

National Commission for Health Education Credentialing. (n.d.). *Home.* www.nchec.org/

Office of Disease Prevention and Health Promotion. (2022). *Healthy People 2030: Physical activity.* https://health.gov/healthypeople/objectives-and-data/browse-objectives/physical-activity

Partnership for a Healthier America. (2022). *Healthier Campus Initiative.* www.ahealthieramerica.org/search?q=Healthier+campus+initiative

Polacek, G.N., Erwin, T.D., & Rau, J.G. (2013). The longitudinal impact of an undergraduate general education wellness course in early adulthood. *Journal of Health Education Teaching, 4*(1), 15-23.

Seabert, D., McKenzie, J.M., & Pinger, R.R. (2022). *McKenzie's an introduction to community and public health* (10th ed.). Jones & Bartlett Learning.

Small, M., Bailey-Davis, L., Morgan, N., & Maggs, J. (2013). Changes in eating and physical activity behaviors across seven semesters of college: Living on or off campus matters. *Health Education and Behavior, 40*(4), 435-441. https://doi.org/10.1177/1090198112467801

Strange, C.C., & Banning, J.H. (2021). *Designing for learning: Creating campus environments for student success* (2nd ed.). Jossey-Bass.

SUNY Cortland. (2019, February 11). News detail. Pioneering Digital Start-up launches from Campus. *The Bulletin.* https://www2.cortland.edu/news/detail.dot?id=a9b508b7-99ab-45a4-a4b9-6c1a6d188e87

SUNY Cortland, Institute for Civic Engagement. (2015). *Institute for Civic Engagement News, 8*(3). https://www2.cortland.edu/dotAsset/4c7b4b7c-dd88-4bdc-be2d-f914a4c659e6.pdf

The Jed Foundation & Education Development Center. (2017). *A guide to mental health action planning.* www.jedfoundation.org/wp-content/uploads/2017/11/campus-mental-health-action-planning-jed-guide.pdf

The NAPA Group. (2018). *Trends in alumni relations.* https://napagroup.com/2018/01/02/trends-in-alumni-relations/

The NAPA Group. (2021). *Trends in alumni relations in the post-pandemic era.* https://napagroup.com/2021/05/trends-in-alumni-relations-and-advancement-in-the-post-pandemic-era/

U.S. Department of Agriculture. (n.d.). *Nutrition at college.* www.nal.usda.gov/fnic/nutrition-college

Wattick, R.A., Hagedorn, R.L., & Olfert, M.D. (2021). Impact of resilience on college student mental health during COVID-19. *Journal of American College Health, 71*(7), 2184-2191. https://doi.org/10.1080/07448481.2021.1965145

The Need for a WSCC-Based School Health Research Agenda

Michael J. Mann

Over the years, I have had the privilege of speaking to a wide range of audiences about the value of school health. Prior to almost any talk, someone asks me about my interest in schools as an influence on health and well-being. Their question typically boils down to some polite version of "Does what happens in schools really matter?" My response is always an unequivocal and emphatic "yes," and understanding why schools matter seems like a good place to start a discussion on the pressing need for a high-quality, carefully planned, and strategically targeted research agenda based on the Whole School, Whole Community, Whole Child (WSCC) model.

The Importance of School Health and School Health Research

Schools exert tremendous influence on young people, including their health and well-being, both while they are students and long after they end their studies. At a minimum, the large amount of time students spend in schools with educators and other school personnel suggests an inescapable impact. The average U.S. student spends six to seven hours per day at school for 240 days per year for 13 years of their lives, not including time spent on school buses, in extracurricular programs, or attending summer school. All this time spent in schools suggests young people are likely to be influenced by the accumulation of these experiences and that understanding them is important, especially considering that they occur during a formative period of growth and development.

The influence of schools on student health is especially easy to see when we think about health and well-being from a multidimensional perspective. We can easily imagine school-based situations that undermine social health (e.g., bullying or social exclusion), mental health (e.g., exchanges that diminish motivation and self-efficacy), and physical health (e.g., exposure to viral pathogens or regulations related to accident prevention and management). Although it may be somewhat harder, we can also imagine school-based situations that promote social health (e.g., establishing a safe, supportive, and respectful class environment that accelerates student learning and growth or a school-based club or team that provides a sense of identity and belonging), mental health (e.g., participation in academic projects that build self-confidence and self-esteem), and physical health (e.g., being provided nutritious meals or receiving treatment at a school-based health center).

Schools also exert a tremendous influence on the communities they serve, including the health and well-being of the community members. Schools reflect the communities they serve and each community's values, priorities, and investments in their children's futures and the future of their community. Likewise, communities reflect how well schools have prepared their students for life in their community. In this way, the quality of schools themselves can serve as a leading indicator of community health—one that indicates not only current levels of academic performance but also the emerging prospects of the communities themselves.

Finally, schools increasingly need to better understand how to navigate social issues that unavoidably affect student and community health and well-being. For example, school shootings are at the center of debates related to existing and proposed gun policies, especially as they relate to how to best ensure children's safety in schools. In addition, schools are currently caught in the crossfire of disagreements related to racial and social justice; the needs of sexual and gender minority students, educators, and community members; and the value of social-emotional learning and the mental health of students, especially in the post–COVID-19 era. Navigating these issues can be difficult in many communities, and school personnel often need help assembling strong evidence from trusted sources that can inform and guide unbiased, fact-based debates and decision-making.

Taken together, all schools have an impact on the total health and well-being of their students and the communities they serve. Sometimes the impact is positive and serves students and communities well. Sometimes the impact is negative and serves students and communities poorly. In either case, there is no escaping the fact that what happens or fails to happen in schools represents an opportunity to make a difference in health, well-being, and opportunity that is realized or squandered. What happens in schools matters. Understanding how to ensure the best outcomes for every student in every school every day demands the type of deep understanding that only careful and comprehensive research can provide.

The Promise of the WSCC Model

From my perspective, the WSCC model represents the most promising means of achieving the systems change necessary to ensure the health of prekindergarten through grade 12 students in the United States today. I also believe it can be used to frame a comprehensive research agenda designed to maximize our impact on student health in schools. Detailed descriptions of the WSCC model and its 10 components can be found elsewhere in this edited book, on the Centers for Disease Control and Prevention website, and throughout the current professional literature related to school health. Thus, I refrain from providing a detailed summary of the actual model here.

However, for the purposes of this perspective, it is important to note that the WSCC model is built on a strong theoretical foundation and based on years of research related to previous models of coordinated school health. The WSCC model, like the Coordinated School Health model that preceded it, is grounded in socioecological theory and recognizes multiple influences on health and learning that originate from multiple levels of society. The WSCC model also includes individual components associated with well-established constructs known to contribute to healthy child development, such as nutrition, physical activity, psychological health, social and community connection, and access to adults able to model healthy living and lifelong learning. From an organizational and systems theory perspective, the WSCC model begins to more thoroughly integrate responsibility for student health and readiness to learn into the professional expectations for all educators and school health professionals.

The WSCC model further advances preceding models of coordinated school health by more explicitly delineating the relationship between enhancing readiness to learn; promoting the health, growth, and development of the whole child; and academic achievement. The model more clearly situates each school and its corresponding WSCC components within the context of its community and more clearly articulates linkages between communities, schools, families and caregivers, and students. The WSCC model also explicitly highlights the importance of making connections between policy, process, and practice, all essential keys to promoting the scalability of the model and securing pathways to implementation (Rasberry et al., 2015).

Outstanding Questions Shaping the Future of WSCC-Based School Health Research

Although it is built on theory and sound evidence, many research questions related to the WSCC model remain, especially questions related to the generalizability and scalability of the full WSCC model. Moreover, although the WSCC model is built on the foundation of previous models of comprehensive school health, broad commitments to the widespread implementation of the full WSCC model may be somewhat ahead of the evidence, because to date rigorous long-term applications of the full model have not been comprehensively tested and replicated across diverse settings.

In fact, there appear to be few rigorous, high-quality, long-term investigations of fully implemented models of coordinated school health in general. More commonly, evaluations of preceding models of coordinated school health and the WSCC model itself tend to focus on one component or partial implementations of the model and short-term results focused on narrow sets of outcomes (Willgerodt et al., 2021). These limitations are somewhat understandable, because these are comprehensive, nonprescriptive, and multilevel models. As a result, proper evaluations are likely to be complex, costly, and conducted over long periods of time. However, overcoming these challenges is essential to understanding the actual value of the WSCC model.

In 2019, while writing more broadly about school health as a strategy that can improve both public health and public education, Dr. Lloyd J. Kolbe suggested the following seven areas that require future research, all of which apply to the WSCC model and frame outstanding questions crucial to advancing school health:

1. Illuminating causal pathways and the interactive impacts of school health programs designed to affect both school health and academic achievement on longer-term population health, education, and economic outcomes
2. Improving the efforts of health agencies to work inside schools to support health and academic outcomes
3. Improving surveillance systems established to monitor each of the 10 components of the WSCC model and their impact on health and education outcomes
4. Assessing and increasing the effectiveness of each of the 10 components of the WSCC model, as well as combinations of components, to improve health, academic, and economic outcomes
5. Engaging cross-disciplinary teams of scientists and practitioners in improving all aspects of the model
6. Assessing and improving school health operational infrastructures, strategic plans, policies, funding mechanisms, and advocacy at all levels (local, state, national, and international)
7. Generating public health and public education workforces that are more ready to implement, evaluate, and improve school health and each component of the WSCC model

Each of these seven suggestions for future research highlights promising opportunities to better understand and improve both the WSCC model specifically and the broader strategy of using school-based health promotion to promote student health, academic achievement, and life success.

I would also humbly add a few other examples of opportunities to fill gaps in our knowledge specific to the WSCC model itself, especially as they relate to the impact and feasibility of the model as a whole:

1. Evaluations that investigate efforts to create conditions that support the adop-

tion and successful implementation of the model by community members, policymakers, educational leaders, educators and other school support staff, families, caregivers, and students

2. Evaluations of the fully implemented model that include all 10 components, assessments of each component, and assessment of the model as a whole

3. Evaluations of large-scale implementation at the district and state levels, not just in single schools, and especially not involving only highly motivated schools and school leaders that do not represent common challenges to implementation, including initial and ongoing resistance to change

4. Comparative evaluations of the model that occur across diverse settings and answer questions related to the generalizability and portability of the model, especially comparisons of schools and school systems that are small and large or rural, suburban, and urban

5. Evaluations that include a range of anticipated short- and long-term impacts of exposure to the full model, such as outcomes related to health, education, economic, and civic benefits

6. Because the WSCC model represents more of a conceptual road map than a detailed, step-by-step intervention, we need meticulous process evaluations that include careful descriptions of exactly how the model was implemented at each site, including how schools prepared for implementation (e.g., planning and engaging in preimplementation training and setting up systems designed to accomplish model goals), coordinated implementation of the full model (e.g., communicating among component leaders and with school and district educators), and integrated the model into school operations and the school community as a whole (e.g., building educator, family and caregiver, and community support and enhancing participation from all groups)

Answering big questions such as these will require focused effort and attention on a scale not routinely seen in the school health research community or commonly funded by sponsors of school health research. To advance our understanding of what drives effective school health, including the efficacy of the WSCC model, we will need to organize, mobilize, and coordinate our research efforts like never before. Doing so will require school health researchers to work together more effectively and to engage in team science with a host of new researchers from a range of interdisciplinary fields. It will also require us to prepare the next generation of school health researchers to conduct extremely complex, interdisciplinary research and to deploy sophisticated methods likely to provide evidence across a range of long-term outcomes related not only to health but also to education, economics, and readiness for civic life.

The Promise of a WSCC-Based Research Agenda for School Health

Recognizing the level of complexity required to answer these outstanding questions and the new ways we need to prepare ourselves to address them can help us begin framing ideas about how we might rise to these challenges. From my perspective, developing a WSCC-based school health research agenda represents an essential strategy for helping us do so. If this is done well, this research agenda could provide the backbone that supports a range of well-coordinated, collaborative research activities and funding.

Formally developed, profession-wide research agendas have long been used to advance entire disciplines by focusing research in critical areas necessary to solve pressing problems, meet urgent needs, or grow a given profession (Mann & Lohrmann, 2019). Research agendas catalog existing knowledge, identify gaps in knowledge, prioritize new knowledge that needs to be obtained, suggest studies that need to be replicated, and direct research efforts toward those priorities.

Research agendas also help identify what does not require further study at this time. They help differentiate between what has been well established (low-priority research) and what new knowledge is essential to advancing the field now (high-priority research). They provide a solid rationale for new studies and promising lines of inquiry for emerging researchers eager to make a difference. They help researchers avoid investing in low-leverage research likely to go unpublished or to be published without advancing knowledge in a substantial manner.

Conversely, research agendas accelerate progress by identifying widely agreed-on, high-leverage research questions and asking what it will take to answer them. Research agendas help researchers recognize the need for new methods, skills, tools, and partners that may be necessary to address questions that have eluded previous researchers. They also help us identify areas in which we need to build the capacity required to conduct large-scale studies beyond the scope of traditional research teams. Research agendas can encourage us to prepare ourselves and our students to meet the challenges of the future instead of repeating the studies of the past.

Perhaps most important, developing a WSCC-based school health research agenda would create opportunities for both profession-wide and interdisciplinary dialogues that—in and of themselves—are likely to strengthen our field. Doing this type of work draws us out of our offices and into new conversations about the direction of our profession and our collective contributions as researchers. It also offers opportunities to invite new collaborators from different fields to join us in our work and to engage emerging researchers in shaping the future of the field in a manner that generates high levels of ownership and long-term commitment. This will expand our cadre of school health researchers in a manner that has become especially important as graduate programs, especially doctoral programs, devoted to advancing school health research have been decreasing for decades while threats to students in schools have been increasing.

Elements of an Effective Process

Ensuring an effective process represents one of the most important ways to reduce barriers to adoption (Mann & Lohrmann, 2019). An inclusive, respectful, and meaningful process offers to generate not only a higher quality research agenda but also a research agenda that the whole school health community feels invested in and that represents the full perspectives of the group. A research agenda derives its full value from being widely used. Therefore, adopting a comprehensive process that supports widespread ownership of the research agenda and that fuels agenda-related action seems vital.

The breadth and complexity of the WSCC model pose real challenges to implementing an effective process. The model was originally developed by the Centers for Disease Control and Prevention and ASCD. One or more national professional organizations represent key constituents for each of the 10 core components. State governments, local school districts, and local schools play the most critical roles related to implementation of the model. School health researchers can be found in a range of institutions across the United States and internationally. In addition, other key stakeholders, including the U.S. Department of Education, appeared to be absent from the development and initial rollout of the model that, if possible, should be included now. Moreover, we should certainly engage the voices of diverse students, families, and community-based policymakers in this work as well. Ensuring an effective process will require us to involve representatives from each these key institutions in the development of the process itself and to coordinate their work in a thoughtful manner that strengthens partnerships between those dedicated to advancing school health (Willgerodt et al., 2021).

Conducting this work well will require a great deal of time, skill, and a holistic perspective that values each of the 10 components of the WSCC model and the model as a whole. Most likely, a convening organization will need to coordinate this complex enterprise. To me, the American School Health Association (ASHA) seems like a good choice because it represents school health as a whole and not any single component of the WSCC model. ASHA is uniquely positioned to convene a coalition of national organizations representing each WSCC component and national, state, and local education and public health leaders invested in advancing school health research and research related to the WSCC model.

With ASHA or a similar organization acting as a convener, this national coalition could work together to achieve five key goals. First, the national coalition would be responsible for developing a research agenda that poses questions related to the WSCC model as a whole (i.e., the questions posed by Kolbe and myself previously) and assesses the long-term impacts of the model across a range of possible outcomes (e.g., health, academic, economic, and civic outcomes at the individual and community levels). Achieving this goal will require the coalition to facilitate new connections, both among the organizations that are members of the coalition and with newly invited organizations, researchers, and practitioners from other disciplines, especially systems thinking, public policy, implementation science, and change management. The national coalition would also be responsible for addressing cross-disciplinary issues that are not easily placed within a single WSCC component or clearly addressed in the model itself (e.g., mounting effective responses to pandemics, addressing gun violence in schools, and meeting the needs of minoritized and marginalized members of the school community).

Second, the national coalition could develop consistent standards and criteria that each national organization would use to develop the portion of the research agenda dedicated to the WSCC component it represents. For example, a national association dedicated to providing school-based counseling services could use these standards and criteria to submit its draft of the counseling, psychological, and social services portion of the WSCC research agenda. Selected organizations representing each component of the WSCC model could do the same. In cases in which more than one organization represents a model component, each organization could submit its draft and ASHA could work to combine the drafts and reconcile differences. These standards and criteria should include requirements for a process that meaningfully engages all participants and that elevates the importance of both (1) evidence-based practice, which often reflects research perspectives and expertise, and (2) practice-based evidence, which often reflects practitioner and community perspectives and expertise (Green, 2006). Ensuring the strength of each WSCC component should be an important goal for the research agenda, because doing so maximizes the strength of the model overall.

Third, the national coalition, in collaboration with the convener, would be responsible for creating a cohesive, combined document that included detailed research agendas for the WSCC model as a whole as well as for each of the 10 core components. In addition, the national coalition would be responsible for the dissemination of the full WSCC-based school health research agenda across all partner organizations, as well as among university and practice-based school health researchers, using multiple, coordinated communications strategies.

Fourth, the national coalition would be responsible for initiating efforts to increase funding related to school health research, especially priority studies necessary to advance the research agenda and comprehensive, large-scale, and long-term evaluation projects. Linking funding directly to the research agenda in this manner is also likely to promote more widespread adoption of the agenda and to fuel increased agenda-related research activity.

Fifth, the national coalition, with support from the convening organization, could be responsible for supporting the ongoing dissemination, translation, and adoption of research agenda–based findings. This work could take numerous forms and include activities such as publishing findings in scientific journals, presenting at conferences, integrating findings into professional preparation and continuing education programs, preparing policy and practice guides, and collaborating with a range of advocacy groups devoted to advancing various aspects of school health. Although robust dissemination-related activity is bound to occur independent of the national coalition, maintaining the coalition and transitioning its work to providing ongoing, cross-disciplinary support for the dissemination and adoption of key research agenda findings would provide a comprehensive dimension to the process likely to maximize the overall impact of the research agenda and to more deeply engage participants at all levels.

Imagining the Future of WSCC

The nature of research is to extend knowledge, not to build a fortress of support around an unchangeable idea or concept. Thus, from the beginning we should accept that new evidence will likely give way to new and improved iterations of the WSCC model or possibly to entirely new models of school health promotion built on what we have learned from our WSCC-based research agenda. Failing to accept these possibilities for change would require us to accept a bias in favor of the model that is not in keeping with ethical research practice. Therefore, we must remember that we are proposing that we use the WSCC model to frame our research in school health, not to build support for the model itself. A welcoming of continuous improvement to the WSCC model and to our strategies for implementing effective school health should characterize our work and be enthusiastically applied to the research agenda itself as it evolves with our newly emerging knowledge base.

As promising as the WSCC model is, like any other model, it is not perfect. For example, from a theoretical point of view, I would argue that the model could be improved by directly addressing the following:

1. Equity and the unique needs of minoritized and marginalized members of the school community
2. School safety, including gun violence, infectious disease management, injury prevention, and transportation services
3. Civic education and fostering the social skills required to participate in a vibrant democracy with a diverse citizenry
4. Often forgotten child development needs, such as opportunities for breaks, rest, and unstructured time to play and socialize

From an operational point of view, I would argue that the WSCC model should go further in integrating school health and the operations of the school itself. Instead of presenting the WSCC model as something separate from and in addition to other, perhaps more fundamental, school operations, we should reconceive of WSCC as a model of schooling itself (i.e., a model of the basic expectations of all schools or how to do school right). Doing so would require us to make goals related to graduation and academic achievement more explicit (Baldwin, 2018) and to integrate other academic subjects into the model (Mann, 2017). A WSCC model revised in this manner could provide a comprehensive structure for our teacher preparation, continuing education, and educational leadership programs and present a more integrated, holistic, and honest vision of what society really expects schools and school professionals to provide for the students, families, and communities they serve.

Opinions may vary regarding the specific examples or suggestions I have provided here. However, if we are to maximize the opportunities associated with a WSCC-based school health research agenda, then we must do so while remaining open to new possibilities for growing and extending the model based on new evidence and as informed by new deliberations within the research, practice, and policy communities.

Summary

I started this perspective by describing a question I am often asked in my travels but want to conclude our discussion by considering a question I often ask in return. When parents and other caregivers ask me whether schools matter, I often ask them what their deepest hopes are for their children and how they know their children are headed in the right direction. No one ever mentions high test scores. They also do not share concerns about how many widgets their child will be able to produce in the future or their child's likely impact on the national gross domestic product. Most parents and caregivers describe hoping that their children will be safe, happy, and healthy—now and in the future. To me, delivering on these hopes represents one of the truest promises of an effective WSCC-based school health research agenda.

Sadly, even briefly considering our existing evidence base and current events suggests that we still have a lot to learn. The COVID-19 pandemic, its corresponding student mental health challenges, unrelenting gun violence in schools, and emerging school-focused policies directed at marginalizing the life experiences of racial and sexual minority students all threaten the health and well-being of students and the educators who serve them. In each case, we have more questions than answers about what needs to be done next. Even when we know what needs to be done, there are numerous questions about how to best go about doing it. Solving these types of problems demands new research and new types of research that are as nuanced, sophisticated, and comprehensive as our problems are socially and technically complex (Mann, 2022).

In this perspective, I am advocating for accelerating our capacity to conduct the types of research necessary to address the problems students, educators, and communities are facing today. To me, developing a comprehensive and collaborative WSCC-based school health research agenda represents a crucial opportunity to advance our efforts to build that capacity; conduct much-needed research; and aid schools in their efforts to support the health, well-being, and success of each member of their school communities. In this way, we will do our part to help schools realize the hope of every parent, caregiver, and educator—safe, happy, and healthy children, now and in the future.

REFERENCES

Baldwin, S. (2018, January 3-6). *Implementation of the WSCC model in Buffalo Public Schools*. International Conference on the Health Risks of Youth, Clearwater, FL, United States.

Green, L.W. (2006). Public health asks of systems science: To advance our evidence-based practice, can you help us get more practice-based evidence? *American Journal of Public Health, 96*(3), 406-409.

Kolbe, L.J. (2019). School health as a strategy to improve both public health and education. *Annual Review of Public Health, 40,* 443-468.

Mann, M.J. (2017, October 11-13). *Healthy, high-achieving, and hopeful: The full promise of school health*. American School Health National Conference, St. Louis, MO, United States.

Mann, M.J. (2022). *Journal of School Health* editorial transition and research priorities for 2022-2024. *Journal of School Health, 92*(1), 7-10.

Mann, M.J., & Lohrmann, D.K. (2019). Addressing challenges to the reliable, large-scale implementation of effective school health education. *Health Promotion Practice, 20*(6), 834-844. https://doi.org/10.1177/1524839919870196

Rasberry, C.N., Slade, S., Lohrmann, D.K., & Valois, R.F. (2015). Lessons learned from the Whole Child and coordinated school health approaches. *Journal of School Health, 85,* 759-765. https://doi.org/10.1111/josh.12307

Willgerodt, M.A., Walsh, E., & Maloy, C. (2021). A scoping review of the Whole School, Whole Community, Whole Child model. *Journal of School Nursing, 37*(1), 61-68. https://doi.org/10.1177/1059840520974346

WSCC: A Future Perspective

What the Future Holds for WSCC, and What WSCC Holds for the Future

Sean Slade

A Model for Our Times

There are times when a model or an approach both encapsulates the need for the times and also provides a direction for the future. This was true in 1987 when Lloyd Kolbe and Diane Allensworth wrote their seminal paper "The Comprehensive School Health Program: Exploring an Expanded Concept" (Allensworth & Kolbe, 1987) outlining the Coordinated School Health model. It provided both a structure for school health services and functions to work better together and a direction for further collaboration. The Coordinated School Health model was subsequently promoted by, and integrated into, the U.S. Centers for Disease Control and Prevention's (CDC) school health functions, services, and grants.

It was also true of the Whole Child initiative launched by ASCD in 2007, which recast the definition of

> a successful learner from one whose achievement is measured solely by academic tests, to one who is knowledgeable, emotionally and physically healthy, civically inspired, engaged in the arts, prepared for work and economic self-sufficiency, and ready for the world beyond formal schooling. (ASCD, 2007, p. 4)

By using Abraham Maslow's hierarchy of needs as a frame, the Whole Child approach established the need for health, and a healthy environment, to be foundational, not just for health but for learning.

I believe the Whole School, Whole Community, Whole Child (WSCC) model, jointly developed and launched by the CDC and ASCD, does something similar. It places health directly within the purview of education—and makes clear the need for healthy environments for healthy learners. It positions both sectors in the context of the local community and extols the need for joint policies, processes, and practices. Moreover, it calls out the common focus of both sectors and services: the child. The WSCC model has allowed a myriad of school and community health and education stakeholders to see themselves in the model, with various entry points and varying rationales for alignment. It sets the scene for integration and direction. Both fortunately and unfortunately, it has provided a response framework for what has occurred since early 2020 with the COVID-19 pandemic.

> Health and well-being have, for too long, been put into silos—separated both logistically and philosophically from education and learning....
>
> Health and education affect individuals, society, and the economy and, as such, must work together whenever possible. Schools are a perfect setting for this collaboration....
>
> The WSCC model responds to the call for greater alignment, integration, and collaboration between health and education to improve each child's cognitive, physical, social, and emotional development. (ASCD & CDC, 2014, pp. 3, 7)

Pandemic as a Cure

Sometimes it takes a crisis for us to see what has been in front of our eyes for a while. Whether it has been because of the absolute necessity for the sectors and community to work together, or whether it was the needed focus on health and well-being as a precursor to learning, the pandemic of 2020 to 2023 has forced us as a society, and as local communities, to integrate the sectors better than they were before. Health and education, especially in the school setting, are natural and needed partners.

Or perhaps, somewhat ironically, it was the time and reflective space that many of us found ourselves in during the pandemic that allowed us to reconsider what is important. The term *well-being* has become ubiquitous as greater attention is directed toward health and harmony (PwC, n.d.). The pandemic made us reappraise our own health and that of our families. It reestablished in many the need for nature, physical exercise, and switching off. The virus reminded us that our health is paramount and had us reappraise actions, apart from the virus, that made us unwell. We are less prepared or willing to do things that are unhealthy and make us unwell.

One example of this can be seen in the Great Resignation of 2022. Although a range of factors play into resignations, resignations can be attributed partly to people moving out of toxic or unhealthy work situations (Ceron, 2022). People are less prepared to endure stress and have realized that they have a choice.

> *A toxic corporate culture is by far the strongest predictor of industry-adjusted attrition and is 10 times more important than compensation in predicting turnover. Our analysis found that the leading elements contributing to toxic cultures include failure to promote diversity, equity, and inclusion; workers feeling disrespected; and unethical behavior.... the important point is that a toxic culture is the biggest factor pushing employees out the door during the Great Resignation. (Sull, 2022, para. 12)*

The Rise of WSCC

Even before the pandemic the WSCC model was growing in use and adoption across the United States (Society for Public Health Education, 2019). It has become the frame for all CDC school health grants and the preeminent school health model in state departments of education and health; has been adapted to suit the local community requirements of numerous states, including Ohio, Michigan, Louisiana, and California; and has even been recast outside the United States, including in Quebec (Canada) and the Philippines. It has been adapted to suit key themes, including the implementation of social-emotional learning and mental health initiatives, and adopted by the majority of school health organizations in the United States, including the American School Health Association, SHAPE America, the Society for Public Health Education, the National Association of State Boards of Education, the National Association of School Nurses, the Alliance for a Healthier Generation, and Action for Healthy Kids.

In the past few years since the start of the pandemic, the need for and interest in both the model and a more holistic, health-infused approach to education continue to grow.

> *Now, two years into the pandemic, school closures have resulted in significant learning loss, social isolation, and poor mental health. A 2021 survey commissioned by The Hunt Institute found that six in ten parents (63 percent) said COVID-19 has been disruptive to their own children's education and their mental health and emotional wellbeing. As the country continues to transition into a new normal, it is critical that schools and educators adopt a "whole child" approach to education, incorporating teaching methods that account for the ways that children grow and learn in their relationships, identity, emotional understanding, and overall wellbeing. (Wise & Siddiqi, 2022, p. 2)*

Federal policy and funding have targeted the health and well-being—social, emotional, mental, as well as physical—of students, their teachers, and their schools. Both the Elementary and Secondary School Emergency Relief Fund as well as the American Rescue Plan highlight the need to focus on health, well-being, and the integration of services. In addition, in 2022 the U.S. Congress awarded $68 million in funds for the expansion of community schools that aim to provide services for health, well-being, and other supports to schools (U.S. Department of Education, 2022). The WSCC model—and the themes that underlie it—is growing in terms of interest, need, and adoption.

Where We Are Going

Regardless of whether—or more likely when—there will be another pandemic, the understanding that health is a prerequisite for learning has become part of the educational dialogue. A more holistic, learner-centered direction in which well-being is highlighted and called out has become commonplace across global organizations planning for future education policies and directions. Take a look at any of the more recent global forecasting and policy publications from key leading organizations and you will find references to health and well-being, not only as a frame for effective education but also—as has been most clearly pointed out by the Organisation for Economic Co-operation and Development (OECD)—as an education outcome in its own right.

> *OECD Education 2030: A Shared Vision*
>
> *We are committed to helping every learner develop as a whole person, fulfil his or her potential and help shape a shared future built on the well-being of individuals, communities and the planet …*
>
> *Need for broader education goals: Individual and collective well-being*
>
> *Unless steered with a purpose, the rapid advance of science and technology may widen inequities, exacerbate social fragmentation and accelerate resource depletion. In the 21st century, that purpose has been increasingly defined in terms of well-being. But well-being involves more than access to material resources, such as income and wealth, jobs and earnings, and housing. It is also related to the quality of life, including health, civic engagement, social connections, education, security, life satisfaction and the environment. Equitable access to all of these underpins the concept of inclusive growth. (OECD, 2018, pp. 3-4)*

> *United Nations Educational, Scientific, and Cultural Organization Chair for Global Health and Education*
>
> *There is an emerging evidence base that shows that learning outcomes are improved, social and emotional wellbeing are increased, and health risk behaviours are reduced in response to more holistic or whole school approaches. Such approaches are typically based on coherence between the school's policies and practices that promote social inclusion and a wider commitment to education and health. The World Bank Human Capital Project recognises that the intersection of good health, nutrition, and education can drive economic growth, and that investment in children and adolescents brings substantial effects and high economic returns.*
>
> *Schools are not the only options for investment—we do not want to exclude others, including peer-led community interventions—but schools offer a basic and globally consistent setting for promoting health and wellbeing …*
>
> *Notwithstanding these efforts to promote health, greater cooperation and mutual support of local health and education professionals is essential to achieve our global ambition for schools to be the means through which the world's children and adolescents develop the capabilities for lifelong health, wellbeing, and success. (Jourdan et al., 2021, paras. 6, 23)*

> *World Innovative Summit on Education—Agile Leaders of Learning Innovation Network*
>
> *[The Agile Leaders of Learning Innovation Network] seeks to increase the quantity of future-fit school leaders to support schools and systems in their transitions toward resilient and future-thriving learning environments that maximise learner outcomes and wellbeing, for a brighter, more equitable, and inclusive future for our children and our world….*
>
> *There is a strong need to emphasise their wellbeing as part and parcel of the education system. When we talk about teacher professional development and ongoing training,*

facilitating the mindsets and social and emotional competencies that foster wellbeing must be central.

The education system has left wellbeing as a side track, hoping it may come as a secondary effect of schooling. This omission has high costs in the lives of educators and children alike. The pandemic has evidenced the fact that lacking the capacity to have a healthy relationship with oneself, others and with life's challenges – such as isolation, stress, illness, loss and the unknown – in an ever more uncertain world, is an onerous oversight. We can learn from the current mental health crisis and strive to uproot its causes. (Centre for Strategic Education, 2022, pp. 4, 34)

A Culture of Well-Being

It is too soon for us to fully realize the impact of COVID-19 on our systems and society. We are still too close to the pandemic for us to clearly understand its lasting influence. It will likely take several more years before we can effectively look back to understand the change or changes that it made and is making to our systems. However, we can gauge the difference already. Pro-child policy is on the rise. Sectors are being encouraged to work more closely together. Communities and their stakeholders are being asked to take on greater roles. Finally, the focus on health and well-being is at the fore. These aspects are all core to the WSCC model. It is a model that was perhaps seven years ahead of its time, or rather a model that provided a basis for our systems and services to work closer together and for the child, which became more apparent in 2020.

If there is one area that perhaps needs to be added to the model to ensure its potential is reached, however, it is the role of establishing a culture of health and well-being. Culture is pervasive; it disrupts sound strategy and often derails intention—good or poor. Establishing a culture of health and well-being is key to sustainable implementation of the WSCC model.

Without such a culture the model and its intentions become another top-down model for consideration—or worse, a temporary initiative that will soon be rolled back. Culture is dominant, and to establish a coherent and common culture across the school and its community the school leader (the superintendent, principal, or assistant principal) must step forward. The school leader provides educational credibility for any initiative. This person allows others to see the venture as part of their own role as a teacher or support professional. The school leader is also able to bring together diverse stakeholders across the school and its community. Highlighting the need to embrace culture and the role that leaders play in establishing such a culture may boost or supplement the original WSCC model. Too often we discuss frames and models in terms of entities or functions, and too infrequently do we highlight the role that people—each of us—play in their success. A depiction of the addition of culture and leadership to the WSCC model is presented in figure 10.2.

How do we move toward such a culture? We increase the value of well-being among education leaders as a fundamental part of any functioning school. We advocate for the spread of health and well-being across the whole school and community so it becomes another part or facet of the school—albeit a foundational part. Such a move has occurred across Tacoma, Washington, where they have adopted and utilized the WSCC model to implement the Tacoma Whole Child initiative. Launched at the same time the WSCC model was released in 2014, the initiative has sought to embed health, well-being, connection to the community, and a Whole Child approach into and across area schools and their instruction, assessments, and mission. It is not surprising that it was led by the deputy superintendent, Dr. Josh Garcia. His voice and authority gave it educational credibility. Without committed leadership, and educational leadership in particular, such approaches wither and are soon replaced. Leadership helps form the culture, and the culture ensures that such initiatives remain embedded despite later changes in leadership.

232 Promoting Health and Academic Success: The WSCC Approach

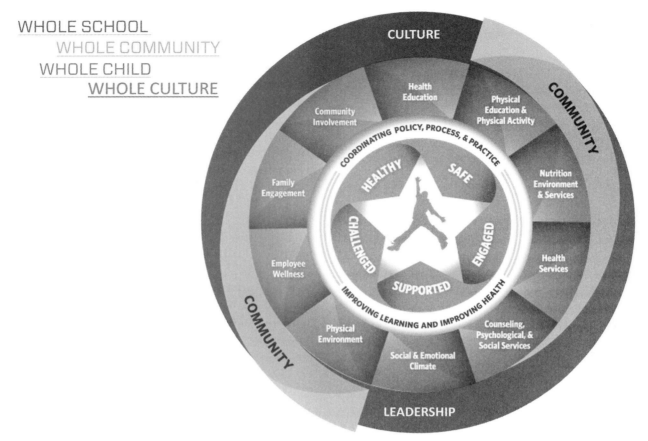

FIGURE 10.2 Whole School, Whole Community, Whole Child, Whole Culture (WSCC+C).

Toward a Healthy Future

The WSCC model has established itself as the preeminent school health model across the United States and is quickly establishing itself as a model for combating the harm caused by COVID-19. Collaboration of function, alignment of services, and integration of policies, processes, and practices across the whole school and its community allow us to strengthen our learning environments and prepare for a likely subsequent pandemic.

However, collaboration, alignment, and integration do more than support health outcomes—they also aid and boost learning. For our children and our communities, both are needed. Dr. Gene Carter, then chief executive officer and executive director of ASCD, said the following on the release of the WSCC model:

The Whole School, Whole Community, Whole Child model developed by ASCD and the CDC takes the call for greater collaboration over the years and puts it firmly in place. For too long, entities have talked about collaboration without taking the necessary steps. This model puts the process into action. (ASCD & CDC, 2014, p. 8)

The pandemic has now put the need to focus on health and well-being clearly into focus.

REFERENCES

Allensworth, D.D., & Kolbe, L.J. (1987). The Comprehensive School Health program: Exploring an expanded concept. *Journal of School Health*, 57(10), 409-412.

ASCD. (2007). *The learning compact redefined: A call to action.* https://library.ascd.org/m/21e2f544234c3e97/original/WCC-Learning-Compact.pdf

ASCD & Centers for Disease Control and Prevention. (2014). *Whole School, Whole Community, Whole Child: A collaborative approach to learning and health.* https://files.ascd.org/staticfiles/ascd/pdf/siteASCD/publications/wholechild/wscc-a-collaborative-approach.pdf

Centre for Strategic Education, Victoria. (2022). *Education reimagined: Leadership for a new era.* Retrieved December 28, 2022, from www.wise-qatar.org/app/uploads/2022/03/cse-wise-education-reimagined-leadership-for-a-new-era-final.pdf

Ceron, E. (2022, January 11). *What's driving the great resignation? Toxic culture is a bigger driver than pay.* Bloomberg. Retrieved December 28, 2022, from www.bloomberg.com/news/articles/2022-01-11/what-s-driving-the-great-resignation-toxic-culture-is-a-bigger-driver-than-pay

Jourdan, D., Gray, N.J., Barry, M.M., Caffe, S., Cornu, C., Diagne, F., El Hage, F., Farmer, M.Y., Slade, S., Marmot, M., & Sawyer, S.M. (2021). Supporting every school to become a foundation for healthy lives. *The Lancet Child & Adolescent Health*, 5(4), 295-303. https://doi.org/10.1016/s2352-4642(20)30316-3

Organisation for Economic Co-operation and Development. (2018). *The future of education and skills: Education 2030.* www.oecd.org/education/2030/E2030%20Position%20Paper%20(05.04.2018).pdf

PwC. (n.d.). *Redefining wellbeing in a post-pandemic world.* Retrieved December 28, 2022, from www.pwc.com/mt/en/publications/humanresources/redefining-wellbeing-in-a-post-pandemic-world.html.

Society for Public Health Education. (2019, April 25). *Implementing the WSCC model: Five years later* [Video]. YouTube. www.youtube.com/watch?v=Cjk2gN_qn4k

Sull, D.C.S. (2022, January 11). Toxic culture is driving the great resignation. *MIT Sloan Management Review.* Retrieved December 28, 2022, from https://sloanreview.mit.edu/article/toxic-culture-is-driving-the-great-resignation/

U.S. Department of Education. (2022, July 12). *Education Department announces $68 million in grants to support students through full-service community schools.* www.ed.gov/news/press-releases/education-department-announces-68-million-grants-support-students-through-full-service-community-schools

Wise, R., & Siddiqi, J. (2022). *Whole Child education: Supporting students' learning and development.* The Hunt Institute. Retrieved December 28, 2022, from https://hunt-institute.org/wp-content/uploads/2022/02/HI-CC-Report-2-2022-v3.pdf

LEARNING AIDS

APPLICATION ACTIVITIES

1. The first two perspectives in chapter 10 describe the involvement of ASHA and SOPHE in supporting and advancing the WSCC model. Review either the December 2020 issue of ASHA's *Journal of School Health* (*JOSH*) or SOPHE's WSCC Team Training Modules initiative and analyze examples of the organizations' WSCC activities. Present your review in a WSCC perspective approximately 250 words in length. Directions for the two options are as follows:

    Option 1: If you select the *JOSH* review, scan the abstracts of all articles in the issue. Then present your thoughts on (1) the importance of the overall issue as a resource for presenting important information that will assist schools in implementing WSCC and (2) the relevance of the information in promoting WSCC in multiple states and school districts. Read one article and present your reaction to its content in your WSCC perspective. The December 2020 issue of *JOSH* is accessible at https://onlinelibrary.wiley.com/toc/17461561/2020/90/12.

Option 2: If you select the WSCC Team Training Modules review, look over the project website (https://elearn.sophe.org/wscc) to gain an idea of the overall content of the modules. Focus your WSCC perspective on the three WSCC fact sheets. In your perspective, present your thoughts on the value of each fact sheet for advancing and supporting WSCC in schools. The fact sheets are accessible at https://elearn.sophe.org/wscc-fact-sheets.

2. Write a letter to the editor of the campus newspaper or a blog post presenting a rationale for your campus adopting a WSCC approach to support students' health and overall well-being.
3. Analyze Michael J. Mann's research perspective, then identify what you perceive to be the five most important WSCC research priorities. Develop an 8- to 10-minute PowerPoint presentation that describes the priorities. In the presentation, present a brief rationale for each of the identified priorities.

INDEX

Note: The italicized *f* and *t* following page numbers refer to figures and tables, respectively.

A

AAP (American Academy of Pediatrics) 87*f*
ABP (American Board of Pediatrics) 87*f*
absenteeism, chronic 63-65
ACA (American Counseling Association) 87*f*
academic achievement and health 25
    adult health and 64
    adverse childhood experiences 62-63
    chronic absenteeism 63-65
    CSH model and 3
    early childhood 62
    emotional/mental health and school climate/culture 67-68
    family and parental engagement 69
    health-risk behaviors 60-62, 61*f*
    health services and school-based health centers 68-69
    nutritional services 69-70
    physical education and physical activity 70-72, 71*f*
    school connectedness 65-67, 66*f*
    WSCC approach and 65-72, 66*f*, 71*f*
ACES (Association for Counselor Education and Supervision) 88*f*
active transport 39
administrative and policy diagnosis 122*f*, 123
administrative leadership 108, 145
administrative support 171
adverse childhood experiences 62-63, 166
advisory boards 172
Agile Leaders of Learning Innovation Network 230-231
alcohol use 61*f*
Allensworth, Diane 2, 16
Alliance for a Healthier Generation 152
alumni, parent, and visitor engagement, campus 213*t*, 214-215
American Academy of Pediatrics (AAP) 87*f*
American Board of Pediatrics (ABP) 87*f*
American Counseling Association (ACA) 87*f*
American Public Health Association (APHA) 87*f*
American School Counselor Association (ASCA) 88*f*
American School Health Association (ASHA) 5, 16, 88*f*, 198-201, 206, 225-226
anti-racist teaching 90-91
anxiety 68
APA Task Force on Psychological Practice With Sexual Minority Persons 87*f*
APHA (American Public Health Association) 87*f*
ASCA (American School Counselor Association) 88*f*
ASCD 3, 24-25
ASCD's nine levers of school change 106-107, 106*f*
ASHA (American School Health Association) 5, 16, 88*f*, 198-201, 206, 225-226
ASHA WSCC Award 199
assessment tools, WSCC-related 119-120, 119*f*
asset assessment 131
Association for Counselor Education and Supervision (ACES) 88*f*

B

biking 217
biological factors, and premature death 14, 14*f*
breakfast 69-70, 113
Brockton Healthy Schools Team (Massachusetts) 110
budgetary constraints 109
Buffalo (NY) urban school case study 170-174
Building Healthy Communities: A School Leader's Guide to Collaboration and Community Engagement 148
bullying 63, 67, 84

C

CAEP (Council for the Accreditation of Educator Preparation) 206-207
campus–community relations 213*t*, 215
CBPR (community-based participatory research) 94
CDC (Centers for Disease Control and Prevention) 3, 16, 18, 19, 168
CDC Healthy Schools 5-7, 207
Center for Communities That Care 104
Center of Excellence for Protected Health Information 200
Centers for Disease Control and Prevention (CDC) 3, 16, 18, 19, 168
challenged (Whole Child tenet) 24, 33, 34*f*
change, school 106-107, 106*f*
childhood, health and education in early 62
Child Nutrition Act of 1966 15
Child Nutrition and WIC Reauthorization Act 125
children of color 81
Chinese Journal of School Health (CJSH) 180
classroom-based physical activities 38-39
climate, school 44-45, 63, 67-68, 119*f*
collaborations
    ASCD's nine levers of school change 106-107, 106*f*
    barriers and challenges to 107-110
    implementing and sustaining 111-112
    recruiting partners for 110-111
    sample operating agreement 112
    school–family–community 102-103
    socioecological framework 105-106, 105*f*
    successful 103-105
Collaboratory on School and Child Health 7
college, Whole Campus model. *See* Whole Campus model

College Student Mental Health Survey 215
communicable diseases 2
communication issues 108
communication of efforts and outcomes 157, 157f
community, as overarching WSCC concept 50-52
community-based participatory research (CBPR) 94
Community Eligibility Provision 70
community involvement 48-50
   and DEI promotion 93-94
   needs assessment 171
   professional development 194
   role of teachers and leaders 156t
   school–family–community collaborations 102-103, 107-110
   strategies for improvement 154t
   and Whole Campus model 213t, 215
Community Toolbox (University of Kansas) 148, 148f
connectedness, school 65-67, 66f, 90
Coordinated School Health (CSH) model 2-3, 12, 12f, 16-20, 221, 228
coordination, collaboration, and communication (3Cs) 171, 172
Council for the Accreditation of Educator Preparation (CAEP) 206-207
counseling, psychological, and social services 42-44
   professional development 194
   roles of teachers and leaders 156t
   strategies for improvement 154t
   and Whole Campus model 213t, 216
counseling and mental health services, campus 213t, 216
counseling services 16
COVID-19 pandemic 162, 163, 207, 228-229, 231
critical race theory (CRT) 91-92
CSH (Coordinated School Health) model 2-3, 12, 12f, 16-20, 221, 228
cultural humility 92
culturally responsive teaching 90
culture of well-being 231, 232f
curricula, health-promoting 15
cyberbullying 63, 67, 84

D

DASH (Division of Adolescent and School Health) of CDC 3, 16, 18
data, and their use 130-132
DEI. *See* diversity, equity, and inclusion (DEI)
depression 68
disabilities, children with 83-85
district-level WSCC program implementation 147f, 171-172
diversity, equity, and inclusion (DEI) 85-86
   anti-racist teaching 90-91
   children of color 81
   community involvement and 93-94
   critical race theory 91-92
   cultural humility and 92
   culturally responsive teaching 90
   disabilities 83-85
   family engagement and 93
   homelessness/housing instability 82-83
   immigrant status 83
   LGBTQ+ children 83
   organizational position statements 87f-89f
   poverty 81
   social justice–oriented schools 89-92
   students with disproportionately poor education outcomes 80-85
   and Whole Campus model 214
Division of Adolescent and School Health (DASH) of CDC 3, 16, 18

E

early childhood, health and education in 62
educational attainment 21
education and health 22f, 25
Education Commission of the States 164
Education for All Handicapped Children Act (P.L. 94-142) 15-16
education support professionals 110-111
Elementary and Secondary Education Act 15, 162
Elevance Health Foundation 200
emergency operations plans 45-46
emotional climate 44-45
emotional/mental health 67-68
employee wellness 46-47
   roles of teachers and leaders 156t
   SHI use to improve 51
   strategies for improvement 154t
   and Whole Campus model 213t, 214
engaged (Whole Child tenet) 24, 33, 34f
environmental factors, and premature death 14, 14f, 20-21, 21f
epidemiological, behavioral, and environmental assessment 121f, 122-123
Erika's Lighthouse 200
European Conference on Health Promoting Schools 179
Every Student Succeeds Act (ESSA) 24, 162-163, 204

F

family engagement 47-48, 69
   DEI promotion through 93
   needs assessment 171
   professional development 194
   roles of teachers and leaders 156t
   school–family–community collaborations 102-103, 107-110
   strategies for improvement 154t
   and Whole Campus model 213t, 214-215
family issues 108
federal government, role in education 162-163
federal support for CSH programs 19-20
Fit, Healthy and Ready to Learn 18
focus groups 128-129, 129f
Focusing Resources on Effective School Health (FRESH) framework 178
formative evaluation 133, 133f, 134f
Framework for Safe and Successful Schools, A 155-156
FRESH (Focusing Resources on Effective School Health) framework 178

G

Global School-Based Student Health Survey 179
Go for Health 15
Great Resignation of 2022 229
Great Society programs 15
Growing Healthy 15
Guide for Developing High-Quality School Emergency Operations Plans 45-46

H

Head Start 15, 62
health and academic achievement
   adult health and 64
   adverse childhood experiences 62-63

chronic absenteeism 63-65
early childhood 62
emotional/mental health and school climate/culture 67-68
family and parental engagement 69
health-risk behaviors 60-62, 61f
health services and school-based health centers 68-69
nutritional services 69-70
physical education and physical activity 70-72, 71f
school connectedness 65-67, 66f
WSCC approach and 65-72, 66f, 71f
health and education 22f, 25
health behaviors, individual 14-20, 14f
health care factors, and premature death 14, 14f
health care services 213t, 215-216
health disparities 149-150
health education 2, 13, 36-37
national standards 36f
professional development 192-193
role of teachers and leaders 156t
strategies for improvement 154t
and Whole Campus model 213t, 216
Health Is Academic: A Guide to Coordinated School Health Programs (Marx) 18
Health-promoting schools framework 177-178, 177f
health promotion stages
addressing individual behaviors 14-20
addressing infectious diseases 13
addressing social determinants of health 20-24
health-risk behaviors 15, 18, 60-62, 61f, 150
health services 2, 41-42, 68-69
professional development 193-194
roles of teachers and leaders 156t
strategies for improvement 154t
HealthSmart 173
healthy (Whole Child tenet) 24, 32, 34f
Healthy People 2020 (USDHHS) 21
Healthy People 2030 163
Healthy People initiative 19-20
Healthy Schools Toolkit (Health Equity Works) 7, 111, 207
high-risk behaviors 15, 18, 60-62, 61f
Historically Black Colleges and Universities 201

HIV (human immunodeficiency virus) 16, 18, 25, 165
homelessness/housing instability 82-83
H.O.P.E. Buffalo 173-174
human immunodeficiency virus (HIV) 16, 18, 25, 165
human right, education as 166
humility 92
hygiene. *See* health education

I

IJSH (International Journal of School Health) 180
immigrant status, families with 83
Individuals with Disabilities Education Act (IDEA) 167
infectious disease prevention 13
informant interviews 127, 127f-128f
Institute of Education Sciences 15
institutionalization of action plans 143
integrated student services (ISS) 22-23, 23f
International Commission on the Futures of Education 181
international efforts to improve school health programs 176-177
FRESH framework 178
future of 180-182
health-promoting schools framework 177-178, 177f
International School Health Network 179
journals of school health 180
Research Consortium for School Health and Nutrition 180
Save the Children 180
Schools for Health in Europe Network 180
United Nations Children's Fund 179
United Nations Educational, Scientific, and Cultural Organization 179
World Bank 179
World Health Organization 178-179
WSCC framework 177
International Journal of School Health (IJSH) 180
International School Health Network 179
interscholastic sports 40
intersectionality 91
intramural sports 40

ISS (integrated student services) 22-23, 23f

J

Japanese Journal of School Health (JJSH) 180
Journal of School Health (JOSH) 3, 5, 6, 16, 17, 35, 180, 199-200
journals of school health 180

K

Keys to Excellence: Standards of Practice for Nutrition Integrity 40-41
Know Your Body 15
Kolbe, Lloyd 2, 16

L

Lalonde report 14
leadership by state education agencies 164-166
learning and skills for life, work, and sustainable development 182
LEAs (local education agencies) 162, 168
LGBTQ+ children 83, 84, 93, 94
lifestyle factors, health and premature death 14-15, 14f
local education agencies (LEAs) 162, 168
logic models 132, 132f

M

Making the Connection: Health and Student Achievement 19
Maslow's hierarchy of needs 33, 34f
Medicaid 15
mental health 67-68, 109, 155, 213t, 216
minority students 81
mission statements 149
Monitoring and Evaluation Guidance for School Health Programs 178
Multitiered System of Supports (MTSS) framework 166-168, 167f

N

Namaste Charter School 149
National Association of Chronic Disease Directors (NACDD) 7
National Association of Secondary School Principals (NASSP) 88f
National Center for Health Education (NCHE) 203
National Committee on the Future of School Health Education 200, 206

National Future of School Health Education Expert Panel 206
National Health Education Standards: Achieving Health Literacy (NCSHE) 203
National Health Education Standards: Model Guidance for Curriculum and Instruction (NCSHE) 36-37, 36f, 192, 203-204
National PTA 88f
National School Breakfast Program 15, 69-70
National School Lunch Program 40
NCHE (National Center for Health Education) 203
needs assessment 120, 123-130, 124t, 171-172
No Child Left Behind Act 162
nurses/nursing, school 15, 16, 41-42, 68-69, 193-194
nutrition environment and services 40-41
   implementation 69-70
   professional development 193
   roles of teachers and leaders 156t
   strategies for improvement 154t
   and Whole Campus model 213t, 214

O

OECD Education 2030: A Shared Vision 230
Organisation for Economic Co-operation and Development (OECD) 230
organizational chart, WSCC 170, 171f
Organizing Schools for Improvement 22
Our Child, Our Future (Ohio) 86
outcome evaluation 133-134, 133f, 134f

P

parental literacy 93
parent engagement 47-48, 69
   DEI promotion through 93
   needs assessment 171
   professional development 194
   roles of teachers and leaders 156t
   school–family–community collaborations 102-103, 107-110
   strategies for improvement 154t
   and Whole Campus model 213t, 214-215
Partners for Breakfast in the Classroom 113
partnerships, community 48-50
physical education and physical activity 13, 16, 37-40
   high school student participation rates 61f
   implementation 70-72, 71f
   national standards 38f
   professional development 193
   roles of teachers and leaders 156t
   strategies for improvement 154t
   and Whole Campus model 213t, 217
physical environment 45-46
   professional development 193
   roles of teachers and leaders 156t
   strategies for improvement 154t
   and Whole Campus model 213t, 217
physicians 42
policies, programs, and practices (3Ps) 171, 174
poverty 20-21, 81, 93
PRECEDE–PROCEED framework 120, 121f-122f, 123-130, 124t, 127f-128f, 129f
premature deaths 14, 14f, 21f
process evaluation 133, 133f, 134f
professional development 155-157, 173-174, 191-194
professional preparation 206-207
Promoting Health Through Schools: Report of a WHO Expert Committee on Comprehensive School Health Education and Promotion (WHO) 178
psychological services 42-44
psychologists, school 16, 43
PTA, National 88f

R

racism
   anti-racist teaching 90-91
   critical race theory 91-92
   culturally responsive teaching 90
Raising Healthy Children 174
RAPID actions for education recovery 179
Ready to Learn and Thrive: School Health and Nutrition Around the World 179
recess 38
Reducing the Risk 173
Registries of Programs Effective in Reducing Youth Risk Behaviors (CDC) 153
research, school health, WSCC-based 220
   elements of effective process 224-226
   future of WSCC 226-227
   importance of 220-221
   outlook of 223-224
   promise of WSCC model 221-222
   topics for investigation 222-223
Research Consortium for School Health and Nutrition 180
resource identification 148-149
resources, WSCC 5-7, 195
Rhode Island 162, 164-165
Role of Districts in Developing High-Quality School Emergency Operations Plans, The 45-46
Role of the School Physician 42
Rudd Center for Food Policy and Obesity 7

S

SABER (Systems Approach for Better Education Results) 179
safe (Whole Child tenet) 24, 32, 34f
sanitary inspections of schools 13
Save the Children 180
Say Yes to Education Buffalo 174
school-based health centers (SBHCs) 42, 68-69
school change 106-107, 106f
school connectedness 65-67, 66f
school health
   evolution of 2-3
   journals of 180
   leadership by SEAs in 164-166
   WSCC-based research agenda 220-227
School Health Action Congress 200
school health advisory councils (SHACs) 25, 34, 145-147, 146f
School Health and Nutrition Health Education Manual 180
school health coordinator 142-144, 144f
school health improvement plan 150-153, 152f
School Health Index (SHI) 51, 125, 126, 143, 151, 170, 172, 192
School Health Index (SHI) Self-Assessment and Planning Guide (CDC Healthy Schools) 5, 45, 50, 192
School Health Profiles 165
School Health Resource Guide (NACDD) 7
school health teams 25, 34, 145-147
school nutrition program (SNP) 15, 40-41
Schools and Health: Our Nation's Investment (IOM) 18
Schools for Health: Foundations for Student Success—How School Buildings Influence Student Health, Thinking and Performance 45

Schools for Health in Europe Network (SHE) 180
SEAs (state education agencies) 163-166, 168
Seaside Conference 15
sedentary behaviors, and academic achievement 61*f*
SEL (social-emotional learning) 44
sexual health education 173
sexual risk behaviors 82
SHACs (school health advisory councils) 25, 34, 145-147, 146*f*
SHAPE America (Society of Health and Physical Educators) 37-38, 89*f*
Shattuck report 13
SHE (Schools for Health in Europe Network) 180
SHI (School Health Index) 51, 125, 126, 143, 151, 170, 172, 192
Shine Light on Depression 200
siloing 107
SMART goals 151
SNP (school nutrition program) 15, 40-41
social and emotional climate 44-45
　professional development 193
　roles of teachers and leaders 156*t*
　strategies for improvement 154*t*
　and Whole Campus model 213*t*, 216-217
social determinants of health 20-24, 21*f*, 22*f*, 23*f*, 104, 166
social-emotional learning (SEL) 44
social justice–oriented schools, DEI and 89-92
social services 42-44
social workers, school 43-44
Society for Public Health Education (SOPHE) 3, 5-7, 88*f*, 187, 200, 202
　accomplishments and milestones 203-204, 204*t*-205*t*
　early years 203
　future efforts and plans 207-208
　WSCC and 206-207
　WSCC Team Training Modules 39, 207
Society of Health and Physical Educators (SHAPE America) 37-38, 89*f*
Society of State Leaders of Health and Physical Education 200
socioecological framework for collaborations 105-106, 105*f*
solution-focused approach 111
SOPHE. *See* Society for Public Health Education (SOPHE)

Southwest Educational Development Laboratory 104
sports, school 40
staff diversity 94
staff professional development 191-195
stakeholder engagement 134-135, 172-173
Starting Healthy 203
state education agencies (SEAs) 163-166, 168
student health education and promotion, campus 213*t*, 216
summative evaluation 133-134, 133*f*, 134*f*
supported (Whole Child tenet) 24, 33, 34*f*
Systems Approach for Better Education Results (SABER) 179

T
teacher education programming 186-189, 188*f*, 190*f*
teachers, teaching, and the teaching profession 182
teacher wellness 46-47, 51
Teenage Health Teaching Modules 15
3Cs (coordination, collaboration, and communication) 171, 172, 174
3Ps (policies, programs, and practices) 171, 174
tobacco product use 61*f*
Transforming Education Summit (2022) 181
transportation 45
Tritsch, Len 15
trust 103

U
United Nations Children's Fund (UNICEF) 178, 179
United Nations Educational, Scientific, and Cultural Organization (UNESCO) 178, 179, 230
universal health care 20
universal precautions 18
urban school case study 170-174
U.S. government, role in education 162-163

V
Virtual Healthy School 187
vision, common 108
vision statements 148, 148*f*, 149

W
walking school bus 39
well-being 229, 230, 231

wellness 46-47, 51
wellness champions 171
wellness policies 171
WellSAT WSCC tool 7, 126, 151
What Works Clearinghouse (Institute of Education Sciences) 15
White House Conference on Child Health and Protection (1930) 13
WHO (World Health Organization) 166, 178-179
Whole Campus model 210, 211*f*
　alumni, parent, and visitor engagement 213*t*, 214-215
　campus–community relations 213*t*, 215
　components of 213*t*, 214-217
　counseling and mental health services 213*t*, 216
　employee wellness 213*t*, 214
　family engagement 213*t*, 214-215
　health care services 213*t*, 215-216
　health education and promotion 213*t*, 216
　nutrition environment and services 213*t*, 214
　parent engagement 213*t*, 214-215
　physical activity 213*t*, 217
　physical environment 213*t*, 217
　social and emotional climate 213*t*, 216-217
　student health education and promotion 213*t*, 216
　whole college student 211, 212*t*
Whole Child approach 3
Whole Child tenets 3, 24, 32-34, 34*f*
Whole College Student tenets 212*t*
Whole School, Whole Community, Whole Child (WSCC) model. *See* WSCC model
Whole School, Whole Community, Whole Child Model, The (NACDD) 7
windshield tours 125
World Bank 178, 179
World Health Organization (WHO) 166, 178-179
World Innovative Summit on Education 230-231
WSCC model 2, 3-5, 4*f*, 228
　ASHA role in advancing 198-200
　case study 188*f*
　components of 35-50, 188*f*, 190*f*, 192
　cross-disciplinary coordination 200
　and culture of well-being 231, 232*f*
　evolution of 12*f*, 24-25

WSCC model *(continued)*
  as expansion of school health model 16-19
  and federal support for CSH programs 19-20
  overview 32-35, 33*f*, 34*f*
  research agenda for school health based on 220-227
  resources 5-7, 195
  rise of 229-230
  summary sheets 189, 190*f*
WSCC program evaluation 132-133
  formative evaluation 133, 133*f*, 134*f*
  planning for 134-136, 134*f*, 135*t*
  plan review and implementation 155
  sample evaluation plan 135*t*
  summative evaluation 133-134, 133*f*, 134*f*
WSCC program implementation 142, 143*f*
  administrative support and commitment 145
  communication of efforts and outcomes 157, 157*f*
  evaluation plan review and implementation 155
  implementation 153-155, 154*t*
  outcomes 149-150
  professional development 155-157
  resource identification 148-149
  school health advisory council and teams 145-147, 146*f*
  school health coordinator 142-144, 144*f*
  school health improvement plan development 150-153, 152*f*
  timeline 153
  tips for district-level 147*f*
  vision statements 148, 148*f*
WSCC program in practice
  future opportunities 168
  leadership by state education agencies in school health 164-166
  and Multitiered System of Supports framework 166-168, 167*f*
  role of federal government 162-163
  role of states in education 163-164
  urban school case study 170-174
WSCC program planning 118
  assessment tools 119-120, 119*t*
  data and their use 130-132
  focus groups 128-129, 129*f*
  informant interviews 127, 127*f*-128*f*
  needs assessment profile data collection 123-130, 124*t*
  program evaluation planning 134-136, 134*f*, 135*f*
  review WSCC implementation 126-130, 127*f*-128*f*, 129*f*
  school and community understanding 124-125
  school district health and wellness profile 118-123, 121*f*-122*f*, 124*t*, 130
  wellness policy review 125-126
WSCC Team Training Modules 39

Y

Youth Risk Behavior Survey (YRBS) 18, 60-62, 61*f*, 125, 150, 165, 170, 172
Youth Risk Behavior Survey (YRBSS) 82, 119*t*, 121*f*, 165

ABOUT THE EDITORS

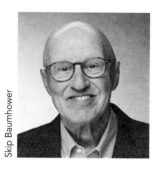

David A. Birch, PhD, is a professor emeritus in the department of health science at the University of Alabama. He served as a professor and the department chair from 2011 to 2018 and was coordinator of the doctoral program from 2018 to 2020. He previously served as a professor and the chair of the department of health education and recreation at Southern Illinois University–Carbondale and as a faculty member at Indiana University and Penn State University.

Birch is a past president of the American Association for Health Education (AAHE) and the Society for Public Health Education (SOPHE). He has served on the board of directors of AAHE, the American School Health Association (ASHA), and the National Association of Health Education Centers as well as on the SOPHE board of trustees. He is currently a board member of the Foundation for the Advancement of Health Education (FAHE) and is on the editorial board of *Health Education & Behavior*. He is a former editorial board member for the *Journal of School Health, Pedagogy in Health Promotion: The Scholarship of Teaching and Learning,* and the *American Journal of Health Studies*.

Birch is a charter fellow of AAHE and an ASHA fellow. He has received the highest professional award from three organizations—the ASHA William A. Howe Award (2019), the SOPHE Distinguished Fellow Award (2018), and the Eta Sigma Gamma Honor Award (2015)—along with numerous other professional awards. He was Illinois State University's 2008 Ann E. Nolte Scholar in Health Education. As a faculty member at Indiana University, he received the Trustees' Teaching Award and the Teaching Excellence Recognition Award.

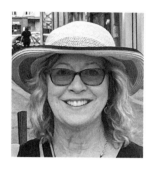

Donna M. Videto, PhD, RMCHES, is a SUNY distinguished service professor and professor emerita of health. She has worked in school health education and pedagogy for over 40 years. She has worked with school districts in Pennsylvania, Virginia, and New York to advance school health and the WSCC model, and she taught K-12 health education early in her career. Currently she works in international education, developing courses and teaching in Italy and the Czech Republic.

Recently retired from SUNY Cortland, where she taught graduate and undergraduate students in health education and education, Videto also served as the coordinator of student teaching in health education and the director of the faculty development center. She has written over 30 publications, including the books *Promoting Health and Academic Success: The Whole School, Whole Community, Whole Child Approach* and *2011 Needs Assessment and Program Planning for Health Education and Health Promotion*, and she has made over 150 national, regional, and state-level presentations at conferences and as part of her committee work for SOPHE, AAHE, and ASHA. An AAHE fellow and recipient of the Delbert Oberteuffer Mortar Board for excellence in school health education preparation, she recently completed her position as the vice president of the Foundation for the Advancement of Health Education (FAHE) and currently serves as a scholarship application reviewer for that foundation.

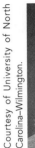
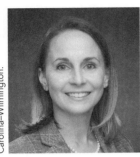

Hannah P. Catalano, PhD, MCHES, is an associate professor of public health at University of North Carolina–Wilmington (UNCW). She currently serves on the board of directors for the American School Health Association (ASHA) and cochairs the ASHA Research and Publications Committee. She is an editorial board member for the *Journal of School Health*, a member of the National Committee on the Future of School Health Education, and a member of the SOPHE Think Tank work group that provides strategic direction on the Institute for Higher Education Academy.

Catalano is a founding faculty fellow of the UNC-UNCW Research Collaboratory in the College of Health & Human Services at UNCW. She also founded and currently leads the university's Whole School, Whole Community, Whole Child Research Collaboratory (WSCCRC), which is a unique initiative to engage college students in scholarly discussions around WSCC and to facilitate meaningful research on the model. She previously served as a member of the National Consensus for School Health Education's Expert Review Group and is a former Future Leaders Academy Fellow of ASHA and NextUp Leadership Development Fellow of UNCW.

ABOUT THE CONTRIBUTORS

Diane DeMuth Allensworth, PhD, has 40 years of experience in school health. She started her career as a professor of health education at Kent State University for 20 years. While on the faculty at Kent State University, she began working with the American School Health Association, ultimately serving as the executive director for two years. In 1997, she became branch chief for program development and services in the Division of Adolescent School Health of the Centers for Disease Control and Prevention (CDC). From 2001 to 2005, she was on loan from the CDC to HealthMPowers, a nonprofit focusing on nutrition and physical activity for preschool through secondary students and their families. She served as the organization's first executive director, a board member for 20 years, and a consultant from 2017 to 2022. She has written or coauthored numerous refereed articles and books and served on the committee that wrote the Whole School, Whole Community, Whole Child model for the CDC and ASCD.

Randi J. Alter, PhD, has served as the executive director of the American School Health Association since 2018. Prior to this, Dr. Alter was a research associate and lead evaluator for Prevention Insights at Indiana University. Her primary projects involved providing technical assistance and evaluation services to addiction prevention professionals and grassroots coalitions. Over the course of her tenure at Indiana University, she was active in the field, in the classroom, and in scholarship. Her research interests include the evaluation of prevention initiatives, coordinated school health programs, and psychosocial factors related to health.

M. Elaine Auld, MPH, MCHES, is the chief executive officer, emerita, for the Society for Public Health Education (SOPHE). As SOPHE's chief executive officer from 1995 to 2021 she oversaw the organization's portfolio in professional preparation, professional development, research, publications, and advocacy. Over her more than 40-year career, Ms. Auld has published some 50 journal articles and book chapters on the profession's role in community and school health education, health equity, national and international workforce development, and public policy. With regard to the Whole School, Whole Community, Whole Child model, Ms. Auld was principal investigator on several Centers for Disease Control and Prevention cooperative agreements that provided training and materials development for professionals, promoted the model as part of the National Task Force on the Future of School Health Education, and helped establish SOPHE's School Health Teacher Education Standards used in credentialing.

Sue Baldwin, PhD, MCHES, FASHA, has worked as a health educator for more than 25 years designing, implementing, and evaluating health education programs and curricula. She has taught at the collegiate and high school levels for nearly two decades. Dr. Baldwin has been the Buffalo Public Schools district wellness coordinator for seven years and in 2020 was appointed the supervisor of health and physical education in Buffalo, New York. Under her direction the Whole School, Whole Community, Whole Child (WSCC) initiative was implemented across 60 schools. The program was awarded the 2019 American School Health Association WSCC District Wide Implementation Award, recognition from the Centers for Disease Control and Prevention with a district site visit, and urban district recognition from ASCD for the district's use of the WSCC model. Dr. Baldwin has received numerous awards for her work in school health. She received her bachelor's from Gannon University, her master's from Slippery Rock University, and her doctorate from Kent State University. Moreover, she completed a master's in educational leadership and policy at SUNY Buffalo and obtained her school building and school district leader certifications in New York.

Alexis Blavos, PhD, MCHES, is an associate professor at SUNY Cortland and member of the Division Board for Certification of Health Education Specialists of the National Commission for Health Education Credentialing. Her academic and work experiences include 15 years of service in the public health field as a practitioner and researcher. Among her many research interests are college health, advocacy, health policy, and the responsibilities and competencies of health education specialists.

Bonni C. Hodges, PhD, a SUNY Distinguished Service Professor and professor in the health department at SUNY Cortland, has been working in school and community health for more than 30 years. She has a particular interest in the intersection of school and community health practice. She has published in such journals as *Health Promotion Practice,* the *Journal of School Health,* the *American Journal of Health Education,* and the *Health Educator.* She was the director of the five-year School Health Systems Change Project and is currently codirector of the Institute for Division III Athlete Well-Being and Athletic Leadership. She earned her bachelor's in physical education/athletic training from Ithaca College, her master's in exercise science from Northeastern University, and her doctorate from the University of Maryland–College Park.

Lloyd J. Kolbe, PhD, is professor emeritus of applied health science at Indiana University School of Public Health–Bloomington. He conducts public health policy research and development to improve child and adolescent health and education in the United States and in other nations. Dr. Kolbe has held senior positions across private-sector, government, and academic institutions and has written more than 160 scientific publications on the health and education of young people, school health programs, and public health policies. His appointments include member of the U.S. Public Health Service Senior Biomedical Research Service, chair of the World Health Organization Expert Committee on School Health Promotion, chair of the Centers for Disease Control and Prevention (CDC) Board of Scientific Counselors, and founding director of the CDC's Division of Adolescent and School Health.

Michael J. Mann, PhD, FASHA, spent almost 20 years working as a teacher, principal, regional director, operations leader, and program founder in the alternative school setting. Currently, he is an associate professor in Boise State University's School of Public Health and Population Science. His teaching and research are focused on promoting child and adolescent health, especially in schools and through school–community partnerships. Michael is currently the editor of the *Journal of School Health.* He is also a former board member for the American School Health Association and has served on a wide range of national committees devoted to advancing the fields of school health and health education. He completed his doctorate in health and human behavior at the University of Florida in 2007.

Elisa Beth McNeill, PhD, is currently a clinical professor of pedagogy in the School of Public Health at Texas A&M University (TAMU). She serves as the coordinator of the Health Education Teacher Certification Program. Beth is a 35-year teaching veteran with experience with middle school, high school, and at-risk pregnant and parenting adolescents. She earned her master's degree and principal certification in educational administration and her doctorate in health education from TAMU. Beth is known for her innovative instruction. She teaches courses in human sexuality, elementary and secondary school health pedagogy, technology for teachers, and community and school health methodology. She is a coauthor of the textbook *Health Education: Creating Strategies for School and Community Health.* On the national level, Beth has served on committees to update the Health Education Code of Ethics, the Health Education Specialist Practice Analysis II project with the National Commission for Health Education Credentialing, and the Health Education Terminology project and most recently cochaired the committee to update the National Health Education Standards (3rd ed.).

Lori Paisley, the senior director of coordinated school health in the Tennessee Department of Education, has 29 years of experience in education. Lori taught special education for four years, then started a system-wide program for students with emotional disturbance, which she led for five years before serving her school district in special education leadership for 11 years. Her school district was one of 10 pilot sites for coordinated school health in Tennessee. When coordinated school health expanded statewide in 2007, she led this work for her district until 2012, when she began working for the Tennessee Department of Education. During her 11 years with the department, she served as the state contact for alternative education, dropout prevention, school counseling, and school safety until 2014, when she began leading coordinated school health as executive director. Although working with students with disabilities led her to the field of education, her passion is school health and ensuring that students are healthy and ready to learn.

Rosemary Reilly-Chammat, EdD, is the associate director of school health and extended learning in the Office of Student, Community and Academic Supports in the Rhode Island Department of Elementary and Secondary Education (RIDE). She has served in a variety of roles in RIDE over the past 10 years. In addition, she worked for 26 years in the Rhode Island Department of Health, leading a variety of efforts related to student health and health in schools. She is the past president of the Society of State Leaders of Health and Physical Education and is on the board of the American School Health Association (ASHA). She received an ASHA Fellow Award in 2021.

Angelia M. Sanders, PhD, MEd, earned a doctorate in sociology from Kent State University and a master's in educational psychology and bachelor's in psychology from the University of Mississippi. She is currently a professor and the director of the division of health systems management and policy in the School of Public Health at the University of Memphis. Previously, she worked as a faculty member in public health at the University of Kansas School of Medicine–Wichita, Mississippi University for Women, and the University of Alabama. She was also a behavioral scientist and public health advisor at the Centers for Disease Control and Prevention. Dr. Sanders has authored or coauthored numerous publications and conducted research focused primarily on health disparities and health equity.

Sean Slade, MEd, is a global education leader, speaker, and author with three decades of experience in education spanning five countries and four continents. With a strong background in education reform and well-being, he has driven policy change, implemented initiatives, and developed educational leaders to enhance the social impact of education. He currently serves as the head of education at BTS Spark, North America, a not-for-profit practice focusing on developing the next generation of school leaders. He led the development of the Whole School, Whole Community, Whole Child model in 2013-2014 and has been a leading advocate for a Whole Child approach to education. He is an expert on social-emotional learning for NBC's *Today Show*, an advisory member for the Organisation for Economic Co-operation and Development's Future of Education & Skills 2030, a member of the World Innovative Summit on Education—Agile Leaders of Learning Innovation Network, and a founding member of the United Nations Educational, Scientific, and Cultural Organization (UNESCO) Chair Global Health & Education. He has written for the *Washington Post*, *The Huffington Post*, *EdWeek*, and EdSurge. His latest book, *Questioning Education: Moving From What and How to Why and Who*, was published by Routledge in 2022.

Assunta R. Ventresca, MSN, retired, was the director of health-related services for the Buffalo Public Schools (BPS) in New York for 13 years. Assunta's leadership was instrumental in ensuring a nurse in every school, the formation of a district health council, the provision of dental health services for students, and the establishment of numerous committees addressing the health of students and staff. She played a lead role in the development of the BPS wellness policy and the condom availability policy. Assunta's efforts in promoting the Whole School, Whole Community, Whole Child model and her dedication and leadership to the health and well-being of the children of Buffalo resulted in her receiving the 2013 American School Health Association Health Coordinator of the Year Award, the Adolescent Health Alliance of Buffalo's Community Leadership Award, the Planned Parenthood of Western New York Education Award, and the BPS Parent Coordinating Council Parent Partner Award. Born and raised in Buffalo, she earned her associate's degree in nursing from Trocaire College and a BS in Nursing and an MSN in Community Health, both from D'Youville University.

Michele Wallen, PhD, MPH, is an associate professor in and chair of the department of health education and promotion at East Carolina University (ECU). She began her professional career as a teacher in North Carolina public high schools. Prior to joining the faculty at ECU, she worked as a health education consultant for the North Carolina Department of Public Instruction. Michele earned her bachelor's from the University of North Carolina at Chapel Hill and her master's in public health and doctorate from the University of North Carolina at Greensboro. Michele works to advance health education initiatives in schools and has worked on numerous projects to support the preparation and development of public health and education professionals.

Kayce D. Solari Williams, PhD, is a clinical associate professor and internship coordinator in the Health program in the department of psychological, health, and learning sciences at the University of Houston as well as the cofounder and chief executive officer of Be Well Health Resources, LLC, a company focused on employee wellness training and providing equitable access to wellness information and resources. She has been a kindergarten through grade 12 dance and physical education teacher in the Houston, Fort Bend, and Aldine school districts in Texas and is the immediate past president of the American School Health Association. Her current school health work focuses on the employee wellness component of the Whole School, Whole Community, Whole Child model; school dress code policies and disparities in violations based on race, gender, and body type; obesity prevention; and the promotion of an active lifestyle.

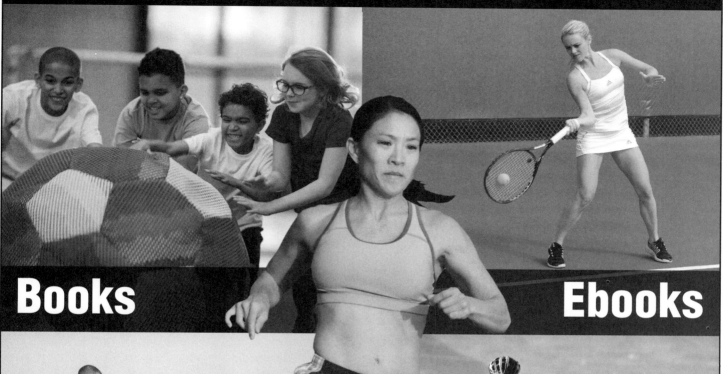